AF540604

2nd Revised and Expanded Edition

Principles of
MEAT TECHNOLOGY

2nd Revised and Expanded Edition

Principles of
MEAT TECHNOLOGY

V.P. Singh
Assistant Professor
Department of Livestock Products Technology
U.P. Pt. Deen Dayal Upadhyay Pashu Chikitsa
Vigyan Vishwavidyalaya Evam Go Anusandhan Sansthan
Mathura – 281 001, U.P.

&

Neelam Sachan
U.P.P.V.S. & Ex. Assistant Professor
Department of Veterinary Public Health
U.P. Pt. Deen Dayal Upadhyay Pashu Chikitsa
Vigyan Vishwavidyalaya Evam Go Anusandhan Sansthan
Mathura – 281 001, U.P.

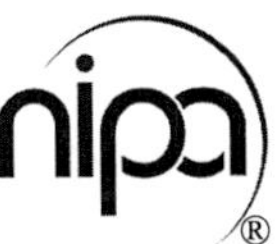

NEW INDIA PUBLISHING AGENCY
New Delhi – 110 034

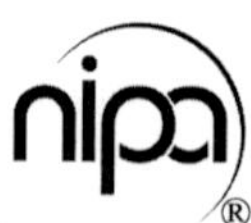

NEW INDIA PUBLISHING AGENCY
101, Vikas Surya Plaza, CU Block, LSC Market
Pitam Pura, New Delhi 110 034, India
Phone: + 91 (11)27 34 17 17 Fax: + 91(11) 27 34 16 16
Email: info@nipabooks.com
Web: www.nipabooks.com

Feedback at feedbacks@nipabooks.com

ISBN: 978-93-83305-79-7

Composed and Designed by NIPA

Dedicated
to
Almighty

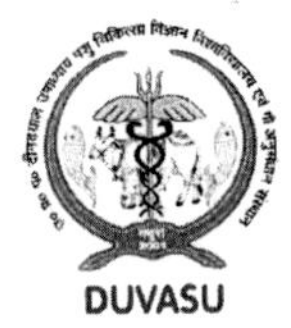

उत्तर प्रदेश पंडित दीनदयाल उपाध्याय पशु चिकित्सा विज्ञान विश्वविद्यालय
एवं गौ अनुसंधान संस्थान, मथुरा - 281001 (उ. प्र.) भारत

U.P. Pandit Deen Dayal Upadhyaya Pashu Chikitsa Vigyan Vishwavidyalaya
Evam Go-Anusandhan Sansthan, Mathura - 281001 (U.P.) INDIA

Prof. A. C. Varshney
Vice Chancellor

Foreword

Meat serves as one of the best sources of animal protein with respect to its higher digestibility and bioavailability. In the next decades to come, meat is going to play the major role in the prevention of protein malnutrition. Meat also possesses high nutritive value among the other available sources of protein. In the last few decades the production of meat has been dramatically increased and in near terms it is going to be paced more. Meat demand as a whole in the global market also has been increased.

In spite of a huge population of livestock including poultry, India lags behind in terms of meat production and meat marketing. The non-organised meat processing centres, poor slaughter house facilities, lack of scientific knowledge and hygienic meat processing are the major hurdles of Indian meat industry. The alarming demand for meat both at home and foreign level demands a scientific approach to meat technology. With the global pace, India is marching ahead with all newer technologies and advancements in the field of technology.

I feel immensely happy in seeing the contents and the efforts of the authors in preparing the book titled "*Principles of Meat Technology*" which fulfils the requirements of UG and PG Students of Veterinary Science as well as livestock products technology. This book will also be helpful to the students of food science and food products technology and processing. The book is sufficient enough in gathering update information regarding the science of meat and technology.

I convey my hearty feelings to the hard efforts of the authors as well as wish a grand success.

A.C. Varshney

Preface

To serve the nation in terms of nutritional food security, safety and employment generation is the prime duty of food scientists. To upgrade the national economy with the improvement in the quality, quantity and safety is need of today. Another challenge ahead is to meet out the daunting demand of modern consumers with high quality protein. Meat is one of the most significant and easily available food sources with high biological value protein. Meat industry is also capable to uplift the status of rural people and employment generation in rural areas. However, in India, little attention has been paid to the meat sector though it contributes about Rs 25984 crores every year in total livestock output. This sector is not only important for providing meat and by-products for human utility but also contributes for sustained livestock production and livelihood activities in India. The approach to obtain efficient livestock production, processing and utilization now becomes more stringent due to consciousness of consumers and competitive environment created through trade liberalization by World Trade Organization (WTO).

So keeping all these facts in mind the 2nd edition of the book titled "*Principles of Meat Technology*" is upgraded with the vast material and recent innovations in meat science. Each and every aspect of the meat science right from production of meat to ultimate consumption is very well illustrated and documented. The recent aspects like organic meat production, genetically modified food of animal origin and various types of standards on meat, fish and poultry products are very well incorporated in the present edition. In other words all the requirements of the today's students of veterinary science, food science, meat technology and other related fields are taken up from basics to the modern. Thus it is expected that the veterinary professionals, students, industry personnel and other professionals of allied fields may continue their support for acceptance of the present edition.

The improvement and upgradation is a continuous process. So the critical comments and suggestions on various aspects of this book will help us in improving this manuscript in future.

V.P. Singh
Neelam Sachan

Contents

Dedication .... *v*

Foreword .... *vii*

Preface .... *ix*

1. **Retrospective and Prospective of Meat Industry in India** 1

2. **Structure and Composition of Muscle Including Poultry Muscle** 15

3. **Conversion of Muscle to Meat** 39

4. **Nutritive Value of Meat** 55

5. **Fraudulent Substitution of Meat** 67

6. **Preservation of Meat and Aquatic Foods** 87

7. **Ageing of Meat** 111

8. **Modern Processing Technologies of Meat and Meat Products** 123

9. **Packaging of Meat and Meat Products** 161

10. **Formulation and Development of Meat and Sea Foods** 183

11. **Physico-Chemical and Microbiological Quality of Meat and Aquatic Food and Food Products** 231

12. Basics of Sensory Evaluation of Meat Products 251

13. Nutritive Value, Preservation, Packaging of Egg and Egg Products 265

14. Laws Governing National / International Trade in Meat and Meat Products 283

15. Organic Meat Food Products 329

16. Food Products of Genetically Modified Animals and Marine Origin 337

Colour Plates 347

Index 349

1 Retrospective and Prospective of Meat Industry in India

In spite of big potential of the largest livestock population in the world, meat industry in India is still in nascent stage. It is a business of those who are not trained and very much literate. The industry is primarily based on the raw material that is not reared for meat purpose but serves the secondary role after passing their viable life in primary field. The industry is also facing problem of social prejudice and meat is taboo for certain communities. But scenario is now changing and people are coming forward to organise the sector. Now the society is accepting the facts that meat is an only source of cheap and nutritious food to million of people in India and the good source of animal protein for large segment of Indian population, particularly landless, small and marginal farmers.

India ranks fifth in the world meat production with the annual meat production of about 6.3 million tones which is 2.21% percent of world meat production. In the last two decades meat industry in India has grown @ 4.5% whereas, during the last five years, this segment has been growing very fast at the rate of 27% annually. It has a good future if given proper attention by the Government and Private Entrepreneurs. In total meat production, share of cattle is 17.34%, buffalo 23.3%, sheep 4.6%, goat 9.4%, pigs 5.3%, poultry 36.6% and others 3.4%. The share of various meat types in total Indian meat production accounts buffalo meat 1.5 million tones, beef 1.28 million tones, mutton 0.24 million tones, chevon 0.53 million tones, pork 0.50 million tones, chicken meat 2.20

million tones and duck meat 0.07 million tones. To produce the above quantities, the extraction or slaughter rates in cattle are about 7.9%, buffaloes 11.1%, sheep 47.9%, goat 37.9%, pigs 88.9% and poultry 73.6%. In the world total meat production Indian cattle meat shares 13.1%, buffalo meat 55.8%, mutton 5.7% and chevon 14.9%. However, India is having world's 15.0% (210 million) cattle, 57.0 %(111 million) buffaloes, 7.0 %(74 million) sheep, 17.0 %(154 million) goat and 1.5% pigs. Overall contribution of meat sector in total output of Livestock sector was Rs 25984 crores in the year 2004-2005.

In spite of progressive growth in meat sector, availability of meat in India is very less (5.5 kg/head/annum) in comparison to the world average (42 kg/head/ annum). As per ICMR (Indian Council of Medical Research) recommendations, minimum amount of 30 g of meat/day/ head should be taken which makes 10.95 kg meat/head/annum. Global meat consumption varies enormously from region to region and large differences are visible within region. Overall USA leads by far with over 322 g of meat consumption per person per day (120 kg/annum). However, Australia and New Zealand close behind European consumer with slightly more than 200 g meat (76 kg/annum). Asia's meat consumption is 84 g/ day or 31 kg/annum including China's 160 g/ day and India only 12 g/day.

In spite of several constraints in India, meat industry has shown a tremendous change in the last one decade with the establishment of eco-friendly fully integrated processing plants. It is now expected that in next ten years, there will also be great change with the establishment of the feedlots as a backward integration to the processing plants. To establish the disease free zones in country, Government of India is taking up FMD control programme in three Zones (North, Central and South) consisting of 56 Districts. Several other disease control projects are also underway all over the nation. So it is assumed that India is poised with a major breakthrough in the meat product exports in the international market.

SWOT Analysis of Meat Industry in India

Strengths

1. Round the year availability of raw materials.
2. Availability of huge number of manpower.
3. High animal protein diet at lower prices.
4. Vast domestic market.

Weaknesses

1. High requirement of working capital.
2. Low availability of new reliable and better accuracy instruments and equipments.
3. Lack of availability of trained and skilled personnel.
4. Remuneration less attractive for talent in comparison to contemporary disciplines.
5. Inadequately developed linkages between R&D labs and industry.

Opportunities

1. Huge availability of raw material in the country offers vast potential for processing activities and value addition in the meat.
2. Integration of developments in contemporary technologies such as electronics, material science, computer, bio-technology etc. offer vast scope for rapid improvement and progress.
3. Opening of global markets may lead to export of our developed technologies and facilitate generation of additional income and employment opportunities.

Threats

1. Competition from global players.
2. Loss of trained manpower to other industries and other professions due to better working conditions prevailing there may lead to further shortage of manpower.

3. Rapid developments in contemporary and requirements of the industry may lead to fast obsolescence.

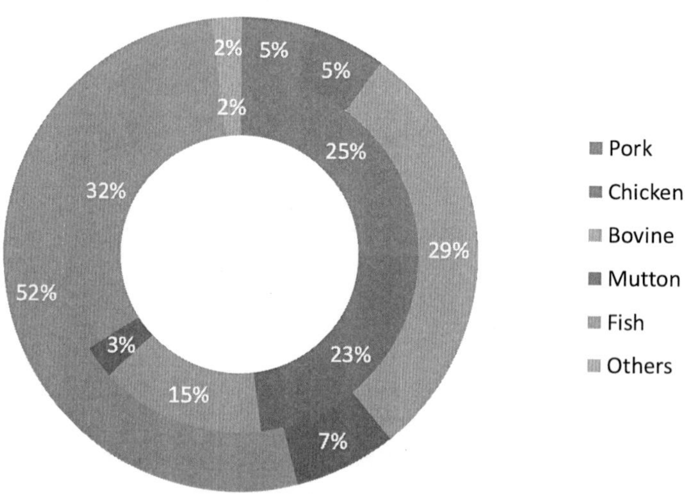

Inner circle represent % share of different meat in year 1994 & outer circle of 2011
(*Source*: FAO,2005 & Worldwatch Institute Report,2014)

Processing of Animal and Fish Products

In our country people are mostly using fresh meat however, very little about 2% of total meat is converted into ready to eat meat products by the processing. However, scenario is entirely different in developed world where more than 60% meat is converted into value added processed products. So to meet the global requirements, efforts are on to develop infrastructure for export of both fresh and processed meat and poultry. The main culprits in development of meat sector are social taboos, scattered production system, unskilled workers, lack of infrastructural facilities, lack of awareness about hygiene, high initial investments in processing etc. However, efforts are being made by the government as well as private entrepreneurs to uplift the sector with the implementation of HACCP and ISO norms. Poultry has done well in rural sector and developed network of marketing in distant remunerative markets. Processed meat products can also help in utilization of underutilized body parts of the animals and meat of the spent animals. The meat from culled birds, goats and buffaloes is tough textured, better suited for processed meat products. There are varieties of processed meat products available such as emulsion meat products, restructured, cured, smoked, enrobed meat products etc.

India is great in its heritage and people of different corners of country like different types of foods to eat. The traditional meat products are not the exceptions so varieties of traditional meat products of India are popular region wise. Gostaba, nate-yakini and Tabak manss are popular in northern region including Kashmir valley, meat curry, mutton dopiyaza, mutton korma, rapka are popular in eastern region, meat rolls, vindaloo, shakudi in western region including Goa, dry salted meat in southern region but some of the meat products are very much popular throughout the country like meat samosa, meat tikka, meat ball or kofta, kabab (seekh, shami, boti), meat pickles etc.

Indian fisheries and aquaculture is an important component of food sector. Indian fisheries globally ranks 3rd while in aquaculture India stood 2nd at global level. Indian fisheries contribute 1.07% to national GDP and 5.3% in agricultural GDP. Presently total fish production in India is 6.4 million metric tonnes in which contribution of Inland fisheries is 3.4 million metric tonnes and rest 3.0 million metric tonnes is obtained from marine sources. The per capita availability of fish in our country is 9.0 kg. The export of fish from India in previous year was around 7,200 crores.

India, with its 8,129 km long coastline and an exclusive economic zone of 2.02 million square km; 1,97,024 km of rivers and canals and 4.4 million hectares of reservoirs and fresh water lakes has an enormous potential for fisheries. In 1999, the country had an estimated 1,81,284 traditional fishing crafts; 44,578 motorized traditional crafts, 53,684 mechanized fishing boats and about 200 deep-sea vessels in operation. At present India is having 1,070 fish hatcheries and producing fish seed around 21000 million fry. About 14 million people are engaged in Fish sector business. Fish processing in India is done almost entirely for export. Open sun dried fish and fish meal are the only major exceptions. At present India has freezing units, cold stores, ice plants, canning units and fish meal plants. Capacity of most of these processing and storage units is small as compared to the facilities in fish processing industry in technologically advanced countries. The fish processing and storage facilities in India are inadequate compared to the potential for fish production and processing. Extensive network of refrigerated handling, transport, storage and retailing has to be put in place. To make the fish processed industry sustainable fish waste and by-products must be utilized in profitable manner.

Now traditional meat processing techniques are being replaced with the function oriented processing techniques. These modern concepts of processing involve definite aim to be achieved along with the new product development or modification of traditionally popular meat products. Some of the ingredients when used in product development lead to a functional change in the meat products. some of these are fat replacers, dietary fibres, salt replacers, fatty acid profile replacers, antioxidants, enzyme in processing, nitrite substitutes, texture modifiers etc. Innovations in processing techniques also involve retort pouch processing, hurdle technology, high pressure technology, active and intelligent packaging, reddening etc.

Export Potential of Indian Meat Industry

At present India is having 30 export oriented modern abattoir and 77 meat processing plants registered with APEDA exporting raw meat (chilled & frozen) to about 65 countries; through which India exported 5, 45,731 tonnes bovine and 52,251 tonnes sheep and goat meat (2009-10) amounting to Rs 5436 crores and Rs 737 crores, respectively. This is expected to grow substantially over the years to come. The major export was of deboned and deglanded frozen buffalo meat, which accounts for 85% of the total meat exports and 23% of the total buffalo meat produced in the country. The rest of the meat exported is from sheep, goat and poultry. Poultry contributes less than 5% of total meat export. Among all the states of India, Uttar Pradesh stood first in buffalo meat export (1/3rd of total buffalo meat export) followed by Maharashtra and Andhra Pradesh. Now India is able to produce meat from animals procured from disease free zones and processed in the state of the art processing plants following world class sanitary and phytosanitary measures and certified with HACCP and ISO-9002.The prospects for the Indian meat industry seem bright in the years to come. This is primarily because of the improving livestock health situation in India. However, India has always been free from mad cow disease and Rinderpest since 1995. With greater thrust on value addition and processed products, India's meat exports are likely to move up the value chain in a significant manner.

According to the statistics, Asia accounts for 40.2% of meat exports, followed by the Middle East (38.5%) and Africa (12.1%). In year 2003, amongst the Asian region, Malaysia imported half of its $249 million worth meat from India alone. In the same year, India was single largest exporter of meat to the Philippines with an export value of $50.6 million with the market share of 38%. However, in year 2011-12 top ten markets for Indian Buffalo meat were Algeria (53,733 tonnes cwt), Philippines (47,452 tonnes cwt), the United Arab Emirates (45,291 tones cwt), Iran (33,982 tones cwt) and Thailand (29,935 tones cwt). The other markets were African countries including Angola (25,730 tones cwt), Congo (15,117 tones cwt) and Gabon (7,275 tones cwt).

Beef particularly carabeef is the single largest meat item exported by the Indian industry. India's Bovine meat exports were worth $360 million in fiscal 2005, accounting for 94% of the overall exports of $383.5 million. In the last six years, the Bovine meat exports have registered a 17.2% annual growth. The high exports have been possible due to competitive pricing of buffalo meat. The Indian buffalo meat is also considered as tender and liked by the Indian ethnic groups residing all over the world.

The global meat consumption stood at 297 million tons in 2011, growing at an annual rate of 2.0%. In overall meat consumption Asia and Pacific credit on top (56%) followed by Latin America and Caribbean (18%), North America (8%), Africa (7%), Europe (7%) and others (4%).

Among all meat types pork was the most popular meat in 2011, at 109 million tones, accounting for 37 percent of both meat production and consumption,. This was followed closely by poultry meat, with 101 million tons produced while production of both beef and sheep meat stagnated between 2010 and 2011, at 67 million and 13 million tonnes, respectively. As per USDA (2013) estimate it was concluded that meat production grew nearly 26 percent in Asia, 28 percent in Africa and 32 percent in South America.

Meat Export Trend

The share of meat export in total agro products during 1995-96 to 2012-13 was as follows:

Duration	Figures in Rs. crores		
	Agro products Export (APEDA)	Meat Export	As % of Agro Products
1995-96	7915	614	8
1996-97	7723	690	9
1997-98	7271	792	11
1998-99	9682	770	8
1999-00	7365	797	11
2000-01	9213	1453	16
2001-02	10169	1177	12
2002-03	13828	1345	10
2003-04	14184	1647	12
2007-08	-	3549	-
2008-09	-	6913	-
2009-10	-	7201	-
2010-11	42437	9817	23
2011-12	83485	14471	17
2012-13	118254	18342	16

Source: APEDA, 2012

Quality Control and Standards Existing in Indian Meat Industry

At present different systems are in operation for production of safe meat and meat products. They are:

a) *Meat Food Products Order 1973, 1994*: Directorate of Marketing and Inspection (Ministry of Agriculture, Govt. of India) would administer this order for safety and quality of meat and meat products during production, processing and distribution. Besides, it has promulgated Raw Meat (Chilled and Frozen) Grading and Marketing Rules (1991) to regulate the hygienic production of meat and meat products. Meat Food Products Advisory Committee formed under this order advises the Government on matters related to meat and meat products.

b) *Export Quality Control and Inspection Act (1963):* This act deals with the promotion of export of safe food products to global markets. The Export Inspection Council has been established to ensure compulsory quality control and inspection of various commodities.

c) *Agriculture and Processed Food Products Exports Development Authority (APEDA):* APEDA operates under Ministry of Commerce, Govt. of India, covering the export of agro and processed food products including meat and meat products. It looks after the development of export trade of food products and strengthens the capabilities related to the quality control systems.

d) *Bureau of Indian Standards (BIS):* The activities of BIS in the field of meat and meat products processing are two folds: a) formulation of Indian standards and b) their implementation through its voluntary and third party certification system. These standards, in general, cover raw materials permitted and their quality parameters, hygienic conditions under which the product is manufactured. It also regulates the packaging and labeling requirements of food products including meat products. Bureau of Indian Standards is a national agency that set standards for a variety of foods including meat and meat products. It operates quality system certification in India.

e) *Ministry of Food Processing Industries (MoFPI):* The Ministry concerns on the development of food industries including meat in the country. It extends financial support for strengthening and upgrading infrastructure facilities in meat industry and support R & D programmes in improving the quality of meat and meat products. With opening up of the Indian Economy due to globalization, most of the restriction on import of different food items including meat have been withdrawn.

f) *GATT and sanitary / phytosanitary measures:* Agreement on the application of Sanitary and Phytosanitary Measures (The SPS Agreement concluded under GATT in 1994) came into effect in 1995 for developing the international standards to ensure the safety of food for consumers and to prevent the spread of pests or diseases in animals and plants. These measures protect human/animal life from risks arising from additive contaminants, toxins or disease causing organisms in their food. The objectives of SPS can be accomplished in several ways as indicated below:

1. Requiring product to come from a disease free area

2. Inspection of products

3. Specific treatment of processing of products

4. Setting allowable maximum levels of pesticide residues or permitting the uses of only certain additives in food.

g) *Food Safety and Standards Authority of India (FSSAI):* Food Safety and Standards Authority of India (FSSAI) is a single window system. The basic aim of FSSAI is to facilitate the food trade business with the harmonization of laws and to make the easy registration and other legal formalities to run or start the new business. FSSAI is an integrated approach of nine different laws and eight different ministries governing the food sector. It is basically a modified version of Food Safety and Standards act, 2006. The basic motto of the comprehensive law is avoidance of overlapping of various laws, removal of multiple regulations, harmonization with international law, framing of regulatory requirements based on science and risk analysis, facilitation to the trade without compromising consumer safety and bringing in innovation in foods etc. The existed laws of the country i.e Prevention of Food Adulteration Act, 1954, Fruit Products Order, 1955, Meat Food Products Order, 1973, Vegetable Oil Products (Control) Order, 1947, Edible Oils Packaging (Regulation) Order, 1988, Solvent Extracted Oil, De-oiled Meal and Edible Flour (Control) Order, 1967, Milk and Milk Products Order, 1992 and any order under Essential Commodities Act, 1955 relating to food are now will be governed by this integrated law. The basic aims of this law are:

i. To ensure that all food meets consumer's expectations in terms of nature, substance and quality and is not misleadingly presents.

ii. To provide legal powers and specify offences in relation to public health and consumers' interest;

iii. To shift from regulatory regime to self compliance through Food Safety Management system.

iv. Science based standards

v. Proprietary food, novel food, GM food, dietary supplements, nutraceuticals etc. brought into the ambit of the new act.

Livestock Health

Livestock health status plays a major role in world meat trade. The livestock health situation in India is definitely improving. India has always been free from the dreaded Mad Cow Disease (BSE) and has been free from Rinderpest since 1995. There has not been a single incidence of Contagious Bovine Pleuro Pneumonia (CBPP) in India during the previous 12 years. Foot and Mouth Disease remains the only issue of concern, though better controlled. However, due to newer developments in vaccination and diagnostics, importing countries are adopting at least a "Lets evaluate the risk" policy. AIMLEA is playing a leading role in this important change in world thinking, through various submissions and data, including through the Office International Des Epizooties (OIE) now known as World Organization for Animal Health (WHO equivalent for all Terrestrial Animals). Importantly, a major programme has been initiated by the Central Government since August 2003 through the FMD-Control Programme (FMD-CP) covering 54 districts across the country. With the Indian Veterinary fraternity's successful accomplishment of eradication of Rinderpest, a more difficult and dreaded disease, it will not be wishful thinking to believe given the right resources, substantial and relevant areas in India could become FMD free, duly recognized by the OIE, in the next 5-6 years. Uttar Pradesh and Maharashtra, the prominent States where Buffalo meat is processed for export, have covered most of the balance districts in their States under Assistance to States for Control of Animal Diseases (ASCAD) where the Centre's contribution is 75%. Already Uttar Pradesh and Maharashtra have not reported FMD for several consecutive months, which is excellent progress. Some specific additional districts need to be covered both under FMD-CP and in 2 states (Andhra Pradesh and West Bengal) under ASCAD. The involvement of AIMLEA and FMD specialists from the private sector can help fine-tune the implementation vis a vis industry's requirements. The vaccine quality also needs to be assessed to confirm efficacy over a prolonged period in the Indian environment.

The future of Indian meat industry is very bright due to availability of raw material and vast man power. In this regard government and non government organisations are showing their interest to uplift the status of poorer country. It is a field in which we can get foreign revenue through export of meat and meat products by the modernisation of infrastructural facilities for abattoir and meat processing plants. There is also an urgent need to aware the public for hygienic meat production and processing techniques. Meat processing technology and value addition in meat may be the key factor in making the meat industry prosperous and viable. The strict sanitary, phytosanitary and qualitative measure must be adopted to take ahead this childhood industry.

References

1. Abraham, J. (2008). Emerging issues of Indian meat sector in relation to food security, safety and health. In: 3rd Convention of Indian Meat Science Association and National Symposium on Safe Meat Food, Good Health and Environment, July 4-5, 2008: 20-24.
2. APEDA (2012). Annual Report published by APEDA in 2012.
3. FAO (2004). Annual Report of FAO, 2004, Rome.
4. FAO (2005). FAO STAT data. Food and Agriculture Organisation, Rome. Accessed in July 2005.
5. FAO (2005). Global Livestock Production and Health Atlas Food and Agriculture Organisation, Rome. Accessed in July 2005.
6. Government of India, Department of Animal husbandry (2003). Annual Report 2002-2003, New Delhi.
7. Government of India,NDC (2002), 10th Five Year Plan, New Delhi.
8. Karim, S.A. (2008). Meat animal production in India. In: 3rd convention of Indian Meat Science Association and National Symposium on Safe Meat Food, Good Health and Environment, July 4-5: 2-8.
9. Kondaiah, N. (2008). Meat production, processing and utilization-Indian scenario and R&D requirements. In: 3rd convention of Indian Meat Science Association and National Symposium on Safe Meat Food, Good Health and Environment, July 4-5, 2008: 9-19.
10. Livestock Industry Report 2005 - CLFMA of India.

11. Sharma, N. (2006). Meat production in India. In: IMSACON-II, Second Convention of Indian Meat Science Association and National Symposium on Prospects and Challenges in Indian Meat Industry, July 27-29: 3-8.

12. Suresh, A., Kavita, B. and Chaudhary, K. R. (2012). India's meat export: structure, composition and future prospects. Indian Journal of Animal Sciences, 82(7): 749-756.

13. Thota, C.K. (2006). Indian Meat Industry and International market. In: IMSACON-II, Second Convention of Indian Meat Science Association and National Symposium on Prospects and Challenges in Indian Meat Industry, July 27-29: 87-99.

14. USDA (2013). Budget summary and annual performance plan. FY 2013.

□□□□

2 Structure and Composition of Muscle Including Poultry Muscle

The word *meat* comes from the old english word *mete,* which referred to food in general. Most often this means the skeletal muscle and associated fat but it may also describe other edible tissues such as organs, livers, skin, brains, bone marrow, kidneys and lungs etc. In other words we can say meat is those animal tissues which are suitable for use as food by the man. It is composed of numerous types of tissues like muscle tissues, epithelial tissues and nervous tissues but the major component of meat is muscle. Particularly skeletal muscle is the principal source of muscle tissue in meat while smooth muscle contributes little to meat. The muscle and connective tissues are the major compositional components and contributes towards qualitative and quantitative characteristics of meat. Broadly muscle can be classified into striated and smooth muscles. Striated muscles have transverse band pattern as seen in skeletal and cardiac muscle. However, smooth muscles do not show such pattern and mainly found as a component of blood vessels.

Skeletal Muscle

Skeletal muscle constitutes about 35-65% of the carcass weight of meat animals with the exception of excessively fat animals. The muscles have direct attachment with bones but some of them are also attached with ligaments, fascia, cartilage and skin. Animal body is made up of more than 600 muscles which vary in their shape, size and activity.

Muscle fiber is a structural unit of skeletal muscle tissue and constitutes 75-92% of total muscle volume. On cross sectional study of muscle fiber it appears in three distinct parts:

1. *Epimysium*: It is connective tissue sheath surrounding the entire muscle.
2. *Perimysium*: A layer beneath epimysium which divide the muscle fibers into small groups or fasciculi. These groups are also known as primary bundles. When few primary bundles come together they form secondary bundles and secondary bundles coming together leads to formation of tertiary bundles.
3. *Endomysium*: The layer beneath perimysium which surrounds each muscle fiber individually. These are very thin strands.

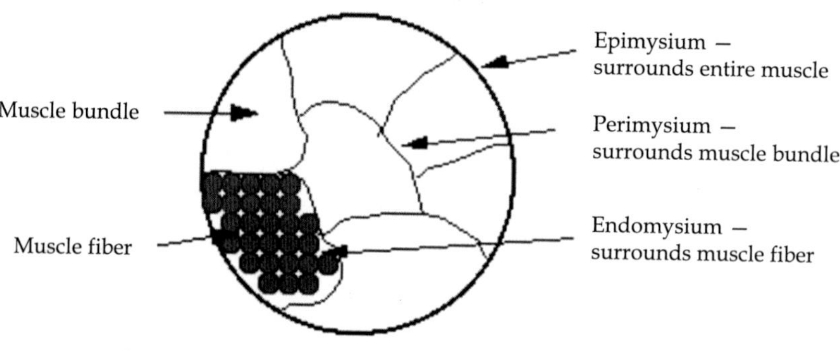

Fig. 2.1.

The epimysium, perimysium and endomysium serve as the structural basis for skeletal muscles. They conduct the vascular and neural supply to and from the muscle. Larger nerves and blood vessels lie at the periphery of perimysium and between the adjacent fasciculi. The size of fasciculi, in fact, has bearing on the texture of the muscle i.e. muscles engaged in lighter activities have fine texture and it is reverse for the heavier muscles or muscles which have to work more.

Skeletal Muscle Fiber

Muscle fiber is a highly specialized cell of skeletal muscle tissue. Muscle fibre makes around 75-92% of muscle volume. The other constituents responsible for muscle volume are blood vessels, nerve fibres and extra cellular fluids. The muscle fibers of meat animals and poultry are long, unbranched, thread like cells and taper slightly at both ends. The diameter of muscle fiber ranges from 10 μm to more than 100 μm. This muscle fiber is a combined structure of sarcolemma, sarcoplasmic reticulum, nuclei, mitochondria, Golgi bodies, T-system and contractile protein fibrils. The membrane surrounding the muscle fiber is known as sarcolemma. It is composed of protein and lipid material and transmits nervous signals along the surface of muscle fiber. It resembles with plasmalemma of other cells of the body in its structure, composition and properties. Transverse tubule is a network of tubules formed by sarcolemma invagination along the length of fiber, its entire circumference and usually referred as T-system or T-tubules. Basically it is a portion of the sarcoplasmic reticulum that stores and releases calcium during contraction and relaxation. The other structures found in microscopic examination include.

Sarcolemma: Sarcolemma surrounds the muscle fibres. It is elastic in nature and composed of fat and protein. Its elastic nature is responsible for its adjustment during contraction, relaxation and stretching.

Myoneural junction: A place where motor nerve endings terminate on the sarcolemma is known as myoneural junction.

Motor end plate: A structure present at the myoneural junction that forms a small mound on the surface of the muscle fiber.

Sarcoplasm: Cytoplasm of muscle fibers contains intracellular colloidal substance in which all organelles are suspended is known as Sarcoplasm. Major constituent of sarcoplasm is water (75-80%) and other constituent of sarcoplasm includes lipids, glycogen, ribosomes, proteins, nonprtein nitrogen substances and inorganic materials.

Nuclei: Nuclei is the brain of the cell. The nuclei of mammalian muscle are multinucleated and located at the periphery of the muscle fiber just beneath the sarcolemma. Nuclei of skeletal muscle fiber are ellipsoidal in shape.

Myofibrils: It is long, thin, cylindrical rods usually 1-2 μm in diameter that run within and parallel to the long axis of the muscle fiber. Myofibrils are embedded in sarcoplasm and extend the entire length of the muscle fiber. The muscle fiber of a meat animal measuring 50μm in diameter contains about 1000 to more than 2000 myofibrils.

Myofilaments : It is comprised of thick and thin filaments. The thick are comprised of myosin and the thin are comprised of actin, troponin, and tropomyosin. The alignment of thick filament is parallel to each other and remains same in entire myofibril while thin filament is aligned across the myofibril, parallel to each other and also with thick filament. In this arrangement thick and thin filaments overlap with each other in certain regions along their longitudinal axes and provide the striated appearance to the myofibril. The density of myofilaments in different regions gives light and dark visibility when visualized with polarized light and give birth to the light and dark bands. Light band is known as I band and it is isotropic in nature while thick band is called A band which is anisotropic in polarized light. The I band is less dense than A band and bisected by a thin band called Z line. The unit distance between two adjacent Z lines is known as sarcomere. It is a basic contractile unit of the muscle because event of muscle contraction and relaxation cycle takes place in sarcomare. It has Z-lines on either end along with A-band or two 1/2 I-bands. The length of sarcomere is varying as per contraction state but in relax state it is 2.5 μm. In the centre of A band there is a lighter region than remaining region in the band. This central lighter region of A band is known as H zone. A line bisecting in the centre of H zone is known as M line. Relatively low density area in H zone on either side of the M line is referred as pseudo H zone.

Thick and thin filaments are different in their dimensions, chemical composition, properties and their position within the sarcomere.

S. No.	Thick filament	Thin filament
1.	Its diameter varies from 14-16 μm and they are about 1.5μm long.	They are 6-8 μm in diameter and extend approximately 1.0 μm on either side of the Z line.
2.	It constitutes the A band of sarcomere.	It constitutes I band of sarcomere.
3.	It consists primarily of myosin protein and known as myosin filament.	It consists primarily of actin protein and referred as actin filament.

H-Zone: H zone of A band is less dense than rest of the A band area and contains only myosin filaments. The width of H zone varies with the state of muscle contraction. The orientation of myosin filament in this zone region of sarcomere is in hexagonal pattern.

Z-line ultrastructure: It is comprised of Z filaments and constitutes the material of Z line. These are the connecting units between sarcomeres. The connection of actin filament is on either side of z line. Each actin filament connects to four Z filaments which pass obliquely through the Z line. This structural arrangement of the Z line shows connection of an actin filament of one sarcomere to the four actin filaments from the next sarcomere. This orientation of actin filament provides zigzag pattern to Z line.

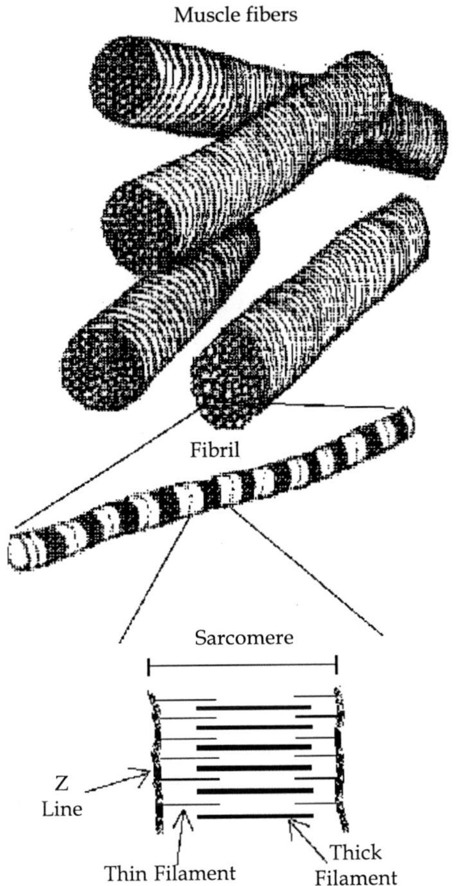

Fig. 2.2 : Structure of meat (*Source:* Robert Burn)

Sarcoplasmic reticulum and T tubules: Sarcoplasmic reticulum is a membranous system of tubules and cisternae (flattened reservoirs for Ca^{++}) that forms closely meshed network around each myofibril. It is intracellular in nature and reticulum membranes of the sarcoplasmic reticulum are the storage site of Ca^{++} in resting muscle fibers. While Transverse tubules commonly known as T tubules are associated with the sarcolemma. Longitudinal tubules of the reticulum are formed by relatively thin tubules oriented in the direction of the myofibrillar axis. These L tubules converge and form a perforated sheet or window like

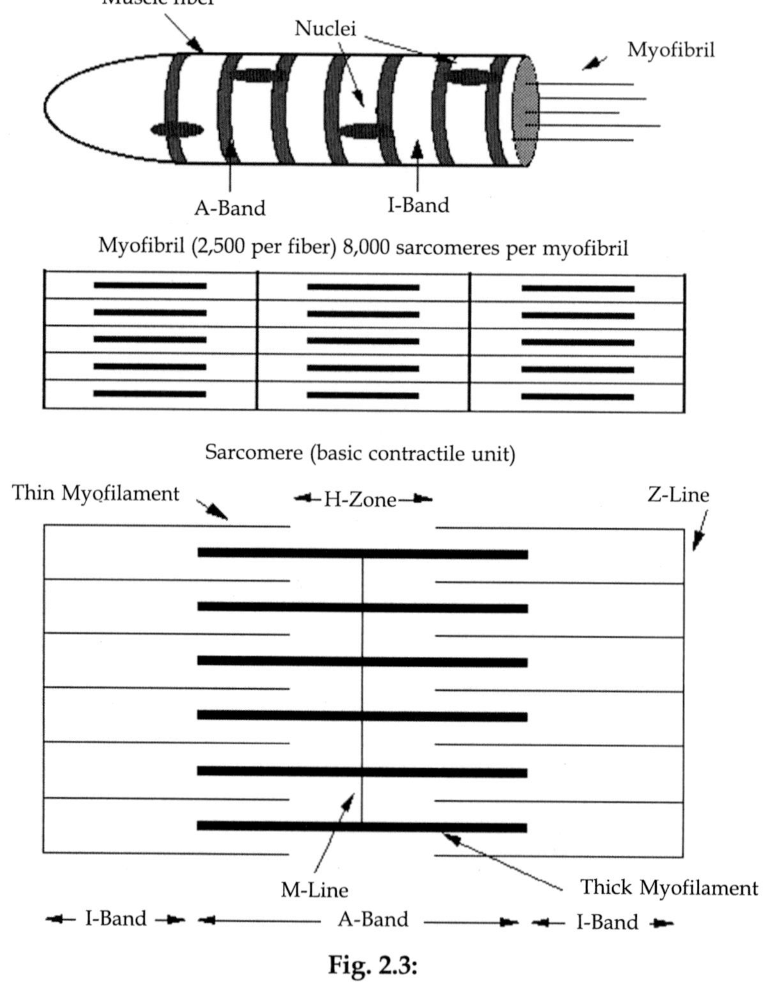

Fig. 2.3:

Source: Growth and Structure of Meat Animals H. J. Swatland, Department of Animal and Poultry Science, University of Guelph, Canada (1&2)

opening known as fenestrated collar in the H zone region of sarcomere. While in the junction of A and I bands these L tubules converge and join with a pair of larger transversely oriented tubular elements known as terminal cisternae. The central T tubules and the two tubular elements of the terminal cisternae collectively form a structure known as Triad. These are two in number in sarcomere and encircle each myofibril at

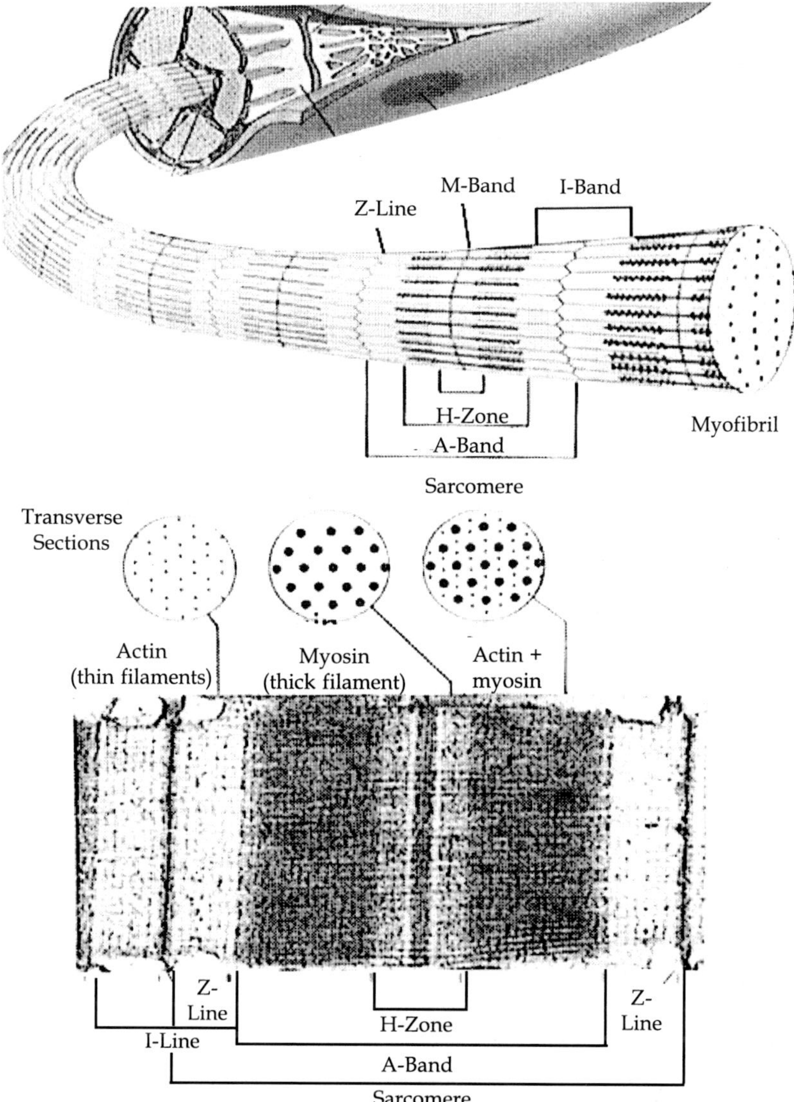

Fig. 2.4 : (*Source:* M.J. Farabee 2007) www.emc.maricopa.edu/faculty/farabee/BIOBK/BioBookMUSSKEL.html

the junction of A and I band in mammals, birds and some fishes. It is estimated that Sarcoplasmic reticulum constitutes approximately 13% and T tubules about 0.3% of the fiber volume.

Mitochondria: It is a powerhouse of the cell and contains enzymes that cell uses in the oxidative metabolism. The mitochondria of the skeletal muscles are abundant in the periphery of the muscle fiber near the pole of the nuclei and myoneural junctions.

Lysosomes: Small vesicles located in the sarcoplasm that contain a large number of enzymes collectively capable of digesting the cell and its contents. The best known of these are the proteolytic enzymes like cathepsins which are used in meat tenderization in the ageing of meat.

Golgi complex: The muscle fiber is a multinucleated cell and contains numerous Golgi complexes which act as a concentrating and packaging apparatus in metabolic production lines of the cell.

Smooth Muscle

Smooth muscle has little contribution to meat and found mainly in wall of arties, lymph vessels, gastrointestinal and reproductive tracts. The smooth muscle fiber is varying in their shape, size and may have spindle or contour shape. The sarcolemma of smooth muscle fibers connects the neighbouring fibers with the help of membrane contact bridges formed by it. Smooth muscle fiber is a single nucleus cell located mainly at the center of the cell. The sarcoplasmic reticulum and myofilaments are less developed than skeletal muscle. Actin and myosin filaments are found in same proportion but they lacks in striations. The myofilaments of smooth muscles are attached with dark zones of sarcolemma and these dark zones are analogous to the Z lines of skeletal muscles. Smooth muscle fibers may be single or in bundles but they are always surrounded by the reticular fibers. They are also have the network of collagenous, elastin filaments and contains ground substance, blood vessels and nerve fibers but supply of blood to the smooth muscle is poor than skeletal muscle.

Cardiac Muscle

Cardiac muscles have the characteristic properties of both skeletal and smooth muscles. It has single centrally located nucleus like smooth muscles and branched muscle fibers as skeletal muscles. It contains numerous glycogen granules in the sarcoplasm as well as numerous large mitochondria's. The myofilaments of cardiac muscles are not organised into myofibrils however, actin and myosin filaments are readily apparent under the microscope and also gives striated appearance. T tubules occur at Z line and are larger in diameter while sarcoplasmic reticulum are less developed and absent in terminal cisternae. The myocardium layer of heart makes the bulk of cardiac muscle and held by reticular and collagenous fibers.

Epithelial Tissue

Epithelial tissues contribute little to the meat because it is usually removed during slaughtering and processing. The epithelial tissue remaining in meat is mainly found in blood, lymph nodes and edible organs such as liver and kidney. These tissues have little intracellular material but maintain intercellular contacts. These tissues are responsible for protection, secretion, excretion, transport, absorption and sense perception.

Nervous Tissue

Nervous tissues contribute only 1% to the meat and the main function of these tissues are immediately prior to and during stunning and bleeding of the animal slaughter. In the central nervous system neuron comprises the bulk of nervous tissues. The other parts of nervous tissues are cell body (polyhedral shaped), axon (long cylindrical structure), neuroplasm (cytoplasm), centrally placed nucleus, dendrites (short branched structure), axon endings etc. Nerve fibers are composed of groups of neuronal axons and the group of fibers alongwith fascicles forms nerve trunks. In peripheral nervous system, nerve fibers are frequently referred as myelinated or unmyelinated because these are surrounded by Schwann cells and larger fibers are ensheathed with myelin cells within the Schwann.

Connective Tissue

Connective tissue is distributed throughout the body as a component of skeleton, connects and holds various parts of the body together i.e. organs, blood, lymph vessels and sheaths that surround tendons, muscle, skin, hide, nerve trunks, muscle fiber and nerve fibers. Connective tissues act as a body barrier against infective agents and plays vital role in wound healing. Connective tissue is composed of various structures some of them are discussed below.

Connective tissue proper: Fibrous connective tissue that surrounds muscles, muscle bundles and muscle fibers. The connective tissue proper alongwith adipose tissue contributes to qualitative and quantitative quality of muscles. This connective tissue proper has distinct fibers thus known as fibrous connective tissue while bone and cartilage are considered as supportive connective tissue. This CT proper is consist of mainly two types of the cells, fixed cells (fibroblasts, undifferentiated mesenchyme cells and specialized adipose cells) and wandering cells (eosinophils, plasma cells, mast cells, lymph cells and free macrophages).

Ground substance: The connective tissue proper is consisting of viscous solution containing soluble glycoproteins where cells and extracellular fibers are embedded are known as ground substance. The ground substance is also contains precursors of collagen and elastin namely tropocollagen and tropoelastin respectively. And among mucopolysaccharides, hyaluronic acid and chondroitin sulfates are the major components.

Extracellular fibers: The extracellular fibers forms dense connective tissue and they all together forms a network known as loose connective tissue. These are primarily comprised of collagen, elastin, and reticulin.

Adipose tissue: It is mainly of two types (white versus brown fat) depending on the developmental stage of the animal life cycle. Most of adipose tissue in meat animals is white fat while brown fat is mostly present around kidneys in animals at birth and starts disappearing with the advancement of age.

Cartilage: Cartilage of adult animal's body is mainly present on the disks of bone joints and composed of cells (chondrocytes) and exracellular fibers embedded in gel like matrix. These are of three types (hyaline, elastic and fibro cartilage) depending upon amount of collagenous and elastin fibers in the matrix. Among them hyaline is most abundant and others are merely modifications of it. Hyaline cartilage is found in surface of bones at joints, ventral ends of ribs, bottons (dorsal tips of thoracic vertebrae), lumber and thoracic vertebrae while elastic cartilage are found on epiglottis, internal and external portions of the ear. The fibro cartilage is found mainly in the association of tendons to bone attachment and capsules of ligaments and joints.

Bone: Bone is also a connective tissue and has all the structures of it but its extracellular matrix is calcified thus provides rigidity and protective properties to the skeleton. In long bones, a hollow cylinder with long, central shaft structure is present known as diaphysis. The enlargements of bones at both ends are referred as epiphyses and a bone covering with a thin membrane of specialized connective tissue is called periosteum. The articulating surfaces of the epiphysis covered with thin layer of hyaline cartilage at the ends of bones are termed as articular cartilage. The articular cartilages of adjacent bones forms joints together contain a specialized connective tissue substance called synovial fluid. Cartilaginous region separating the diaphysis and epiphysis is known as epiphyseal plate. Marrow is a structure found in the central interior of diaphysis, it is primarily red in young animals and yellow in adults and older animals.

Blood and lymph: Blood normally constitutes 7% of the animal body weight in mammals. It is necessary for nutrient, oxygen transport for cell metabolism and removal of waste by-products from the body. It provides defence mechanism against infectious agents and regulates pH and fluid balance in the body. The major blood cells in the body are platelets, erythrocytes and leukocytes.

Muscle and meat classification: On the basis of intensity of colour of muscle fibers meat is mainly classified into red or white. The examples of red meat is beef, buffalo meat, chevon, mutton etc while poultry and fish meat is comes under white category. The only few muscles are composed of only red or white muscle fibers while most of the muscles of meat animals are composed of both red and white muscle fibers. The muscle fibers in between red and white are known as intermediate fibers.

Characteristics	Red muscle fibers	Intermediate muscle fibers	White muscle fibers
Colour	Red due to higher myoglobin contents	Red due to higher myoglobin contents	White due to less myoglobin contents
Fiber diameter	Small	Intermediate	Large
Enzymes for metabolic activities	Higher in oxidative enzymes and lower in glycolytic enzymes	Intermediate in levels of both glycolytic and oxidative enzymes	Higher in glycolytic enzymes and lower in oxidative enzymes
Mitochondria	Numerous and larger in size	Intermediate in number and size	Lesser in number and small in size
Capillary density and lipid contents	Greater capillary density and lipid contents	Intermediate in both contents	Lower in both contents
Sarcoplasmic reticulam and T tubules	Less developed	Intermediate in development	More extensively developed
Mode of action	Tonic (contract slowly but for longer duration of time)	Contract faster than red fibers but less easily fatigued as white fibers	Phasic (contract rapidly in short bursts but easily get fatigued

Source: (Forrest *et al.*)

Composition of Muscle

Muscle is the principal component of meat. It is made up of water and organic compounds such as protein, fat and carbohydrates. The amount of different components varies according to meat type, animal species and age, body configurations etc. Water makes the major components (65-80%) of muscle tissue and among organic compounds protein is a main component and accounts average 19% of total muscle.

Water

Water is a principal constituent of extracellular fluid of muscle and numerous chemical constituents are suspended in it. It accounts approximately 75% of muscle volume. It also serves as medium for transport of substances between muscle fiber and vascular bed. Water, present in the muscle shows polar behaviour and it is associated with electrically charged reactive groups on the muscle protein. In muscle, water exists in three forms i.e. bound, immobilized and free water. Bound water is tightly bound with muscle by the electrically charged reactive groups and it is impossible to remove such water by the application of even severe mechanical and physical forces. It accounts about 4-5% of total water. The immobilized water is also bound with reactive group but as the distance increases from the reactive group on protein its bound is going to weaker thus its removal is dependant on the force applied to remove it. However, free water in the muscle is held by the surface forces only and can be removed easily. The amount of water decreases with the advancement of age of animal due to increase of adipose tissue in adults and older animals.

Proteins

Protein is a principal component of organic compounds or solid matter of muscle and contributes to 16-22% of total muscle mass. Muscle or meat proteins can be classified into three different groups on the basis of functions and solubility. These groups are myofibrillar or salt soluble proteins, sarcoplasmic or water soluble proteins and connective tissue or stromal or insoluble proteins.

Components of meat	In mammalian skeletal muscle (%)	In poultry muscle (%)
Water	75(range 65-80)	60-74
Protein	18.5 (range 16-22)	18.5-20.5
Myofibrillar protein	9.5	-
Myosin	5.0	
Actin	2.0	
Tropomyosin	0.8	
Troponin	0.8	
M-protein	0.4	
C-protein	0.2	
α-actinin	0.2	
β-actinin	0.1	
Sarcoplasmic protein	6.0	-
Soluble sarcoplasmic and mitochondrial enzymes	5.5	
Myoglobin	0.3	
Haemoglobin	0.1	

Contd.

Contd. to page 27

Components of meat	In mammalian skeletal muscle (%)	In poultry muscle (%)
Cytochromes and flavo proteins	0.1	
Stromal or connective tissue proteins	3.0	-
Collagen and reticulin	1.5	
Elastin	0.1	
Other insoluble proteins	1.4	
Lipids	3.0 (range 1.5 -13)	6-19.8
Neutral lipids	1.0(range 0.5 -1.5)	3.2-10
Phospholipids	1.0	2.8-9.8
Cerebrosides	0.5	-
Cholesterol	0.5	60mg/100 g
Non-protein nitrogenous substances	1.5	-
Creatine and creatine phosphate	0.5	
Nucleotides (ATP, ADP etc.)	0.3	
Free amino acids	0.3	
Peptides (anserine,carnosine etc.)	0.3	
Other non protein substances(creatinine, urea, ionosine mono phosphate, nicotinamide adenine dinucleotide, nicotinamide adenine dinucleotide phosphate	0.1	
Carbohydrates and non-nitrogenous substances	1.0 (range 0.5-1.5)	2.0
Glycogen	0.8(range 0.5-1.3)	
Glucose	0.1	
Intermediate and products of cell metabolism (hexose and triose phosphates, lactic acid, citric acid, fumaric acid, succinic acid, acetoacetic acid etc.)	0.1	
Inorganic constituents	1.0	1.0 -1.3
Potassium	0.3	46 (mg/100g)
Total phosphorous (phosphorous and inorganic phosphorous)	0.2	407(mg/100g)
Sulphur including sulphate	0.2	268(mg/100g)
Chlorine	0.1	-
Sodium	0.1	46 mg
Others (magnesium, calcium, iron, cobalt, copper, zinc, nickel, manganese etc)	0.1	Calcium(5.8 mg/100g)

Source: Forrest *et al.* and Sharma B.D

Myofibrillar proteins or contractile proteins: Proteins of myofilament are known as myofibrillar proteins. These proteins are of utmost importance because these proteins have great contribution in water holding capacity, emulsifying capacity and also in tenderness of meat. These are primarily actin and myosin and contribute 75-80% of myofibrillar proteins. Remaining fraction of these proteins is regulatory proteins and has regulatory functions on Adenosin-triphosphate-actin-myosin complex. These regulatory proteins are tropomyosin and troponin within the thin filament, two M proteins, a-actinin , b-actinin, C protein (which surrounds the myosin filaments to form the thick filaments), desmin (which encircles the Z disks and radiate out to connect adjacent myofibrils.

Actin: It is most abundant protein in cytoplasm of mammalian cells and contributes about 20 to 25% of myofibriller proteins. These are low charge proteins and have isoelectric pH around 4.7. It is rich in proline amino acid and imino group of this amino acid makes folding among the polypeptide chain and forms globular shape known as G-actin. The longitudinal polymerization of G-actin produces fibrous nature of actin known as fibrous actin (F-actin).

G-actin is a spherical monomer of two domains (large and small) and present at low ionic strength. The nucleotide (ATP or ADP) binding in cleft between domains occurs and each actin can bind to 4 other actins. G-actin molecule contains a high-affinity myosin head binding site. Another two types are also expressed in muscle especially in skeletal and cardiac muscles. These G-actin are linked together in strands in F-actin like the beads on a string of pearls and two F-actin are spirally coiled around each other and forms a characteristic super helix of actin filament.

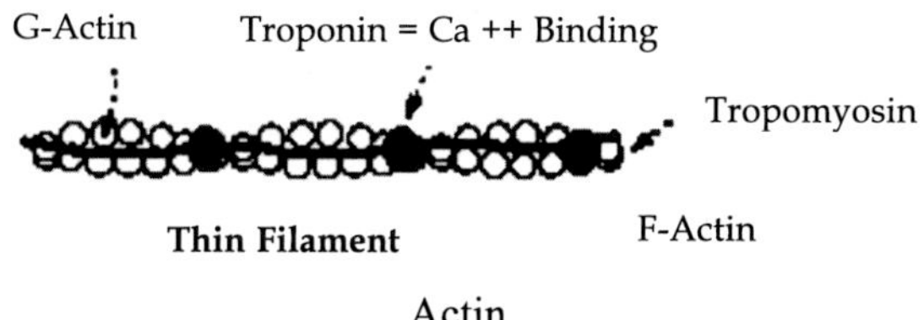

Actin

F-actin are helical polymer and are associated with head to tail polymerization of asymmetric monomers, at physiologic ionic strength, hydrolysis of ATP to ADP speeds polymerization and imposes polarity, steady- state flux of subunits through F-actin.

Myosin: Myosin is a most abundant (50-55%) protein of myofibrils. It is a fibrous and highly charged protein and has isoelectric pH around 5.4. Structure wise it is elongated rod shaped divided into three parts like head, neck and tail. By the action of enzyme trypsin in neck region of myosin, it breaks into two fractions which differs in their molecular weight known as light chain (light meromyosin) and heavy chains (heavy meromyosin).

Myosin light chains are of four types and each has molecular weight of 20000. It is divided two chemical classes and heads associated with one of each. Its C-terminal half forms a helical and N-Terminal makes globular head. It is responsible for isozymes activity of skeletal and cardiac muscles. These are DTNB light chain (phosphorylatable) and alkali light chain (non-phosphorylatable). These chains have high affinity to bind Ca^{++} and the myosin light chain kinase is responsible for changes conformation of myosin heads, potentiates actin-myosin interaction at low Ca^{++}, regulates myosin's ATPase activity and myosin assembly into thick filaments.

Myosin

In the contraction stage of muscles, head attaches to G–actin molecule of actin filaments and forms crossbridges. In this crossbridges formation phenomenon, a chemical complex known as actomyosin is formed which leads to the rigor mortis stage (rigid and inextensible condition in post mortem muscle).

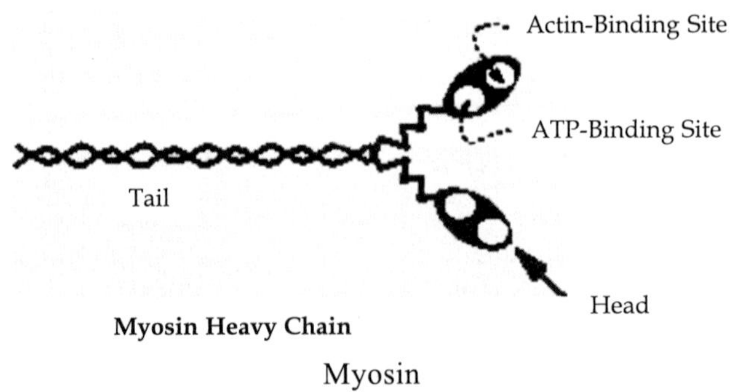

Myosin

Regulatory Proteins of Myofibrils

Tropomyosin: It is a highly charged protein molecules, fibrous in nature due to less proline contents and its isoelectric point occurs at pH 5.1. The contribution of tropomyosin in total myofibrillar proteins is 8 to 10%. It is a long thin filamentous strand formed with two coiled peptide chains (two stranded a-helical coiled-coil protein) attaches each other at end to end. This strand of tropomyosin attaches with actin filament on the surface of each of two coiled chains of F-actin. It contains two subunits a and b and among them b tropomyosin binds head to tail along length of actin filament. It regulates the Ca^{++} dependent muscle contraction alongwith troponin. In relaxed state of muscle it probably interferes with actin-myosin interaction.

Troponin: It is a calcium ion receptive globular protein, rich in proline and contributes 8-10% to the total myofibrillar proteins. Its major function is calcium sensitivity in actomyosin-tropomyosin complex. Structure wise it is present in the grooves of actin filament near the end of tropomyosin molecules. It is found in actin filament in a fashion that one molecule of troponin is attached at every 7 or 8 G-actin molecule. It is also made up of three subunits Troponin-T (TN-T), Troponin-C (TN-C) and Troponin-I (TN-I). TN-T binds with tropomyosin so it is known Tropomyosin binding subunit. It also makes its attachment with F-actin filament. TN-C is one of the most highly conserved proteins binds with Ca^{++} at low and high affinity sites. TN-I exits in skeletal and cardiac both muscles and prevent the actin myosin interaction in relaxed stage.

M-protein: It is a protein found in M line substance and binds tails of myosin together in muscles. It has 4% share in myofibrillar proteins. It is responsible for the maintenance of myosin filament.

α-actinin: It is made up of 97 kD subunits arranged in anti-parallel direction. It exists mainly in two forms i.e type-2 and type-3. Type-2 is generally present in all muscle fibers while type-3 is found in types- ii fibers only. These proteins are found in Z lines and are Ca^{++} insensitive but forms strong complex with F-actin. It is a globular protein and contributes 2-2.5% in myofibrillar proteins.

β-actinin: It is also a globular protein and founds in last part of actin filaments. Its main function is to maintain the constant length (1μm) of actin filament in each half sarcomere.

C-protein: It is a single polypeptide chain of 140,000 molecular weight and normally found in middle one third of each half of A-band. It is of three types MYBPC1, MYBPC2 and MYBPC3. It binds with myosin at tail region and it is responsible for maintenance of thick filaments in bundles of 200 to 400 molecules. It is also known as cytoskeleton protein.

Desmin: It circles the periphery of Z line and it is responsible for link of Z lines with adjacent myofibrils. It is also responsible for integration of contractile apparatus with sarcolemma and nucleus. Desmin protein is also considered as cytoskeleton type protein.

Sarcoplasmic proteins: These proteins are generally found in sarcoplasm of muscle and commonly referred as water soluble proteins. These proteins are readily extractable in water or low ioninic strength (0.06) salt solution. These proteins are soluble sarcoplasmic and mitochondrial enzymes, myoglobin, haemoglobin, cytochrome and flavoproteins etc. These proteins are effective emulsifiers of fat and are considered superior to myofibrillar proteins. Myoglobin is a major component contributes to colour of meat while haemoglobin, cytochrome enzyme and flavoproteins contributes little to meat colour. Haemoglobin stores oxygen in RBC's and bringing it to tissues however, myoglobin stores oxygen in muscles which is used in different metabolisms. The content of myoglobin differs in different animal species, age, sex and specific muscle for example muscles of cattle and buffalo (0.5%) have more myoglobin than pigs (0.06%). It is more in adults sheep than lamb, more in bulls than cows and also more in more active muscles (diaphragm) than passive muscles. In this protein there are numerous enzymes are found in sarcoplasm which can be broadly classified into proteolytic, amylolytic and lypolytic.

Structural Proteins

Connective tissue proteins: These are also known as stromal or insoluble proteins. These proteins makes supporting framework for living body. These proteins are mostly fibrous in nature which includes collagen, elastin and reticulin.

Collagen is a principal structural protein and is a major component of tendons and ligaments and lesser extents of bones and cartilage. It is also considered as most abundant (contributes 20-25% of all proteins of mammalian tissues) protein in the animal body and greatly influences meat tenderness. Collagen is basically a glycoprotein but also contains small quantities of galactose and glucose. Among the amino acids found in collagen, glycine is most abundant (contribute 1/3 of the total amino acids) while hydroxyl proline and proline account for another 1/3 of the amino acids. Amount of hydroxyl proline is almost constant (13-14%) in collagen and does not occur to any significant extent in other animal proteins. Tropocollagen molecule is the structural unit of collagen fiber and found in collagen in overlapping fashion. Collagen fibers are almost inextensible and individual fiber is colourless but after aggregation as in muscle sheaths and tendons gives white colour. The collagen fibers consist of intermolecular cross linkages which decide the relative solubility and tensile strength of the fibers. Due to the solubility pattern of collagen fibers meat of younger animals are tender than older ones because they have less cross linkages in collagen fibers and higher solubility. Collagen fibers are insoluble in dilute acid or alkali solution or concentrated solutions of neutral salts and non electrolytes unless they have denatured previously by heat or urea. But can easily be digested by pepsin and collagenase but are resistant to trypsin and chymotrypsin digestion. It is composed of unusual amino acids like glycine, hydroxyproline, alanine, proline, hydroxylysine etc.

Name of amino acids	Contribution in collagen protein (in %)
Glycine	> 33
Hydroxyproline	10
Alanine	11
Proline	12
Hydroxylysine	< 1
Tyrosine, histidine and sulphur containing amino acids	<1

Elastin as the name indicates it can easily stretched and return to normal length after release of tension. It is less abundant connective tissue protein than collagen and mainly found in ligaments, walls of arties and in the framework of different organs including muscles. It has yellow appearance and fluoresces as bluish white fibers under ultraviolet light. The large strand of elastin is found in ligament nuchae supporting the neck of ruminants and it also have characteristic yellow colour. Elastin contains different amino acids among them glycine is greater (1/3 of the total amino acids) in quantity and other amino acids are hydroxyproline (1-2%), tryptophane, tyrosine. It has lesser quantity of sulphur containing amino aids than collagen but posses two characteristic amino acids like desmosine and isodesmosine. In the nutritive value of meat it contributes very little or nothing because it is extremely insoluble and highly resistant to the digestive enzymes.

Reticulin is structures of small fibers which forms the delicate network around cells, blood vessels, neural structure, epithelium etc and also support them to hold in place. It is chemically similar to collagen but quit different than collagen in their morphological and histological characteristics. Reticulin fibers are fine, wavy, branched and appear black shinning threads on staining with ammonical silver solutions while mature collagen stains brown in this solution.

Adipose tissue is a specialized type of connective tissue in which fat storage cells are located. It is a site of accumulation of numerous adipocytes. There are two types of fat or adipose tissues generally recognized in mammalian muscles- white and brown. White type is found in meat animals while brown type is seen at birth and mostly found around the kidneys.

Lipids

Lipid is extremely variable component ranging from 1.5 to 13% of carcass and an inversely proportional to water contents of meat. The main lipids of animals are neutral lipids or triglycerides and phospholipids. The other forms of lipids are found mainly intracellular in muscle fibers i.e. cerebriside, cholesterol etc. In muscles, fat is generally present in two forms i.e. intramuscular and intermuscular.

Intramuscular fat is also known as marbling, in which fat is deposited within the loose networks of the perimysial connective tissue septa in close proximity to the blood vessels. However, intermuscular fat is called as seam fat; it is present in between the individual muscles inside the connective tissue septa. Another form of fats in meat is subcutaneous fat (finish), it is generally found inside the skin and visible after skin removal while fat stored around heart, kidney and in the pelvic canal areas is known as adipose tissue. Hard fat around kidneys and other glandular organs of cattle and sheep is referred as suet.

Neutral lipid or triglycerides are one of the major components of meat. These are glycerol esters of long chain fatty acids. Animal lipids commonly consist of simple triglycerides which have fatty acids of even carbon atoms but beef and mutton are mostly mixed triglycerides and contains branched chain fatty acids with odd number. In the animal lipids, saturated and monounsaturated fatty acids are mainly found. The predominant unsaturated fatty acids are palmitic and stearic which are of molecules with chains of 16 and 18 carbon atoms respectively. Likewise predominant unsaturated fatty acids in meat fats are oleic, lenoleic and lenolenic. Among them oleic acid is a principal fatty acid found in animal body.

Phospholipids are generally found in muscle tissues in form of phosphoglycerides but it also exist in different other forms like phosphatidyl choline, phosphatidyl ethanolamine, phosphatidyl serine and sphingomyelins. Phospholids are principal structural and functional constituents of cell membrane and are responsible for flavour and shelf stability of meat products. Fat also contains some essential fatty acids which are considered as precursor material for synthesis of phospholipids in cell membrane.

Cholesterol is an unesterified or free form of sterol found in cell membranes of animal tissues. Generally lean meat is low in cholesterol but in veal cholesterol contents are more even it is low in fat. Cholesterol comes under bad fat category that's why its minimum quantity is desirable.

Carbohydrates

Immediately post mortem, muscles normally contain 1% glycogen (most abundant carbohydrate in muscles) and most of which disappears before completion of rigor mortis. In animal body approximately half of the carbohydrate are found in liver (2-8% of fresh liver weight) in the form of glycogen and rest half is found in whole of the body like muscles (in glycogen form), in blood (in glucose form), organs and glands. Some other carbohydrate compounds are also found in animal bodies which are intermediates of carbohydrate metabolism and mucopolysaccharides of connective tissues. The role of carbohydrate in animal body is energy metabolism and in the structural tissues. The amount of glycogen present in the muscle decides the ultimate pH. Physical properties of meat like water holding capacity, tenderness and colour are also depend on rate and amount of glycogen breakdown.

Inorganic Substances

Muscle contains a variety of inorganic substances like physiologically important cations and anions, calcium, magnesium, potassium, sodium, iron, phosphorous, sulphur and chlorine. The main role of inorganic substances is in rigor mortis but it also controls pH, water holding capacity and also contributes in meat colour and tenderness. The contribution of inorganic substances in muscle is about 1% and among all potassium alone contributes 0.3% in inorganic substances.

Vitamins

Vitamin is a most variable factor in muscles and it is dependant on species and age of animals, degree of fatness and type of feed given to the animals. The greatest variation is found in vitamin-B complex. As it is 5-10 times more in pork than beef and mutton. Vitamins found in muscles can be classified into water soluble i.e. vitamin-B complex and vitamin C and fat soluble vitamins (vitamin A, D, E and K). Among them water soluble are mainly found in lean and fat soluble in fatty tissues. Overall meat is a good source of vitamin-B complex and poor source of fat soluble vitamins and vitamin C but some organs like liver and kidney contains appreciable amount of theses vitamins. Generally meat vitamins are relatively stable during heating and processing but thiamine and vitamin B_6 is heat labile. Among vitamin B_6 and thiamine, vitamin B_6 is more heat stable.

References

1. Bourne, G.H. (1960). The Structure and Function of Muscle, Academic Press, New York, Ist ed. Vol.3.
2. Forrest, J.C., Aberle, E.D., Hedrick, H.B., Judge, M.D. and Merkel, R.A. (1969). Structure and Composition of Muscle and Associated tissues. In: Principles of Meat Science, W.H. Freeman and Company, San Francisco, pp 27-89.
3. Lawrie, R.A. (1966). Chemical and biochemical constituents of muscle. In: Meat Science, Pergamon Press, New York, Ist ed., pp 66-115.
4. Meat science university Texas A&M University internet source, google.
5. Murray, J.M. and Weber, A. (1974). The Cooperative Action of muscle Proteins. Scientific American, Vol. 230, No. 2, pp 58-71.
6. Panda, P.C. (1976). Formation, structure, food value and chemical composition of eggs. In: Text Book On Egg and Poultry Technology.Vikas Publishing House Pvt. Ltd., New Delhi, pp 9-46.
7. Sharma, B.D. (1999). Structure, composition and nutritive value of meat tissues. In: Meat and Meat Products Technology (Including Poultry Products Technology), Japee Brothers Medical Publishers (P) Ltd, New Delhi. Pp 8-22.
8. Vaclavik, V.A. and Christian, E.W. (2003). Meat, Poultry, Fish and Dry Beans. In: Essentials of Food Science, 2nd ed. Springer (India) Pvt. Ltd. New Delhi, pp 147-156.

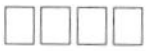

3 Conversion of Muscle to Meat

Conversion of muscle to meat is a complex process in which several physical and chemical changes takes place over a period of several hours or even days. The major changes which take place during this process include fall in muscle pH and temperature as well as muscle shortening which further leads to proteolysis or ageing. These changes during conversion of muscles to meat are variable and have great effect on meat quality (tenderness, juiciness, flavour, colour etc.) and also on certain processing characteristics like emulsification, binding properties and yield of the products. To know this complex process it is necessary to understand the process of energy production and metabolic pathway shifting in live animals.

Pre Slaughter

In the living animal, aerobic metabolism is used to obtain energy. The source of energy at this stage is either free fatty acids or blood glucose or muscle glycogen. In this process total 38 ATP molecules are produced from single glucose or glycogen molecule by the complex processes known as glycolysis, oxidative decarboxylation and oxidative phosphorylation. However, under stressful situations, anaerobic metabolism may be used and lactic acid is produced. Lactic acid is usually transported from the muscles to the liver, where it is re-synthesized into glucose and glycogen, or to the heart, where it is metabolized to carbon dioxide and water.

Post Slaughter

After slaughter, aerobic metabolism begins to fail due to the stored oxygen supply being depleted. To maintain homeostasis, anaerobic energy metabolism starts producing lactic acid, consuming the glycogen stored in the muscles. Thus, the structural integrity of the cells is maintained for a period of time although less energy in the form of ATP is produced.

In the exsanguinated animal, the circulatory system is not capable of removing metabolites so that lactic acid remains in the muscle and increases its concentration during the post-mortem period until the glycogen stored in muscle is consumed. The drop in pH and the ultimate pH of muscle will be different depending on the type of muscle metabolism either glycolitic or oxidative. Glycolitic muscles produce higher amounts of lactic acid than oxidative ones because they use the glycolitic pathway to produce energy rather than the oxidative pathway. For instance, in Semimembranosus, Longissimus dorsi and Biceps femoris muscles, the pH declines quicker and to a greater extent in muscles such as Semispinalis capitis, Psoas major, Serratus ventralis and Quadriceps femoris.

Process of Conversion of Muscle to Meat

The series of changes take place during conversion process from muscle to meat which may be summarized as:

Immobilization and Exsanguination: Immobilization is a process in which animal is rendered unconscious prior to bleeding while in exsanguination blood is removed from the animal body as much as possible. As soon as bleeding starts, series of post mortem changes also begins. First change is drop in blood pressure so to adjust blood pressure heart functions increases and peripheral blood vessels start constricting to maintain the blood pressure and supply of blood to the vital organs. However, only 50% of the blood can be removed from the animal body and remainder being helds in the vital organs. The presence of blood in the vital organs makes them vulnerable for bacterial growth and spoilage. Due to this reason bleeding should be as much as possible.

Loss in homeostasis: Homeostasis is a process of maintenance of physiologically balanced internal environment. This includes pH, temperature, oxygen concentration and energy supply. Homeostatic system is regulated by nervous systems and lost within 4-6 minutes of exsanguination. In this condition animal becomes unable to cop up with the surroundings and physiological functions of the body. The homeostasis is an important step in the conversion of muscle to meat because reactions and changes during conversion of muscle to meat are result of loss of homeostasis. It is also important because pre-slaughter conditions may alter post-mortem changes and thereby have bearing on quality of meat.

Failure of circulatory system and essential nutrients to the muscles: After exsanguination, the circulatory system for carrying the essential nutrients to muscles and waste material away from the muscles ceased. As a result oxygen supply to the muscles depleted because of non-functioning of aerobic pathway through citrate cycle and cytochrome system. Then the energy metabolism is shifted to anaerobic pathway but it produces less ATP. However, the energy required for structural integrity and temperature control of muscle cells can be maintained anyhow. In normal live animal lactic acid is produced in anaerobic pathway, is circulated to liver and then is converted it into glucose and glycogen and then in the presence of sufficient oxygen they produces energy to the muscles. But, in exanguinated animals, lactic acid starts accumulating in muscles until the glycogen stored in muscles is fully depleted. This process of lactic acid accumulation and depletion of glycogen in muscles leads to drop in pH which is fully dependant on the amount of glycogen reserve in the muscle at the time of post mortem.

Post-mortem heat generation and dissipation: soon after exsanguination, muscle temperature rises because due to circulatory seizure heat from deeper parts of body comes out to the lungs and surfaces of the body. The generation of heat and its dissipation from body surfaces is depending upon type of muscle, metabolic difference of body parts and muscles, external parameters like scalding and seinging in pigs and poultry, the temperature of slaughter room, time expands between slaughter and dressing operations.

Post-mortem pH decline: Post-mortem pH decline has a tremendous impact on the colour of meat – whether normal, dark or light. In living muscle, energy is stored as glycogen which provides energy by conversion of glycogen to glucose to pyruvate. Whereas, after slaughter of animal energy is also stored in muscles in the form of glycogen but the energy conversion into glucose and pyruvate is lost so in dying muscle, lactic acid accumulates and lowers pH. The conversion of glycogen into lactic acid and its irreversible accumulation in muscles within 24 hours after death may be summarized as:

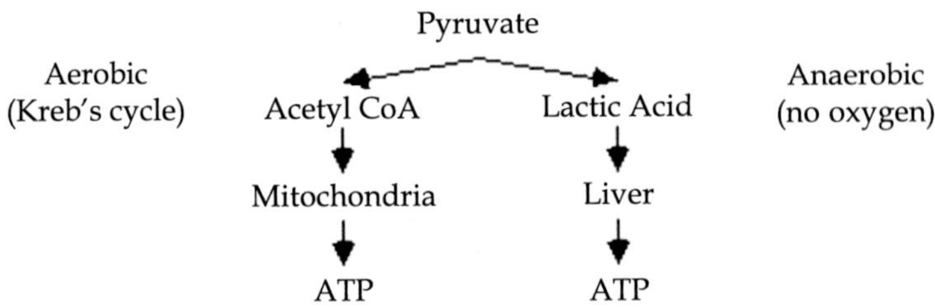

(1) Glycogen $\rightarrow$ lactic acid+2ATP (By anaerobic metabolism)

(2) Muscle pH falls from 7.0 $\rightarrow$ 5.6 (because of lactic acid)

(3) Muscle colour also changes from purple to bright red or pink due to exposure to air.

pH is an important factor in determining the water-holding capacity of meat (the ability of meat to retain its water during application of external forces such as cutting, heating, grinding, or pressing). The water-holding capacity will be lowest at isoelectric point where the number of positively and negatively charged groups of the myofibrillar proteins is equal. Thus, the charges cancel out and no charge is available to hold the bound and immobilized water.

Gross steps in the conversion of muscle to meat

Conversion of muscle to meat is a process which has a sequence of events and changes as given below:

Animal slaughter

↓

Exsanguination

↓

Loss of homeostasis

↓

Drops in blood pressure

↓

To maintain the blood pressure and ensure blood supply to vital organs pumping of heart increases and peripheral vasoconstriction takes place

This situation leads to stoppage of nutrient supply to muscle and removal of waste products from the muscles due to loss of oxygen supply to muscles

↓

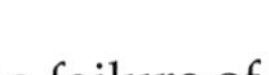

Temperature of carcass rises due to failure of temperature control mechanism

Myoglobin stores little oxygen which lost in short period of time as a result stored oxygen is depleted

Energy process is then shifted to anaerobic metabolism leading to production of lactic acid

By this way muscle can produces less energy which is only sufficient to maintain structural integrity and temperature

Lactic acid starts accumulating (irreversibly) in the muscles until all the glycogen reserve is lost

Drop in pH takes place which depend on amount of glycogen in the muscle at the time of exsanguination

Rigor mortis development

Loss of structural integrity and denaturation of protein leads to loss of defence mechanisms thus muscle becomes susceptible to microbial invasions

From the above sequence of events it becomes clear that the fall in pH and rise in temperature are both results of the same events .This is one of the critical point in conversion of muscle to meat where important measures are required to be taken.

Rigor mortis: Rigor mortis is a Latin word which means "stiffness to death" and generally referred as stiffening of muscles after death. It is due to formation of permanent cross bridges between actin and myosin filaments in muscles. Actually rigor mortis starts when ATP level falls below 5 m mol/kg. The phenomenon of cross bridge formation is same as construction in living muscles except the relaxation in last phase due to lack of energy (loss of ATP complex with Mg^{2+}). Development of rigor mortis is not a permanent phenomenon and starts disappearing due to physical degradation of muscle structure particularly in Z-line area of muscles. The resolution of rigor mortis is faster at higher temperature and it is now proved that an increase of 10°C for certain period doubles the tenderness. Among the animals who obtained slaughter maturity sooner provides faster ageing as compared to others. The fastest proteolysis observed in chicken meat and about 80% tenderness can be achieved in this species within 8 hrs as compared to 10 days in beef, 7.7 days in sheep, 4.2 days in pigs and 9.5 days in rabbits. Loss of elasticity and extensibility, shortening and increase in tension are the some physical changes observed in rigor mortis. Rigor mortis has three phases:

Delay phase: It is a state of rigor in which plenty of ATP in the muscle (complexed with Mg^{++}) is present. In this state muscle remains in the relaxed state and no cross bridges between the thick and thin myofilaments will occur.

Onset phase: As stores of ATP in the form of creatine phosphate (CP is used to rephosphoryate ADP to ATP) are used up, rigor bonds between the thick and thin myofilaments are formed. As more bonds are formed, the muscle loses extensibility.

Completion phase: When the entire CP is lost, the muscle has no way of regenerating ATP. Thus, full rigor mortis will set in. In this stage muscles becomes relatively inextensible. In this process sarcomere length is shorten.

Sketch of Rigor Mortis

Depletion of muscle glycogen → creatine phosphate (CP) is used to convert ADP to ATP → Loss of CP → Muscles becomes unable to maintain relaxed state → actomyosin cross bridges begin to form → onset of rigor mortis → Completion of rigor mortis

Difference between normal contraction and rigor shortening

Normal contraction	Rigor shortening
It is a reversible process	It is irreversible muscle contraction
Temporary bonds formation	Permanent bonds formation
No stiffening	Tension develops within the muscles and leads to stiffening
Cross bridges forms at only 20% of the possible binding sites	Nearly all binding sites in the area of overlap between the actin and myosin filaments are utilised

Loss of protection: The protective mechanism of living cells like membrane protection, functions of internal organs, circulatory and lymphatic system is altered during conversion of muscle to meat which ultimately facilitates the proliferation of micro-organisms in the muscles and organs.

Post-Mortem Changes in Muscle Structure

Microscopically rigor muscles have similar structure as in the living muscle but if pH continues to fall it will reach a range where the cathepsins get activated and lead to proteolysis. A normal pH drop should be from pH 7 to 5.6 - 5.7 in 6-8 hrs post-mortem and to an ultimate pH in range of 5.3 - 5.7 in 24 hrs post mortem. In some animals it will remain 6.5- 6.8 during the first hour after exsanguination. An early accumulation of lactic acid is linked with rise in carcass temperature which leads to denaturation of proteins. The level of denaturation of proteins is species specific with pork being more susceptible than beef while fish flesh is more sensitive to protein denaturation than mammalian muscles. Denaturation of proteins in muscles leads to certain conditions like loss of protein solubility, loss of water holding capacity and loss in the intensity of muscles pigment coloration.

The first structural change observed in this process is degradation of Z-disks by proteolysis. Another significant change observed is degradation of desmin. Both these processes lead to weakening and fragmentation of myofibrils. The other alterations observed in the process are degradation of troponin-T, titin and nebulin while most resistant proteins to alterations are myosin and actin.

Effect of Post-Mortem Changes on Physico-Chemical Characteristics of Muscle

Colour: Normal colour of muscle in living animal is bright red due to abundance of oxygen. But in post-mortem there is shortage of oxygen so colour becomes dark purplish red. Fresh meat at the time of cutting has dark red colour but on exposure to atmospheric air within few minutes it changes into brighter red colour. It is due to oxygenation of myoglobin pigment in the muscles.

Proteins: Solubility of muscle proteins changes due to denaturation of proteins by cathepsin and other factors like low pH and high temperature. Action of cathepsin enzyme in ageing of meat breaks collagen connective tissue proteins.

Water binding capacity: Water binding capacity of the muscles decreases due to fall in pH and denaturation of proteins. The change in water binding capacity in the muscle during conversion of muscle to meat is greatly influenced by rate and extent of pH drop. If pH of muscle remains very high, water binding will also be high and it will be similar to living muscles. Contrary to this, water binding capacity of the muscles will be low in case of rapid drop in pH.

Factors Affecting Post-Mortem Changes

Pre-slaughter factors

Stress: Stress prior to slaughter in animal is an important factor hampering the quality meat production. It may be external or internal stress. It activates homeostatic mechanism of the animal body and generates variable physiological responses. The important changes in meat arising due to stress are change in colour, water holding capacity and pH of meat. These responses are executed through various hormones like epinephrine (breaks down glycogen stored in liver and muscles and also breaks down fat), nor-epinephrine (maintains the blood circulation), adrenal hormones (provide stress resistance) and thyroid hormones (increase metabolic rate). Stress factor is mainly responsible for the conditions PSE, DFD and dark cutting meat.

Environmental effects: the most important environmental factor is temperature. If it is too low, animal is not acclimatized and leads to the conditions like shivering, higher rate of metabolism etc. and if it is too high it will not allow an animal to dissipate body heat leading to ATP splitting and glycolysis. Another important factor is humidity; if it is too high then produces discomfort and if too low then produces weight loss and less tender meat. Other factors are also of equal importance and have great effect on meat quality like light, sound, and space.

Hereditary: The meat quality changes during conversion of muscle to meat are moderately hereditable. However, some of the meat quality parameters like colour, intramuscular fat, tenderness etc. are predominantly decided by the breeds and strains of the particular meat species.

Age and sex: It is now well proven that the collagen content in almost all maturity age groups is almost same. However, the number of intermolecular cross links increases with the age of the meat animals which makes the collagen less soluble and this collagen gives the toughness to the meat. The sex also decides meat colour, tenderness and flavour. It is well known that abnormal meat flavour in pork and some other species is mostly due to male hormone testosterone and its metabolites.

Muscle location and diets: The location of muscle in the meat animal body decides its tenderness. It is also decided by the activity of the muscle, less active muscles are tenderer as compared to more active muscles. Tenderness is also dependent on the amount of connective tissues present. Diet is also important to restore the glycogen level in the muscle and the supplementation of feed with starch and sugar sometimes helps in avoidance of stress conditions in animals particularly in pigs. Similarly the diet rich in carotene contents gives the yellowish tint to the meat by the deposition of this pigment in the fat of that meat species.

Animal handlings: The handling of animals prior to slaughter has great influence on the meat quality. Proper resting, watering, feeding and handling are the key components which need to be given due importance.

Post-slaughter factors

Processing conditions: The way of handling carcasses immediately after slaughter has significant influence on meat quality. The microbiological load of handling place, personnel hygiene of the handlers, equipments used, water conditions etc. are some of the important factors which must be keep ideal to enhance the quality of meat and also to enhance the shelf life of meat.

Temperature: The temperature of carcass during handling as well as during storage has great influence both on quality and shelf life of meat. The handling of meat at 50^0C produces heat rigor in meat due to rapid utilization of ATP and induction of early onset of rigor. Contrary to this if pre-rigor meat is chilled/frozen leads to the conditions like cold shortening and thaw rigor.

Technological interventions: If technological interventions are applied on carcass in proper time and by proper procedures it may alter the meat quality. The most significant intervention is electrical stimulation of carcass to accelerate the conditioning of meat to make the tough meat tender.

Abnormal Post Mortem Changes

PSE (Pale, Soft, Exudative)

In some animals especially in pigs, muscle pH drops rapidly below 5.8 during the first hour after exsanguination or before dissipation of body heat. This kind of meat is termed Pale, Soft and Exudative (PSE). In this case pH decreases twice as fast as normal. It must have increased ATP use for glycolysis to occur rapidly causing pH to fall abnormally fast. Pale colour of this meat is because light is reflected by denatured sarcoplasmic proteins. Softness and exudation from structural damage particularly in areas of super contraction and Z- line loss, increased denaturation of protein. PSE is common in pigs with defective ryanodiine receptors but it is not necessary that all susceptible pigs will exhibit PSE pork. PSE can also occur in normal pigs by improper handling.

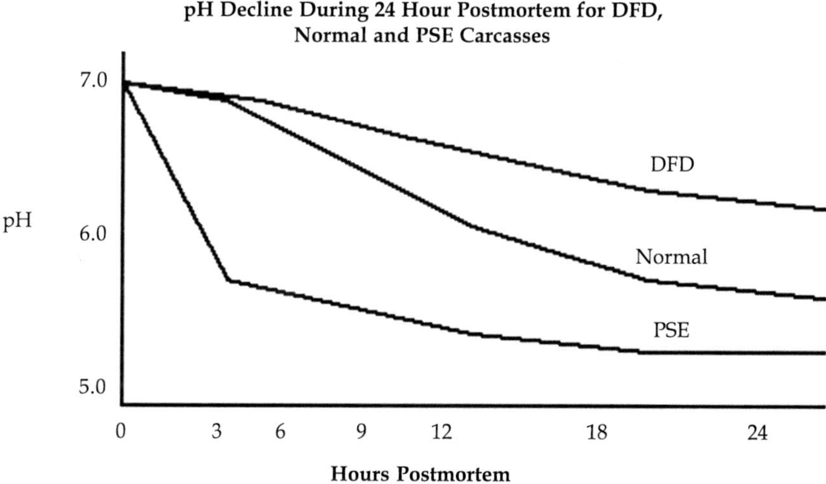

The low pH prevents or retards microbial growth. The rate of pH change post mortem also influences meat quality. Development of low pH (acid) in muscle causes denaturisation of muscle proteins. This denaturisation causes loss of protein solubility, loss of water and protein-binding capacity and loss in intensity of muscle pigment colouration. All these changes are undesirable, whether the muscle is going to be used as fresh meat or subjected to further processing.

The gene that is responsible for PSE meat is the Halothane sensitivity gene (HAL), which is associated with a fast rate of post-mortem decline in pH and which is more likely in stress-susceptible animals. Halothane positive animals are homozygous and they can be detected by exposure to halothane gas which induces the Porcine Stress Syndrome (PSS). However, a more accurate identification of three genotypes is now possible using a direct marker test (DNA Test) developed after the identification of the gene (ryadonine receptor gene, RYR1) and the discovery of the specific mutation.

The pig is not the only animal that can be affected by this kind of defect. Pale meat or exudative meat can be also detected in beef and poultry, but are not necessarily undesirable attributes in these species. Although it is not frequent, exudative meat has been found in carcasses of young bulls. The deviation in quality is generally much less pronounced than that of PSE pork so that PSE in beef has been little investigated. In poultry, particularly turkey, it is common to find pale meat but it is not exudative. Usually it is related to a low haem pigment content of the muscle. PSE can be decreased by rapid post-mortem cooling.

DFD (Dark, Firm and Dry)

In some animals pH drops slightly during the first hour after slaughter and then remains stable at a relatively high level, giving an ultimate pH of higher than 6.00 (6.2-6.5). This condition leads to dark, firm, dry (DFD) meat. In this case muscle appears dark and may be so dry as to be sticky just like pre- rigor muscle because the water is kept tightly bound to proteins. It is mainly due to glycogen depletion at the time of pre-slaughter resulting into little or no lactic acid production post slaughter. In this condition myosin and actin are taken away from isoelectric point. The high pH also enhances microbial meat spoilage. The presence of DFD meat develops mainly in the forequarter, LD and glycolytic muscles of ham for all the species but the frequency is different among species. This condition can be found both in beef and pork. The DFD meat is more prone to spoilage due to higher pH.

PSE meat	DFD meat
Due to short-term hereditary glycogen depletion	Due to long term environmental glycogen depletion
Causes are mainly hereditary but PSE is also associated with swine susceptible to porcine stress syndrome (PSS)	Mainly due to stress conditions during transport-hauling of pigs, without feeding, depletes muscle glycogen.
In this case short-term glycogen depletion prior to death occurs. Then very rapid glycolysis due to excitement (ante-mortem) or due to holding on kill floor a long time before chilling (post-mortem)	Muscles are highly depleted with glycogen and there is limited lactic acid production occurs post-mortem.
Sudden drop in pH below 5.80 during the first hour and then ultimate pH is achieved	Slight drop in pH during the first hour after slaughter and then remains stable at a relatively high level.
PSE is common in pigs with defective ryanodiine receptors but it can also occur in beef and poultry as a less pronounced form	DFD can be found both in beef and pork
Ultimate pH reaches to 5.1- 5.2	Ultimate pH of higher than 6.00
PSE condition leads to loss of colour, firmness and water-holding capacity due to denaturation of proteins	In DFD, meat becomes dark in colour, more firm and high in water-holding capacity
Low pH retards microbial meat spoilage. PSE condition can be decreased by decrease emphasis on selection for heavy muscles.	High pH enhances microbial meat spoilage. DFD condition can be decreased by Feed and rest for 24 or 48 hr prior to slaughter

Chemical basis of PSE and DFD meat

Quality parameters	Normal meat	PSE meat	DFD meat
Muscle colour	Normal	Pale	Dark
Status of glycogen at the time of death	1.0%	0.6%	0.3%
Level of glycogen 24 hrs of post mortem	0.1%	0.1%	0.1%
Lactic acid production	High	Very high	Low
Ultimate muscle pH	5.6	5.1	6.0-6.5

Acid Meat

It is a another kind of pig meat called Acid or Hampshire type meat in which the rate of pH fall within the first hour is normal but the ultimate pH is lower than normal at a value of below 5.5. The RN gene also known as Napole gene is responsible for the Hampshire type meat and affects carcass composition and pork quality, especially in Hampshire pigs. This gene has a favourable effect on carcass length and leanness.

Dark Cutting Beef or Lamb

Dark cutting beef or lamb is caused by long term glycogen or intermediate glycogen depletion which may be of environmental or/ and hereditary in origin. In this case beef stress syndrome (BSS) condition occurs which is a type of alarm reaction of general adoption syndrome. The chemical reaction in this stage can be summarized as:

$$\text{Glycogen} \xrightarrow{\text{Adrenaline}} \text{Lactic acid to liver and pyruvic acid to Krebs cycle}$$

This condition arises due to exhaustion, exposure to cold, excitement, sex (in bullock), sudden feed withdrawal, sickness etc. Incidences of Dark cutting beef or lamb can be reduced by proper handling and prevention of stress to the animals.

Cold shortening and thaw rigor

Cold shortening is a condition which arises when pre-rigor meat is chilled. It is because glycogen remains in the muscles and it is not converted into lactic acid, leads to the irreversible contraction of muscle (shortening of actin and myosin filaments). Cold shortening produces five times tougher meat than normal meat. Cold shortening is generally seen in beef and lamb meat due to higher proportion of red muscle fibres and lesser fat coverings. Thaw rigor is a similar condition in which meat is frozen before onset of rigor mortis. So the glycogen reserve present during thawing induces muscle contraction and meat becomes very tough.

Cold shortening	Thaw rigor
Condition arises when pre-rigor meat is chilled below 15-16^{0}C	Thaw rigor occurs when frozen pre-rigor meat is thawed.
Physical shortening is due to release of Ca^{2+} into sarcoplasm and it may be up to 80% of its original muscle length.	In most of the conditions physical shortening observed in Thaw rigor is up to 60% of the original muscle length
Less severe depending on the release of calcium and failure of calcium pump of sarcoplasmic reticulum	More severe
Most of the times I-band disappears completely	No complete disappearance of I-band

Now with the invention of latest technologies like proteomics, apoptosis etc. the process of conversion of muscle to meat has become more clear. The proteomics is able to provide the information beyond the proteolysis like cleavage sites and degradation patterns of protein during post mortem. Certain markers of tenderness are also identified with the help of proteomics. This is also helpful in identification of PSE conditions. However, apoptosis is related to the muscle atrophy and neuromuscular disorders.

Disorders seen in the conversion of muscle to meat can also be minimized by the due care of animals' pre and during slaughter. The proper handling, rest and other scientific approaches in slaughter practices avoid these abnormal conditions. Some scientific approaches like use of enzymes, high voltage electric stimulation of muscles, proper storage temperature and several other measures are now able to correct these abnormalities up to some extent.

References

1. Hedrick, H.B., Aberle, E.D., Forrest, J.C., Judge, M.D. and Merkel, R.A. (1994). Conversion of muscle to meat and development of meat quality. In: Principles of Meat Science, 3rd edn., Kendall/Hunt Publishing Company, Iowa, pp 95-122.
2. Forrest, J.C., Aberle, E.D., Hedrick, H.B., Judge, M.D. and Merkel, R.A. (1969). Structure and Composition of Muscle and Associated tissues. In: Principles of Meat Science, W.H. Freeman and Company, San Francisco, pp 145-156.
3. Fujii, J., Otsu, K., Zorzato, F., de Leon, S., Khanna, V.K., Weiler, J.E., O'Brien, P.J. and Maclennan, D.H. (1991). Identification of a mutation in porcine ryanodine receptor associated with malignant hyperthermia. Science, 253: 448-451.

4. Garrido, M.D. Banon, S. and Alvarez, D. (2005). Medida del pH. In: Caneque,V and Sanudo,C (Eds), Estandarización de las metodologías para evaluar la calidad del producto (animal vivo, canal, carne y grasa) en los rumiantes. INIA, Madrid, pp. 206-215.
5. Jensen, W.K., Devine, C. and Dikeman, M., (2004). Encyclopedia of Meat Sciences. Oxford, UK.
6. Meat science. Texas A&M University internet source, google.
7. Mendirutta, S.K. (2013). Conversion of muscle into meat-recent concept. In: 5th convention of Indian Meat Science Association and National Symposium on Emerging Technologies Changes to Meet the Demand of Domestic and Export Meat Sector, Feb 7-9: 167-172.
8. Oliver, M.A., Gispert, M. and Diestre, A. (1993). The effects of breed and halothane sensitivity on pig meat quality. Meat Science, 53: 105-118.
9. Sharma, B.D. (1999). Structure, composition and nutritive value of meat tissues. In: Meat and Meat Products Technology (Including Poultry Products Technology), Japee Brothers Medical Publishers (P) Ltd, New Delhi. Pp 8-22.

□□□□

4 Nutritive Value of Meat

Meat is an animal flesh that is used as food. Most often, this means the skeletal muscle and associated fat but it may also describe other edible tissues such as organs, livers, skin, brains, bone marrow, kidneys or lungs. Meat is highly nutritious food because it contains protein, fat and carbohydrates in relative proportion, supply energy as required by the human body, posses ability to build or replace tissues and the substances present in meat are easily absorbed by the human body. Meat is also a good source of B-complex vitamins but fat soluble vitamins are low in meat. It is a good source of phosphorous, zinc and iron but low in calcium. Meat also contains significant amount of copper, sodium, potassium and magnesium but low in carbohydrate contents. Carbohydrate is found mainly in form of glycogen which disappears completely after completion of rigor mortis. In general lean red meat is particularly good source of protein, niacin, vitamin B6, vitamin B12, phosphorus, zinc and iron. About 100g of meat can provide more than 25% RDI of these nutrients. It also provides more than 10% RDI of riboflavin, pantothenic acid and selenium. Of the four meats, mutton is particularly nutrient-dense and the richest source of thiamine.

Functions of Different Nutrients in the Body

Proteins serve as building materials for the growth and repair of body tissues. It acts as component of enzymes and hormones, regulates fluid and electrolyte balance, maintain the acid-base balance and are an integral part of the immune system. Proteins can even be used for energy. Meat is high in both protein quality and quantity. Protein is made up of amino acids. The nine essential amino acids (amino acids that the body cannot make) and must get from food, are found in meat making it a complete protein. Few plant sources are also complete proteins.

Fat is a concentrated source of energy for the body and provides 9 calories energy per gram. It is generally recommended that no more than 30 percent of the total calories consumed ruires from fat. The fat in food provides flavour, aroma and texture as well as increasing the feeling of satisfaction after a meal.

Cholesterol is a waxy, fat-like substance required for cell building, manufacturing hormones and vitamin D and other functions. If no cholesterol is eaten, the body can make all the cholesterol by the metabolism in the body. Blood cholesterol levels are affected by several factors like heredity, age, sex, and type of the foods. It is recommended that consumption of cholesterol through foods should not be more than 200 mg per day.

Iron is a part of the protein haemoglobin and carries oxygen in the blood. It is also a part of the protein myoglobin in muscles which makes oxygen available for muscle contraction. Iron is also important for energy metabolism. It is a nutrient that is necessary for young children experiencing rapid growth, teenagers, and pregnant women, nursing mothers, premenopausal women and athletes. Dietary iron occurs in two forms, heme and nonheme. Heme iron is bound to haemoglobin in blood and myoglobin in muscle tissue. It is found only in meat, fish and poultry and is more easily absorbed by the body than nonheme iron. About 40 percent of the iron found in meat is heme iron whereas; nonheme iron sources include fruits, vegetables, grains, eggs and dairy products. Vitamin-C increases the absorption of iron and the foods inhibiting iron absorption include coffee, tea, red wine, whole grains, bran, chocolate, and legumes.

Zinc is a component of insulin and enzymes. It is an essential component for some physiological functions i.e. growth and reproduction, appetite, taste, night vision and immune system. Good sources of zinc include meat, shellfish, whole grains and legumes.

Phosphorous is an integral part of certain metabolism such as carbohydrates, proteins and fats. It makes the bones and teeth strong in combination with calcium and vitamin D. Phosphorus is found in almost all foods but protein-rich foods such as meat, poultry, fish and dairy products are good sources.

Thiamine, riboflavin, niacin, vitamin B_6 and vitamin B_{12} are found in substantial quantities in meat. Thiamine, riboflavin and niacin are a part of coenzymes used in energy metabolism. Thiamine supports the functions like normal appetite and nervous system. Riboflavin helps in normal vision and skin health and it is widely distributed in animal protein such as meat, poultry and fish. Vitamin B_6 takes part in amino acid and fatty acid metabolism as a coenzyme. It helps in conversion of tryptophan to niacin and also helps in red blood cells formation. Pork is an excellent source of thiamine and vitamin B_6. Niacin is an important component for health of skin, nervous and digestive system. Animal foods are the only sources of Vitamin B_{12} however; body can store excess amounts of it.

Nutritional Status of Meat

Nutritive value of meat can vary widely depending on the species and breed of animal, the way in which the animal is being reared, feeding, anatomical part of the body and the methods of butchering and cooking. For example game animals, birds and deer meat are leaner than meat of farm animals. In general meat has high nutritive value and posses various nutrients required for the growth and development of the human body.

Proteins

In general lean meat contains about 16.5 to 20% protein and it is of high biological value. The protein found in liver and kidneys have very high biological value and are good in replacing and manufacturing the body protein. Body system can absorb about 97% of animal protein while absorption rate of plant protein is only 84%. Animal proteins come under high value category because it contains all essential amino acids (lysine, methionine, cystine, tryptophan, leucine, isoleucine, phenylalanine, valine etc.) in good proportion. Among the proteins found in meat myofibrillar and sarcoplasmic proteins are very good source of essential amino acids while connective tissue proteins are low in tryptophane and sulphur containing amino acids and collagen is poor in lysine.

Comparison of nutrient analysis of100 grams portion of lean meat

Nutrient	Goat	Chicken	Beef	Veal	lamb	Mutton	RDI
General							
Fat , g	14.7	13.6	2.8	1.5	4.7	4.0	-
Protein, g	25.8	27.2	23.2	24.8	21.9	21.5	46-64
Calories,Kcal	239	239	498	477	546	514	6.5-15.8 MJ
Cholesterol, mg	111	88	50	51	66	66	-
Minerals							
Iron, mg	2.6	1.3	1.8	1.1	2.0	3.3	8-18
Calcium, mg	29.8	15.0	4.5	6.5	7.2	6.6	1000-1300
Sodium, mg	90.7	82	51	51	69	71	460-920
Zinc, mg	5	2	4.6	4.2	4.5	3.9	8-14
Magnesium, mg	27.9	23.5	25	26	28	28	310-420
Potassium, mg	362.7	223	363	362	344	365	2800-3800
Phosphorus, mg	68	182	215	260	194	290	1000
Copper, mg	2	0.07	0.12	0.08	0.12	0.22	1.2-1.7
Selenium, mg	-	-	17	<10	14	<10	60-70
Vitamins							
Vitamin-A, IU	40	161.2	<5	<5	8.6	7.8	700-900
Thiamin (B1), mg	0.37	0.06	0.04	0.06	0.12	0.16	1.1-1.2
Pyridoxine (B4), mg	0.2	0.4	-	-	-	-	-
Cobalamin (B12), mg	0.65	0.30	2.5	1.6	0.96	2.8	2.4
Pantothenic Acid, mg	0.35	1.03	0.35	1.50	0.74	1.33	4-6
Niacin, mg	2.96	8.47	5	16.0	5.2	8.0	14-16
Vitamin B6	-	-	0.52	0.8	0.10	0.8	1.3-1.7
Beta-carotene,mg	-	-	10	<5	<5	<5	700-900
Alpha-tocopherol, mg	-	-	0.63	0.50	0.44	0.20	7-10

References: Nutrient Profile information taken from USDA, Human Nutrition Handbook 8-5 and Johnson (1987)

Comparison of Meat, Poultry, & Seafood (Skinless, Lean, Trimmed and Broiled or Roasted)

Food	Calories (kcal)	Carbohydrate (g)	Protein (g)	Fat (g)	Cholesterol (mg)
Pink Salmon	127	0	18-22	4	57
Chicken Breast	142	0	25	3	73
Pork Tenderloin	159	0	16	5	80
Beef Sirloin	171	-	-	7	76
75% lean ground Beef	235	0	32	15	75
95% Lean Sirloin	144	-	-	4	39
95% Lean Hamburger	171	-	-	7	76
Lamb	227	-	27	12	-
Venison loin	139	-	22	5	62
Pork Shoulder	207	-	22	13	82
Veal Cutlet	155		28	4	112

Reference: USDA National Nutrient Database for Standard References (2006)

Amino acid composition of muscle proteins of goat beef, pork and lamb and beef collagen (mg/g protein)

Amino acid	Goat	Beef	Pork	Lamb	Beef collagen
Aspartic acid	-	88	89	85	43
Threonine	48	40	51	49	18
Serine	-	38	40	39	35
Glutamic acid	-	144	145	144	99
Proline	-	54	46	48	114
Glycine	-	71	61	67	187
Alanine	-	64	63	63	74
Valine	54	**57**	50	52	23
Methionine	27	23	25	23	8
Cystine	-	14	13	13	0
lsoleucine	51	51	49	48	15
Leucine	84	84	75	74	28
Tyrosine	-	32	30	32	67
Phenylalanine	35	40	41	39	21
Histidine	21	29	32	27	8
Lysine	74	84	78	76	30
Arginine	75	66	64	69	75
Tryptophan	15	11	13	13	0

References: Extracted from Srinivasan *et al*. (1974) and Pellet and Young (1990).

Raw red muscle meat contains around 20-25g protein/100 g of meat. Cooked red meat contains 28-36g proteins/100 g of meat. It is due to decrease in water content and increase in nutrients concentration during cooking.

Fat

Meat fat is a good source of essential fatty acids like linoleic acid, linolenic acid and arachidonic acid. Animal fat is mainly neutral fat and phospholipids. The most abundant neutral fats are triglycerides which are responsible for calorie value of fat in meat. These are glycerol esters of straight-chain carboxylic acids while phospholipids of meat are normally found in phosphoglycerides form. They are found in less quantity (0.5-1.0%) than triglycerides and are responsible for maintenance of structural and functional components of cells and cell membranes. The main purpose of fat in diet is energy or calorie production. The production of energy is 2.25 times more from fat than carbohydrate and protein. Essential fatty acids like linolenic and linoleic acids are found abundantly in pork and organ meat. Meat fat is absorbed by body system within 5-6 hrs and absorption rate is about 90% and it is much greater than fat of plant origin.

Among all meat fats most abundant fatty acid is oleic acid (monounsaturated fatty acid with one double bond). Most commonly occurring saturated fatty acids are butyric and caproic acid. Saturated fatty acids comprise 40% of total fatty acids in the lean component and 48% in the fat component of red meat. In beef and veal, approximately half of the saturated fatty acids in both the lean and fat component of red meat are palmitic acid and about a third is stearic acid. In lamb and mutton, the proportions of these two fatty acids are more similar. There is little variation between cuts in the proportion of fatty acids. Polyunsaturated fatty acids (PUFA) ranges from 11 to 29% of total fatty acids. Pasture fed beef is a better source of omega-3 fats than grain feed beef. Beef and lamb also have more omega-3 fats than either chicken or pork although fish is still a significantly better source than any of the red meats. Trans-fatty acids found in raw muscle meat vary from as little as 22 mg/100 g in veal to 123 mg/100 g in lamb but is generally less than 3% of the total fatty acid content. Levels in both raw and cooked muscle meat are higher in lamb and mutton than in beef and veal.

Now a day's cholesterol is considered as bad fat for the human body due to the risk of cardiovascular diseases. However, it is proven by many scientists that the dietary intake of cholesterol at the level naturally present in meat is no more related with the blood cholesterol in normal individuals. It is present in minor quantity but makes important component of animal tissues. It exists either in unesterified (free form) or esterified (combined with fatty acid) form. Cholesterol is mostly (90%) found in free form. Total cholesterol content in lean beef, pork and lamb is about 70-75 mg per 100g of fat. It is 300 mg per g fat in liver and 2000 mg per g in brain. Veal contains slightly higher amount of cholesterol than lean beef, pork and lamb.

Fatty acid contents in different meat (percentage of total fatty acids)

Fatty acid	Beef	Lamb	Pork
Palmitic acid	29	25	28
Stearic acid	20	25	13
Palmitoleic acid	2	-	3
Oleic acid	42	39	46
Lenoleic acid	2	4	10
Linolenic acid	0.5	0.5	0.7
Arachidonic acid	0.1	1.5	2

Reference: USDA, handbook No.8 in processed meat by Pearson *et al.* (1968)

Minerals

Meat is a good source of phosphorous and iron but low in calcium. Meat is also the richest source of zinc and is able to fulfill the one third to one half demands of the humans. Meat also contains sodium, potassium, magnesium, copper etc. Contents of fat indirectly influence the mineral contents of meat. Iron is an important mineral readily available through meat. It can serve the purpose of recommended daily allowances (RDA) of about 18 mg per day required for pregnant and non pregnant premenopausal women.

Beef and lamb meat are among the richest sources of the iron and 100g meat can provide at least one-quarter of daily adult requirements. Meat proteins also appear to enhance the absorption of iron from meat. Similarly, absorption of zinc from a diet high in animal protein is greater than from plant foods and the requirements for zinc may be as much as 50% higher for vegetarians. Red meats are also good sources of selenium and provide over 20% RDI per 100g of meat although it is likely that selenium values in meat will be significantly affected by animals feed and the time of the year of sampling. Lean meat is low in sodium but the ratio of potassium-sodium is more than 5. The copper content in raw lean cuts ranges from 0.055 to 0.190 mg/100g in beef and veal, 0.090 to 0.140 mg/100 g in lamb and 0.190 to 0.240 mg/100 g in mutton. Liver and some sea foods are also good sources of copper.

Mineral contents in different meat (mg per 100g of meat)

Mineral	Chicken	Beef (strained)	Lamb (strained)	Pork (strained)	Veal
Calcium	-	8	9	8	10
Phosphorous	129	127	124	130	145
Iron	1.9	2.0	2.1	1.5	1.7
Sodium	263	228	241	223	226
Potessium	96	183	181	178	214

Reference: USDA, handbook No.8 in processed meat by Pearson *et al.*

Vitamins

Meat is an excellent source of vitamin-B complex but low in fat soluble vitamins and lacking in vitamin-C. Red meat is abundant in bioavailable vitamin B_{12}, providing over two-third of the daily requirement from 100g of meat. Up to 25% RDI of riboflavin, niacin, vitamin B_6 and pantothenic acid can also be provided by 100g of red meat. Red meat is a poor source of thiamine as compared with pork. Liver is an excellent source of vitamin-A and rich source of riboflavin and niacin. But the levels in lean muscle meat tissue are low. For all these vitamins older animals tend to have higher concentrations. So the levels in beef are generally higher than those in veal, and mutton has more than lamb. Species wise pork is rich source of thiamin, chicken vitamin B_6 and niacin, beef B_6 and B_{12}. Levels of vitamin D in meat are low and difficult to measure. However, recent assays of meat in New Zealand have reported levels of 0.10 µg vitamin D3 and 0.45 µg 25-OH D3 per 100g in beef and levels of 0.04 and 0.93 µg/100 g respectively in lamb. Given the higher biological activity of the 25-OH vitamin D. This means that 100g of cooked beef could provide 12% of the estimated adequate intake of 10 µg/day for 51 to 70 year old individual. While cooked lamb could provide more than 25%.

Table : Vitamin contents in different meat (mg per 100g of meat)

Vitamin	Chicken	Beef (strained)	Lamb(strained)	Pork(strained)	Veal
Vitamin-A	-	-	-	-	-
Thiamine	0.02	0.01	0.02	0.19	0.03
Riboflavin	0.16	0.16	0.17	0.20	0.20
Niacin	3.5	3.5	3.3	2.7	4.3
Ascorbic acid	0	0	-	-	-

Reference: USDA, handbook No. 8 in processed meat by Pearson *et al.*

Carbohydrates

Role of carbohydrates in nutritive value of meat is almost negligible because amount of glycogen in meat is quite low or even completely absent. At the time of post mortem carcass contains about 1% glycogen (only carbohydrate found in muscle tissue) which disappears with the completion of rigor mortis and has great role in pH of meat.

Meat-Based Bioactive Compounds

In addition to the traditional essential nutrients, meat also contains some bioactive substances like taurine, carnitine, conjugated linoleic acid, endogenous antioxidants and creatines. Taurine is a meat amino acid and found about 110 mg/100 g in lamb and 77 mg/100 g in beef. It is derived through methionine and cysteine metabolism. It is responsible to cope up with immune challenges and may offer protection against oxidative stress. L-carnitine is beta-hydroxy-gamma-trimethyl amino butyric acid found in inner mitochondrial membranes to produce energy during exercise. It is found in skeletal muscle and is particularly abundant in sheep muscle at up to 209 mg/100 g and in beef at around

60 mg/100 g. Conjugated linoleic acid is mostly found in ruminants meat and milk and has as an antioxidant and immunomodulatory properties and may also play a role in the control of obesity and cancers. It is mostly present in the fat component of red meat (approximately 1 g/100 g) but is also found in the muscle meat (10-46 mg/100 g in raw meat and 30-100 mg/100 g in cooked red meat). Meat also contains several endogenous compounds like ubiquinone, glutathione, lipoic acid, and spermine. Coenzyme Q10 (ubiquinone) has antioxidant properties and its level in meat is estimated to be around 2 mg/100 g in both beef and sheep meat. While glutathione is a component of glutathione peroxidase enzymes which have an important antioxidant role in the body. It may also play a role in immune response and enhancing iron absorption by contributing to the meat factor. Glutathione levels in red meat are estimated to be 12-26 mg/100 g in beef and most meats contain approximately twice the level of glutathione of poultry and up to 10 times the content found in fish. Creatine and creatine phosphate play an important role in muscle energy metabolism and muscle performance. Red meat contains approximately 350 mg/100g.

Nutritive Value of Organ Meats

All organ meats (except tripe) are extremely rich in vitamin B_{12} and high in cholesterol especially brains and mostly low in sodium. Liver is a rich source of protein, iron, zinc, riboflavin, niacin, vitamin A and folate. Kidney is rich in protein, thiamine, riboflavin, iron and a source of folate. In addition heart is a good source of iron and zinc but not as good as liver and kidney. In organ meats brains and tripe are not good sources of vitamins or minerals.

Ethics of Eating Meat

Ethical issues regarding the consumption of meat can include objections to the act of killing animals or the agricultural practices surrounding the production of meat. Reasons for objecting to the practice of killing animals for consumption may include animal rights, environmental ethics, religious doctrine or an aversion to inflicting pain or harm on other living creatures. The religion of Jainism has always opposed eating meat and there are also many schools of Budhism and Hiduism that condemn the eating of meat. Some people, while not vegetarians refuse to eat the flesh of certain animals such as cats, dogs, horses or rabbits due to cultural or religious taboo. In some cases, specific meats (especially from pigs and cows) are forbidden within religious traditions. Some people eat only the flesh of animals which they believe have not been mistreated and abstain from the meat of animals reared in factory farms or from particular products such as foie gras and veal.

References

1. Cattlemen's Beef Board and National Cattlemen's Beef Association (2005). Twenty-nine Ways to Love Lean Beef. Retrieved July 23, 2007, from www.kybeef.com/nutrition.htm.
2. Eastridge, J. S. and Johnson, D. D. (1990). The effect of sex class on nutrient composition of goat meat. International Goat Production Symposium, Oct. 22-26, pp. 143-146.
3. Emholm, C., Huttunen, J. K. and Pietinen. P. (1982). Effect of diets on serum lipoproteins in a population with a high risk of coronary heart disease. N Engl J Med., 307:850-855.
4. Forrest, J.C., Aberle, E.D., Hedrick, H.B., Judge, M.D. and Merkel, R.A. (1969). Structure and Composition of Muscle and Associated tissues. In: Principles of Meat Science, W.H. Freeman and Company, San Francisco, pp 27-89.
5. James, N. A., Berry, B. W., Kotula, A. W., Lamikanra, V. T. and Ono, K. (1990). Physical separation and proximate analysis of raw and cooked cuts of chevon. International Goat Production Symposium, Oct. 22-26, pp.22.
6. Lawrie, R.A. (1966). Chemical and biochemical constituents of muscle. In: Meat Science, Pergamon Press, New York, Ist ed., pp 66-115.
7. National Institutes of Health, National Heart, Lung, and Blood Institute (2005). Your Guide to Lowering Cholesterol with Therapeutic Lifestyle Change (NIH Publication No. 06-5235). Washington, DC: U.S. Department of Health and Human Services.
8. Nutritive Value of Foods (1981). Home and Garden Bulletin, Number 72, U.S.D.A., Washington, D.C., U.S. Government Printing Office.
9. Panda,P.C.(1976). Text Book On Egg and Poultry Technology.Vikas Publishing House Pvt. Ltd., New Delhi.
10. Park, Y. W., Kouassi, M. A. and Chin, K. B. (1991). Moisture, total fat and cholesterol in goat organ and muscle meat. J. Food Science 56(5):1191-1193.
11. Pond, W. G. and Maner, J. H. (1984). Swine Production and Nutrition. The Avi. Publishing Company, Inc. Westport, Connecticut.
12. Potchoiba, M. J.,. Lu, C. D., Pinkerton, F. and Sahlu. T. (1990). Effects of all milk diet on weight gain, organ development, carcass characteristics and tissue composition, including fatty acids and cholesterol contents of growing male goats. Small Rumin. Res. 3:583-592.

13. Stromer, M. H., Goll, D. E. and Roberts, J. H. (1966). Cholesterol in subcutaneous and intramuscular lipid depots from bovine carcasses of different maturity and fatness. J. Animal Sci. 28:454.
14. Terrell, R. N., Suess, G. G. and Bray, R. W. (1969). Influence of sex, live-weight and anatomical location on bovine lipids. 2. Lipid components and subjective scores of six muscles. J. Animal Sci. 28:454.
15. U.S.D.A. (1989).A Handbook of USDA, Washington, DC.
16. Vaclavik, V.A. and Christian, E.W. (2003). Meat, Poultry, Fish and Dry Beans. In: Essentials of Food Science, 2nd ed. Springer (India) Pvt. Ltd. New Delhi, pp 179-184.
17. Whitney, E. and Rolfes, S. (2004). Understanding Nutrition. Belmont: Wadsworth Publishing. Clip Art from Microsoft® Clip Art Library. Sandra Bastin, PhD, RD, LD, CCE Extension Food and Nutrition Specialist June 1998; Revised August 2007.

□□□□

5 Fraudulent Substitution of Meat

Fraudulent substitution of meat is the adulteration or mixing of the inferior or cheaper quality meat into superior quality meat. The first case of fraudulent substitution was recorded in thirteenth century A.D. at Florence in Italy. A common fraud in the meat industry in which uninspected meat is substituted for meat that has undergone inspection and been branded as satisfactory. The other frauds are the substitution of meat of another species, e.g. horse for beef especially in Britain and Ireland, beef in kangaroo meat in Australia, cat for chicken or rabbit, goat meat for mutton, mutton for venison, dog meat and cat meat for chevon in other countries including India. As per an estimate about 25-30% of meat sold in India is adulterated. These practices are more common in comminuted meat products. These illegal practices are punishable under PFA act 1955. The choice of method to be applied is depend on the need or condition of meat recovered.

Aim of Fraudulent Substitution Recognitions

1. To safeguard religious taboos.
2. To protect the human health.
3. To prevent the cheating of consumers.
4. To implement the acts and regulations in meat and its products manufacture.
5. It is also important for economic considerations point of view.

Detection of Fraudulent Substitution

1. Physical methods.
2. Anatomical and histological methods.
3. Chemical methods.
4. Biological methods:

   A. Serological methods.

   B. Electrophoretic methods.

   C. Newer biotechnological methods.

1. Physical Methods

The physical methods of fraudulent substitution detection are mainly based on characteristics of flesh and fat of different species.

A. Meat characteristics

S.No.	Meat	Colour	Consistency	Odour	Marbling
1.	Beef	Dark red with slight brownish tinge	Firm and cut surfaces are shiny	-	Present
2.	Buffalo meat	Dark red	Firm	-	Absent
3.	Veal	Pale grey to greyish red	Firm	-	Absent
4.	Chevon	Light red and paler than mutton	Very firm	Goaty odour	Absent
5.	Mutton	Dark red	Firm and dense	Ammonical	Absent to scanty
6.	Pork	Greyish white	Very soft to dark red	Urine like	Present
7.	Poultry meat	White	Firm	-	Absent
8.	Horse meat	Dark red with bluish tinge	Firm with prominent fascia	-	Absent
9.	Camel meat	Red	Fairly firm	-	Absent
10.	Dog	Dark red meat	Firm	Disagreeable and repulsive	Slightly present
11.	Rabbit meat	Pale, grey to grey red	Firm	Pronounced Absent	
12.	Venison	Dark red to brownish red	-	-	Absent or very less

B. Fat identification

S. No.	Fat	Colour	Consistency	Fat type	Bone marrow characteristics	Remark
1.	Beef	Yellowish white	Firm	Intramuscular fat	Pure white to reddish yellow	-
2.	Buffalo fat	Pure white	Slightly firm	No Intramuscular fat	-	-
3.	Veal	Reddish yellow to white	Loose and greasy	No Intramuscular fat	Pink red	-
4.	Chevon	Pure white	Hard, firm and brittle	No intermuscular fat	Firm and slightly red	-
5.	Mutton	Pure white	Hard , firm and brittle	Abundant intermuscular fat	Firm and slightly red	-
6.	Pork	White	Soft and greasy	Subcutaneous but intramuscular also	Pink red and soft	On boiling it turns to whitish grey.
7.	Poultry fat	Yellow	Loose	Mostly subcutaneous	-	-
8.	Horse fat	In young- light gold to yellow In mature -white	Soft and greasy	No intramuscular fat	Waxy, yellow, greasy and soft	On exposure to air turns to blackish
9.	Dog fat	White to whitish grey	Oily and greasy	Slight intramuscular	-	-
10.	Rabbit fat	Whitish yellow	Loose	Fat is absent in muscle and confined to body cavity	-	-

2. Anatomical Methods for Carcass Differentiation

On the basis of anatomical structure of the carcase we can easily differentiate some closely related animal carcases. Some of the basic structural differences in closely related animal species are as follows:

A. On the basis of dental formula

*Cattle and buffalo $2\dfrac{(0033)}{(4033)} = 32$

*Sheep and goat $2\dfrac{(0033)}{(4033)} = 32$

*Pig $2\dfrac{(3143)}{(3143)} = 44$

*Horse $2\dfrac{(3133)}{(3133)} = 40$

B. On the basis of vertebrae and their characteristics

Type of vertebrae	Cattle	Sheep and goat	Horse	Pigs	Chicken	Rabbit
Cervical	7	7	7	7	15-17	7
Thoracic	13	13	18	14-15	7	12
Lumber	6	6	6	6-7	L+S fused	7-8
Sacral	5	4	5	4	14	3-4
Coccygeal	18-20	16-18	15-21	20-30	5-6	14-20

* Cattle and Horse

a. Superior spinous processes of first six dorsal vertebrae
In horse- well developed.
In cattle - not well developed.

b. Transverse processes of last three lumber vertebrae
In horse- articulate with each other.
In cattle- no articulation.

* Sheep and Goat

Lateral border of sacrum In sheep-thickened in form of roll
In goat – thin and sharp

C. On the basis of number of ribs and their degree of curvature

Cattle	-	13
Sheep and goat	-	13
Horse	-	18
Pig	-	14-15
Chicken	-	7
Rabbit	-	12

*Horse and Cattle

a. Ribs are narrower but more markedly curved in horse than cattle.

b. Thoracic cavity is longer (18 ribs) in horse than cattle (13 ribs).

*Sheep and Goat

Thorax- In sheep- barrel shaped
In goat - Laterally flattened

D. On the basis of specific characteristics of long bones

a. In fore quarter

Scapula : In sheep –short and broad, superiors spine, bent back and thickened.

In goat-have distinct neck, spine straight and narrow.

Radius : In sheep-1.25 length of metacarpus.

In goat- twice is the length of metacarpus.

Ulna : In horse- extends half of the length of radius.

In cattle-extends full length of radius and articulates with carpus.

b. In hind quarter

Femur : In horse- third trocanter is present.

In cattle- third trocanter is absent.

Fibula : In horse- extends $2/3^{rd}$ length of tibia.

In cattle- fibula is a small pointed projection.

E. Sex determination on anatomical basis

a. On the basis of gonads and udder.

b. Presence of developed gracilis and bulbocavernosus muscle (erector and retractor penis muscle) in male.

c. On the basis of size of pelvic cavity.

F. Histological methods

i. Fibre length and fibre diameter determination.

ii. Number of fibres in a muscle bundle of a particular muscle.

On the basis of muscle fibre length, diameter, density and pattern we can identify the meat species. Muscle fibre diameter of buffalo meat is smaller than ox meat while number of fibres per mm^2 is more than ox. The striation of muscles in buffalo is more angular as compared to ox while it is horizontal in poultry meat. In poultry, muscle fibres are thinner and density values are greater than other species.

3. Chemical Methods

To determine the meat species, various chemical tests are of immense use in which we can identify different meat constituents and body fat parameters to reach on a particular conclusion.

i) Meat constituent's estimation

In this method we can estimate the glycogen contents, myoglobin contents and some other minerals and vitamins.

a. *Glycogen content*: The glycogen content should be measured as soon as possible after slaughter because it starts diminishing after slaughter and cutting. The glycogen content in the horse flesh is considered as maximum (2.28%) while it is 0.5 to 1.0% in other fleshes of food animals.

b. *Myoglobin contents*: The amount of myoglobin (0.73%) in horse flesh is also significantly higher than other food animals flesh.

c. *Intramuscular fat contents*: Intramuscular fat content is higher in mutton (13.3%) as compared to 2.6% in beef, 0.9% in buffalo meat, 3.6% in chevon and 4.4% in pork.

d. *Fatty acid contents*: The amount of linoleic acid is higher (1-2%) in horse flesh and has practically no stearic acid while flesh of sheep, goat and cattle contains almost nil (0.1%) linoleic acid with large proportion of stearic acid. In hog, fat contains palmitodi-stearin alongwith lauric and myristic acid.

e. *Carotene contents*: Carotene content is absent in buffalo fat while it is present in cow fat in the amount of 0.14 to 0.225 mg per gram of fat. This is the reason of white colour of fat in buffalo flesh and yellow coloured fat in cow and its progeny flesh.

f. *Vitamin-A*: It is absent in buffalo meat, chevon and pork while present in mutton and beef.

ii) Body fat parameters

a. Refractive Index (R.I): In this test fat is liquefied by heat into oil and refractive index of that oil can be estimated. The horse fat oil has maximum R.I of 53.5 as compared to less than 40 in ox and not more than 51.9 in pig fat oil.

b. Iodine Number: This test is based on the amount of iodine absorbed by unsaturated fatty acids present in fat. It is again higher in horse fat (71-86) as compared to 34-46 in ox, 50-70 in pig and 35-46 in sheep fat.

4. Biological Methods

A. Serological or Immunological methods

The prerequisite in this technique is preparation of species specific antiserum, usually antiserum against serum. As an example when we want to test for horse flesh, a rabbit is injected with blood serum of horse periodically. Then rabbit develops antiserum or antibodies specific for horse serum. These antibodies have the quality of precipitating proteins of the horse but not against other animals.

i) Ring Precipitation Test (RPT)

In this method homologous antigen and antibodies reacts together and make a ring at the point of its interaction. For example if the antiserum of horse mixed with filtered extract from the suspected meat in a test tube, a turbidity occurs and forms a definite precipitation ring if sample is positive for horse flesh.

Limitations of the test

a. It is only qualitative test.

b. It is not applicable for heat treated meat.

c. It gives false positive test in closely related species due to cross reactivity.

d. Developed ring is difficult to observe and diffused in a short period of time

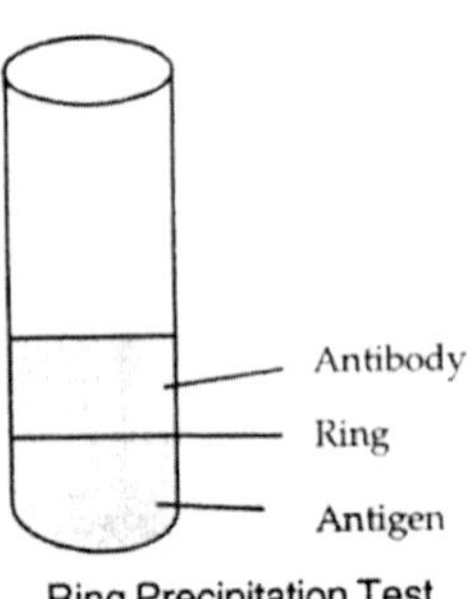

Ring Precipitation Test

ii) Immunodiffusion Test or Agar Gel Precipitation Test (AGPT) or Agar Gel Immunodiffusion Test (AGID)

Initially this test was developed by Ouchterlony in 1948. In this method 2-3 mm thick agar is used and several wells are cut in the gel itself. The sample in form of extract dilutions are filled in wells and tested antisera is also filled in the adjacent wells. These wells are then incubated for 1-2 days and allow diffusion of antigen and antibodies. In case of positive result white precipitate (precipitin band) is formed at the point of its meeting.

To overcome the shortcomings of this test in form of false positive results with non antisera components i.e. citrate and ascorbate etc. Double immunodiffusion test (DID) is invented in which sample is allowed to diffuse in same agar gel and white precipitate is formed in same gel.

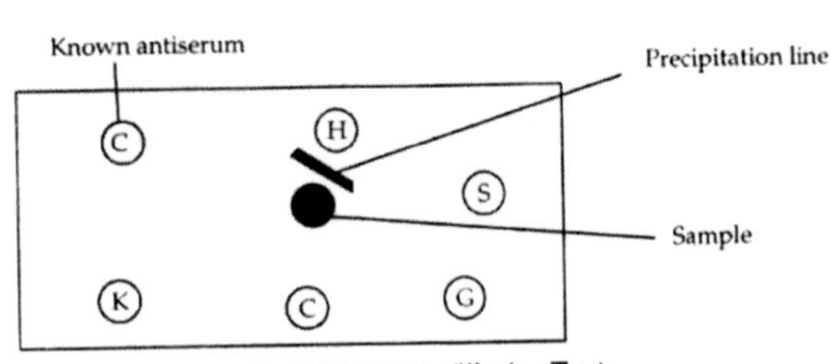

Double Immunodiffusion Test

Advantages

a. It is both qualitative and quantitative test.

b. Adulteration up to 5% can be detected.

c. Cooked meat at 80°C for less than 10 minutes can be detected.

d. It can detect 1:32 dilution of the sample.

e. Slide can be preserved for future use.

Limitations

a. Time taking method and takes about 2-3 days.

b. It is ineffective for thoroughly cooked meat.

c. There is a chance of false positive results in closely related species due to cross reactions.

d. Low sensitivity.

The other modifications of these methods are ORBIT (Overnight rapid beef identification test) for single species identification. In this test three disks i.e blank, disk with beef antigen and disk with bovine antiserum are generally used. The sample fluid is filled in blank disk and directly placed in precast agar gel and allow it to incubate overnight and then observed for precipitation development. The similar test for poultry is known as PROFIT (Poultry rapid overnight field identification test).

Another modification of this test for multispecies identification is MULTI-SIFT (Multispecies identification field test). This test is based on same principle and can be used for beef, pork, poultry, sheep, horse and deer meat.

The use of Dot-blot technique for this purpose is not uncommon in which binding of antigen from the sample takes place in a membrane (nitrocellulose or cyanogen bromide activated nitrocellulose) with a specific antibody. It is a rapid and sensitive test but it is not sufficient method for quantitation.

iii) Enzyme-linked Immunosorbent Assay (ELISA)

It is a rapid, highly sensitive (able to detect 2% adulteration) and most suitable method for handling numerous samples at a time. There are several ELISA techniques are in use depending on the compound fixed first, solid support used and concentrations of antigen and antibodies used. The most common types of ELISA are:

a. Indirect ELISA.

b. Competitive ELISA.

c. Sandwitch ELISA

In Indirect ELISA, species is detected by the antisera that are subsequently used labelled with suitable conjugate while in Competitive ELISA a fixed amount of antigen antibodies are mixed with the meat extract and preincubated. These techniques are mainly based on the polyclonal antibodies against muscle or serum protein. These polyclonal antibodies are limited in production, heterogeneous affinity and needs purification to avoid cross reactions. So the use of monoclonal antibodies is most common in ELISA test because they are specific for a single antigenic site. These monoclonal antibodies can be produced from thermostable proteins of different species or by the hybridoma cell lines.

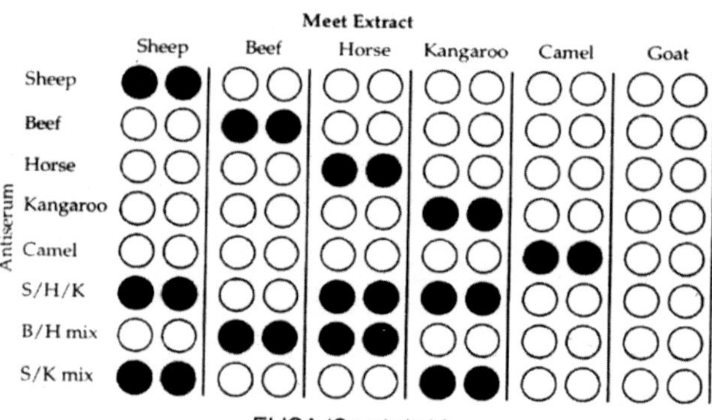

ELISA (Sandwitch)

Steps involve in ELISA techniques are

a. Take a 96 (12X8 wells) multiwell ELISA plate.

b. Either the plate is having already antigen coated micro wells or coats the antigen in micro wells.

c. Addition of sample in the micro wells.

d. Addition of antibodies.

e. Addition of enzyme labelled antibodies.

f. Incubate the ELISA plate.

g. Washing.

h. Addition of substrate solution and incubation for enzyme reaction.

i. Addition of stop solution.

j. Immediate reading of colour in a multiplate reader detector.

k. Make a standard ELISA curve for quantitative results.

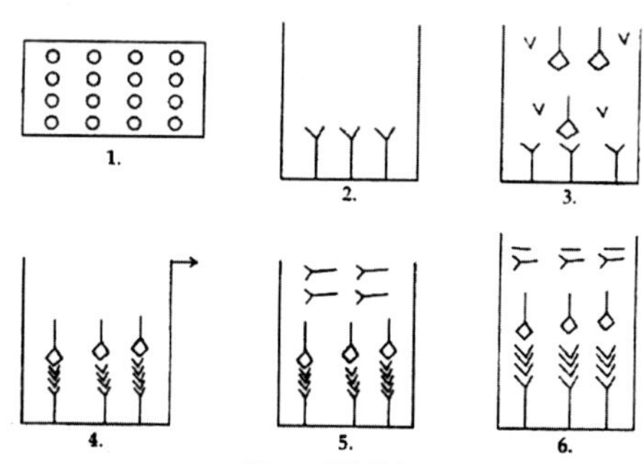

Steps of ELISA

Advantages

a. It is a rapid test and results may be obtained within 2-3 hours.

b. It is a highly sensitive test and it is able to detect even 1-2% adulteration.

c. Meat of closely related species can be differentiated.

d. It is capable for testing numerous samples at a time.

e. It is able to detect pressure cooked meat at 133°C for 20 minutes.

iv) Counter Immunoelectrophoresis (CIE)

It is a type of immunodiffusion test in which electric voltage is used for acceleration of protein movement. In this technique alkaline gel is used which causes electro-osmosis. Under this type of electrophoresis antibodies and proteins from meat extract moves towards each other and in case of homologous condition they forms a precipitation band at the point of its joining. By this technique we can detect one part of species in 300 of meat, it is rapid and more sensitive test.

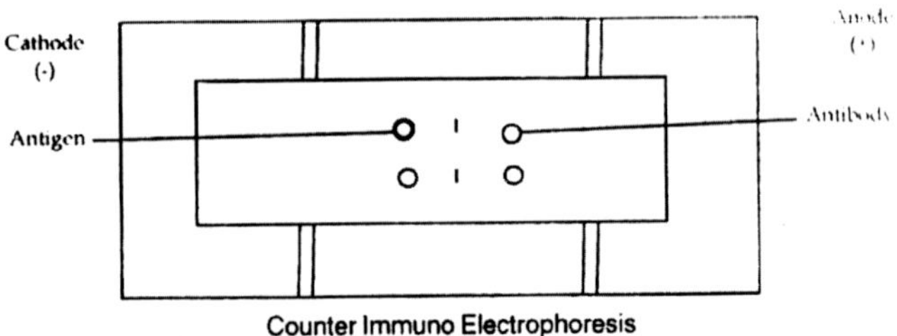

Counter Immuno Electrophoresis

B. Electrophoretic methods

The basic principle involved in this technique is separation of proteins by their differential migration through a supporting medium under the influence of electric field. The protein bands thus resolved are visualised by general, enzymological, chemical or immunological means.

Preparation of sample for electrophoresis

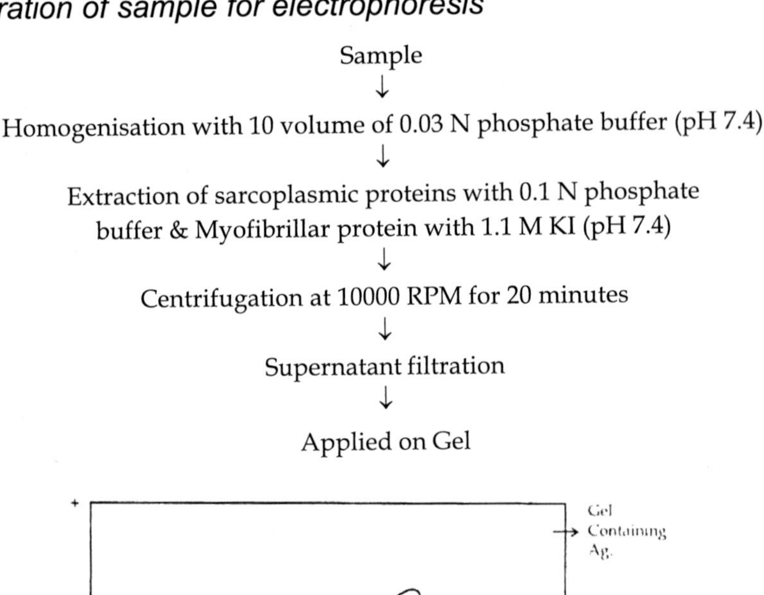

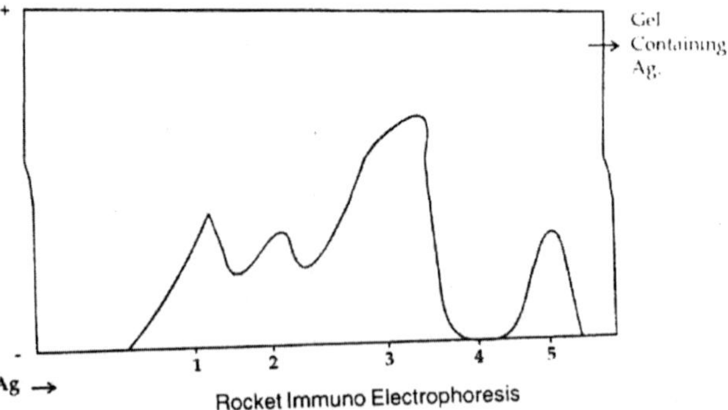

Rocket Immuno Electrophoresis

i) Poly Acrylamide Gel Electrophoresis (PAGE)

Initially disc electrophoresis in polyacrylamide gel was used for meat protein separation on the basis of total protein pattern of different meats. A simple visual differentiation without staining of the species is generally practiced to compare the respective migration rates of the brownish myoglobin bands. But it is a time consuming process and bands diffused early. So the PAGE was shifted to slab gel method. Myoglobin and creatine kinase Isozymes bands obtained in thin layer agarose gels have also been used for detection of beef, pork, chicken and turkey.

But now a days PAGE is carried out in cello gel strips. The process involves three main steps i.e. extraction, electrophoretic migration and staining-destaining. The stain commonly used in this method is amido black. In this process several blue bands formed which may differ in its width and intensity of staining. In a particular species distribution of band and their intensity of staining are stable and characteristic pattern can be examined by naked eyes. On the reading of destained strips through photometer with integrator or pherogram showing different peaks in which width of the bands on the gel and length proportional to the intensity of staining are species specific. This method is useful for fresh as well as for frozen meat identification.

ii) Sodium Dodecyl Sulphate PAGE (SDS-PAGE)

SDS-PAGE is a variant of PAGE is commonly used for separating protein subunits and determining their molecular weights. On heating, polypeptides dissociate and when these polypeptides bind with SDS in the presence of reducing agent 2-mercaptoethanol forms SDS-polypeptides. When this complex is subjected to a sieving polyacrylamide gel, migrate according to the molecular weights of the polypeptides. PAGE-SDS (pH 3-10) can be utilised for identification of beef, mutton, venison, rabbit meat and raw and cooked crustaceans.

Advantages

a. It is a suitable method for heated meat samples up to 100°C beyond which most of the protein bands disappears.

b. This method also has good resolution and reproducibility.

c. It is a good method for closely related meat species.

iii) Isoelectric Focusing (IEF)

IEF is an electrophoretic technique in which charge is utilised at surface of protein to drive it through gradient gel. It is mainly based on the migration of proteins in a pH gradient. The process stops when the surface charges become neutral, the isoelectric point. The subsequent fixing makes the protein precipitated and fixed at the same point as bands. The formation of such bands is species specific and can be utilized for meat species identification by determining the location, density and area of the bands. It is a suitable method for identification of animal species even after cooking at 100°C but not suitable for closely related meat species. It is also not good for frozen meat condition and results are difficult in interpretation and have poor reproducibility.

For better visualization of band patterns in case of lower proportion of contaminants certain enzyme stain can be used. For example coomassie blue for whole muscle samples, phosphoglucomutase for low levels of buffalo, pig or horse meat in beef, adenylate kinase for low levels of kangaroo or horse meat in beef, phosphor gluconate dehydrogenase (PGD) for differentiation of mutton from chevon.

iv) Immobiline gels and Immunoblotting

In this technique electrofocusing is done in immobiline gels contrary to carrier ampholytes in tradition electrofocusing methods. The immobilines are derivatives of acrylamide which produces immobiline pH gradients with the co-polymerization of acrylamide. The covalently bound immobiline gradient allows higher resolution than conventional carrier ampholyte based pH ingredients. The electrophoretic transfer of focussed proteins from polyacrylamide gel to nitrocellulose membrane in order to make them accessible for identifying reaction is known as immunoblotting.

C. Newer Biotechnological Methods

i) Cation exchange chromatography

A simple sample preparation procedure consisting of an extraction step with Milli-Q water as extraction solvent for hemoglobins from meat samples is followed. The filtration is done with a cellulose acetate filter. Then cation exchange chromatographic separation is done and diode array detection obtained. Then different peak patterns for extracted hemoglobins of different species may be obtained. Other heme-group containing proteins like myoglobin or cytochrome C which may also be detected with diode array detection at 416 nm. These may be chromatographically separated from the hemoglobins. By the use of these characteristic peak patterns, the species of the meat can be specified.

a. Chromatograph of pork meat on top, beef on middle and lamb meat at 416 μm.

b. Chromatograms for extracted meat proteins of 80% pork and 20% beef mixture *on top,* 80% cow and 20% pork mixture on middle and 80% beef and 20% lamb mixture on lower at 416 μm.

ii) DNA Hybridization Technique

In this method probes prepared from DNA or cloned DNA are hybridized with target DNA and detected by colour development or audiography. During the early development of DNA sequence analysis, genomic DNA was used as a species specific probe and was hybridised to DNA extracted from meat samples. The subsequent development of probes derived from species-specific satellite repetitive DNA sequences has greatly improved the specificity of the assay, now making it possible to detect admixtures that contribute as little as 5 % or less to a product. An alternative DNA detection system is based on the polymerase chain reaction (PCR) amplification of a segment of the mitochondrial cytochrome *b* gene. Subsequent cleavage by a restriction enzyme gives rise to a species-specific pattern on an agarose gel. This method does not require the development of species-specific probes because it is PCR-based and most suitable for critical samples in which DNA is largely degraded.

Steps involved in this process

a. DNA extraction by alkaline extraction buffer or by common proteinase K/sodium dodecyl sulphate (SDS) procedure.

b. Hybridisation to AP-labelled oligonucleotides.

c. Isolation of double-stranded DNA from meat.

d. Amplification of satellite probes.

e. Hybridisation and detection of probe.

Advantage: By this technique adulteration as low as 0.1% can be detected as compared to 0.4% in CIE, 1% in DID and 5% in IEF.

iii) Polymerase Chain Reaction (PCR)

PCR amplifies a target DNA sequence in an exponential phase, being capable of detecting even a single copy sequence from a single cell sample. It is a qualitative test for meat species specification. The meat of male and female animals can easily be detected by these techniques. The adulteration upto 1% can easily be detected by these techniques. The baseline for meat species specification in PCR is selection of genetic markers. These markers may be nuclear (Growth hormone gene, actin gene, MC1R) or mitochondrial gene markers (Cytochrome-b, 12S and 16S ribosomal RNA subunits, D-loop). Among the gene markers available mitochondrial gene markers are preferred due to easy isolation, multiple copies, stability at adverse environment, ability to detect old samples etc.

Steps involved in this process

a. Extraction of DNA.

b. Denaturation at 96°C for 2 minutes.

c. Annealing with suitable primer.

d. Extension with the help of polymerase.

e. Incubation.

f. Detection of bands.

Advantages

a. It is very quick and sensitive method.

b. Meat of closely related species can be identified.

c. It can discriminate between male and female raw meat.

iv) Polymerase Chain Reaction-Restriction Fragment length polymorphism (PCR-RFLP)

It is a modified form of PCR method in which restriction endonuclease sites are used for PCR products. In this technique PCR amplification of a gene is followed by the digestion with restriction enzymes. Now another version of this technology is known as PCR-RFLP lab on chip technology is readily available.

Key steps of the process

a. Extraction of DNA.

b. Amplification of DNA fragments with the help of DNA polymerase and specific primers.

c. Sequencing of PCR products at restriction endonucleases sites.

d. Digestion with restriction endonucleases.

e. Separation by gel electrophoresis.

f. Detection of stained band.

Advantages

a. It is a suitable method for the analysis of very low amount of meat (1 mg).

b. It is a faster and more sensitive method than DNA hybridization.

c. By this technique two species of animal can be differentiated even after heating at 120°C.

d. Meat from male and female animals can be identified by using PCR by genomic DNA extraction from raw muscles.

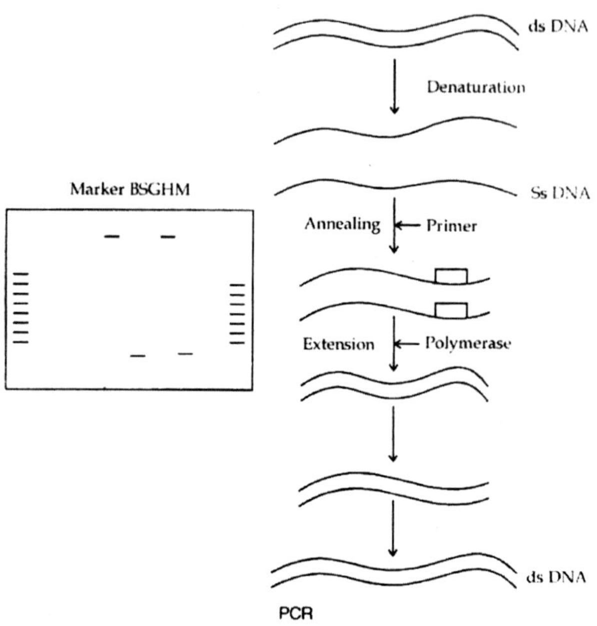

Limitations: It is not hundred percent accurate methods because of existence of some intraspecific variability with in the species as in sheep, turkey and chicken meat.

v) Random Amplified Polymorphic DNA fingerprinting (RAPD)

It is a modified PCR technique in which DNA fingerprints are generated in a very short period of time which can be visualised on gel electrophoresis. In this method prior knowledge of DNA sequencing is not required but known standard has to run each time.

Key steps of the process

a. Sample Selection and DNA Extraction.

b. RAPD amplification using specific primers.

c. Strand denaturation at 94 °C for 1 minutes.

d. Primer annealing at 47 °C for 1 min.

e. Primer extension at 72 °C for 1 min.

f. Electrophoresis (10-μL portion of the amplification is carried out for 45 minutes at 100 V in a 3% agarose gel containing ethidium bromide (1 μg/mL) in TBE buffer (0.045 M Tris-borate and 0.001 M EDTA with pH 8.0).

g. DNA fragments were visualized by UV transillumination

vi) Forensically Informative nucleotide sequencing (FINS) technology

It is a combination of technology in which genetic sequencing is done followed by phylogenetic analysis.

vii) Real time PCR

In this technique early detection and monitoring of early stages is possible. The example of this technology is SYBR Green detection system through which quantification of meat mixtures can be done.

viii) Taq Man assays

In this technique meat species specification is carried out by using species specific primers. The Taq man probes developed by the several scientists for specific purposes can be utilized or species specific primer probes can be generated in this technology to specify the meat samples. This technique is capable for detection of even 0.1% adulteration of meat in meat mixture.

For the detection of meat species no single method is sufficient. Each method has got some advantages and disadvantages. As the physical, chemical and anatomical methods are more suitable for raw meat while minced or comminuted meat requires sophisticated techniques. For this purpose DID, SDS-PAGE, ELISA and IEF are common methods. Among these DID is not sufficient method for closely related meat species, effectiveness of ELISA and SDS-PAGE is hampered by cumbersome process of isolating species-specific proteins, IEF presuppose that the protein composition of meat is similar within species and have differences between the species however, even the electrophoresis patterns of serum proteins and brain proteins could be different within the same species and even the recent technique, fingerprinting has also got limitations of non-reproducibility of band patterns.

References

1. Calvo, J.H., Zaragoza, P. and R. Osta (2001). Random Amplified Polymorphic DNA Fingerprints for Identification of Species in Poultry. Poultry Science 80:522–524
2. Chatli, M.K., Sahoo, J. and Devetkal, S.K. (2005). Detection of adultration. Livestock International, Oct. 2005: 15-19.
3. Chikuni, K., Ozutsumi, K., Koishikawa, T. and Kato, S. (1990). Species identification of cooked meats by DNA hybridization assay. Meat Science 27, 119-128.
4. Dabas, Y.P.S. and Saxena, O.P. (1994). Acts and statutes. In:Veterinary Jurisprudence and Post mortem, International Book Distributing Co. Lucknow, pp 214-219.
5. Gracey, J., Collins, D.S. and Huey, R. (1999). Anatomy, meat composition and quality. In: Meat Hygiene, 10th ed. W.B. Saunders Company Ltd. London, pp 57-65.
6. Lenstra, J. A., Buntjer J. B. and Janssen F. W. (2001). On the origin of meat - DNA techniques for species identification in meat products. Veterinary Sciences Tomorrow - Issue 2, No.14.
7. Matsunaga, T., Chikuni, K., Tanabe, R., Muroya, S., Shibata, K., Yamamda, J. and Shinmura, Y. (1999). A quick and simple method for the identification of meat species and meat products by PCR assay. Meat Science 51, 143-148.
8. Sharma, B.D. (1999). Structure, composition and nutritive value of meat tissues. In: Meat and Meat Products Technology (Including Poultry Products Technology), Japee Brothers Medical Publishers (P) Ltd, New Delhi. Pp 8-22.
9. Sharma, S.D. (2007). Meat judging. In: Universal Meat Hygiene in Public Health Care, International Book Distributing Co. Lucknow, pp 206-208.
10. Singh,V.P. (2009). Fraudulent substitution of meat. In: Training Booklet On Field Related Issues of Livestock Products Technology, DUVASU, Mathura.

□□□□

6 Preservation of Meat and Aquatic Foods

Preservation of foods including meat and aquatic foods is a creation of conditions for the food articles in such a way to stop or greatly slow down the activities of micro-organisms, chemical and enzymatic reactions and physical forces to prevent the meat and aquatic foods from spoilage while maintaining its nutritional value and sensory attributes.

Significance of Meat Preservation

1. Meat and aquatic foods are perishable food items and are very prone to spoilage and rancidity development due to high nutrients, moisture and neutral pH.
2. Once meat and aquatic foods is exposed to microbial contamination, chemical and enzymatic reactions then it will be very difficult to attain asepsis.
3. To enhance the keeping quality of meat and aquatic foods so that it will be available for further processing.
4. It protects meat and aquatic foods from shrinkage, sweeting and other physical forces.
5. To protect human health by providing the wholesome meat and aquatic foods to the consumers.

6. By this way we can minimize utilization of energy in processing of meat and aquatic foods.

Principles of Preservation

The basic principles in preservation of meat and aquatic foods include control of spoilage caused by microbes, enzymes and autooxidation of fat. In the preservation of fish clean sanitation is a prerequisite and to obtain it we generally follow cleaning and gutting of fish before going to adopt actual preservative technique. For that purpose we generally rellie on following principle techniques.

1. Temperature Control
   a. Use of low temperature regime e.g. refrigeration, freezing etc.
   b. Use of high temperature regime e.g. thermal destruction, canning etc.
2. Moisture control e.g. dehydration.
3. Direct microbial inhibition e.g. curing, smoking, irradiation, use of chemicals and antibiotics.

Important micro-organisms responsible for spoilage and infections / intoxications in meat and aquatic foods:

S.No.	Type of bacteria	Temperature Range(°C)	Optimum growth temp. (°C)	Major Spoilage Micro-organisms	Micro-organisms causing infection and intoxication
1.	Psychrophiles	0 to 7	5	*Pseudomonas, Flavobacterium, Acenetobactor*	*Listeria, Aeromonas, Yersinia*
2.	Mesophiles	10 to 40	30-32	*Clostridium, Streptococcus*	*Salmonella Staphylococcus E. coli*
3.	Thermophiles	43 to 80	55-70	*Lactobacillus, Bacillus*	*Clostridium perfringens, Compylobactor*

Methods of Preservation

Preservation of meat and aquatic foods are mainly based on the purpose for which we want to preserve these items i.e. colour and flavour development, protection of bloom etc. Various methods for preservation of meat and aquatic foods are in practice but no single method is sufficient to preserve all type of meat and aquatic foods. So it is a common practice of utilizing more than one preservation technique at a time. This concept of preservation is commonly known as hurdle technology. Some common methods for preservation of meat and aquatic foods are :

1. Chilling or Refrigeration.
2. Freezing.
3. Drying.
4. Salting and curing.
5. Thermal processing.
6. Smoking.
7. Canning.
8. Irradiation.
9. Chemicals preservation.
10. Antioxidant preservation.
11. Antibiotics preservation.

1. Chilling or Refrigeration

Chilling is a process of reducing the temperature to about 0°C to prevent putrefaction and extend the shelf life of meat and aquatic foods. It is a good method for short term storage and it should be practiced just after slaughter of the animals and catching of the fish and continued till its consumption. The basic aim of chilling is to slow down and nearly stops the microbial, enzymatic activities and chemical reactions; reduce the weight loss and discolouration of the surface owing to the haemoglobin oxidation. For chilling of meat especially poultry meat and fish we generally use ice layers but ice alone is not effective for long term preservation because melting water brings about a sort of bleaching of valuable flesh which are responsible for flavour. Icing is a most suitable method for storage of aquatic foods which will remain in good condition for about 3 to 15 days depending on species and other factors. For icing of fishes bulking, shelving, boxing and insulated boxes can be used. The quality of ice must be soft in nature to avoid the mechanical damage to the muscle tissues. The block ice, flake ice, plate ice, tube ice, soft ice may serve the purpose.

Air chilling in form of refrigeration may be the preferred method for preservation of meat and aquatic foods. In this method we use refrigeration temperature of 2 to 5°C with air speed of 0.25 to 3.0 m/s during entire practice from holding to ultimate use. In this practice relative humidity must be about 90% to reduce the shrinkage. The proper spacing between the carcasses and chunks of meat as well as the aquatic foods is necessary for uniform chilling through air circulation. The shelf life of meat and fish is depend on the initial load of the micro-organisms on the carcase. In general it is a most suitable method for the storage of meat and aquatic foods for about a week to 5 weeks depending upon initial load of micro-organisms and kind of meat. In this method chance of cold shortening in the carcases especially in mutton and beef may be seen if we allow the pre-rigor meat to chill below 10°C or lower. So to reduce the chances of cold shortening (toughness of the muscles) we keep the carcases first at 15°C to dissipate the body heat and then passed to cold rooms maintained at 2 to 5°C.

2. *Freezing*

Freezing is generally practiced in sub zero temperature and it is a most preferred method for long term storage of meat and aquatic food. It is a method of choice for fishes which are intended for canning i.e. Tuna, Salmon etc. In freezing of food items like meat and fishes we generally prefer temperature range in between -10 to -30°C. However, meat and other products of animal origin can very well stored for months together at -10°C but most preferred temperature is -18°C because at this temperature almost all water present in meat tissues freezes. In frozen state beef and buffalo meat has a storage life of about 12 months, veal slightly less, mutton and lamb about 8 months, pork and poultry about 6 months without any marked deteriorative changes. Freezing stops the microbial growth, retards the action of enzymes and chemical reactions but preserves the nutritive value of meat and aquatic foods. Although a very little loss of nutrients does occur during thawing of meat. When we thaw the frozen meat or other tissues then it weeps or drips. The drip is a watery blood stained fluid consisting of mainly water, salt, extractives, protein and damaged blood corpuscles.

Considerable Points in Freezing

(i) The loss of weight due to weep or drip is more in beef (about 3%) as compared to mutton and pork.

(ii) In freezing of meat or other animal tissues before completion of rigor mortis, there is a marked contraction on thawing (thaw rigor) and excessive drip unless the muscle is held taut.

(iii) The prerequisite in freezing of animal tissues or meat is its packaging otherwise meat will undergo freezer burn. This is an abnormal state of meat which occurs due to excessive drying of the surface of meat when unprotective meat is comes in contact of freezer or refrigeration pipes. In such condition meat depicts yellowish- brown or whitish discolouration in its surface due to formation of condensed layer of muscular tissue just under the surface.

(iv) Freezing and thawing of young chicken may lead to a bone darkening condition due to leaching of haemoglobin to adjoining tissues from the marrow of porous chicken bones.

Methods of Freezing

Meat quality during freezing is affected by the type of ice crystal formation. As in slow speed of freezing there will be more damage to the muscular tissues due to large ice crystal formation as compared to fast freezing. The temperature range in between -1 to -4°C is the most suitable temperature range in which ice crystals reaches their maximum size and that range is called 'zone of maximum ice crystal formation'. On the basis of speed we can categorise the freezing into two broad categories:

S.No.	Slow freezing	Fast freezing
i.	As per International Institute of Refrigeration speed of freezing should be below 1 cm/h.	Speed of freezing should be above 5 cm/h.
ii.	Extracellular water freezes out of muscle cells.	Intracellular water freezes within the muscle fibres.
iii.	There is formation of large ice crystal due to separation of solution and migration of water out of the muscle cells.	Numerous small ice crystals formation within the muscle tissues uniformly and reduces water migration and separation of solutions.
iv.	More muscular damage due to large ice crystal.	Less muscular damage due to small ice crystal.
v.	More drip loss, shrinkage and distorted appearance of meat.	Less drip loss, shrinkage with desired light colour.

Techniques of Freezing

A. Brine Freezing

Brine freezing system is generally adopted for aquatic foods especially for fish preservation. In this system of preservation saturated brine is used in a tank in which fishes are held. This brine can attain a temperature as low as -21°C before it starts freezing. It is a rapid method because brine comes in direct contact of fishes and removes their heat. The salt used in brine solution in form of hypertonic concentration inhibits the growth of certain micro-organisms. To control excessive penetration of salt in the fishes we can use a mixture of glucose or corn syrup along with salt as a freezing medium. Time taken in freezing depends upon temperature and size of meat chunks but in ideal conditions it will take 15-20 minutes.

B. Plate Freezing

In this method of freezing a series of refrigerated metal plates are used. The meat and aquatic foods are held in trays and refrigerant is passes through the plates to reduce the surface temperature to -10°C. By this technique we can freeze the meat and other aquatic foods of size 3-5 cm within 2-3 hours.

C. Blast Freezing

In this freezing technique tunnels or chambers are used for intense air circulation. In these chambers cooled air is circulated with the speed of 3-5 m/s to achieve the temperature -35 to -40°C. The relative humidity is maintained at 95% or above with 150-300 air circulation coefficients inside the chambers. This is a quick technique for freezing of large sized cuts of meat and the time taken in freezing depends on size of chunks. This technique is now a days used in large meat plants for quick freezing of hot meat immediately after slaughter without any previous chilling.

3. Drying

The basic principle of drying is the reduction of water content in the meat or aquatic foods to an extent in which it will not be available for microbial growth within the food. In meat water is present about 75% and in fishes about 80% when this water content is reduced to 25%, bacterial action stops and below 15% can prevent the mould growth. It is important to prevent the growth of pathogens and spoilage organisms because all organisms require moisture to live and multiply and food enzymes cannot work without a watery environment.

The extent of water availability to the micro-organisms growth and activity is called water activity (a_W). Water activity is a ratio between the water vapour pressure on the meat surface (P) and water vapour pressure of distilled water (P_0) at same temperature. The formula for expressing this relationship is $a_W = P/P_0$ .The fresh meat and fish has a water activity above 0.95. So the reduction of water activity below 0.95 inhibits the microbial activity especially gram –ve rods, below 0.91 inhibits activity of most spoilage bacteria, 0.88 for most yeasts and 0.80 for moulds and *Staphylococcus aureus.*

Three basic methods of drying are used today: *sun drying*, a traditional method in which foods dry naturally in the sun; *hot air drying*, in which foods are exposed to a blast of hot air; and freeze-drying, in which frozen food is placed in a vacuum chamber to draw out the water. In *freeze-drying*, frozen food is placed in a special vacuum cabinet. There, water escapes from the food by sublimation, a process in which ice changes from a solid directly to a vapour without first becoming a liquid. Freeze-dried foods retain their original flavour, texture, and nutrients upon rehydration but must be packaged in moisture-proof, hermetically sealed containers. *Flash freezing* is a process of supercooling foods to temperatures of -195°C (-320°F) through the use of liquid nitrogen. The process reduces cellular deterioration and increases retained moisture so that foods are tastier when they are unfrozen.

4. Salting and Curing

Salting and curing is one of the oldest forms of food preservation. It is used to preserve meat and fish, yielding common products such as bacon, ham, frankfurters, and corned beef. Preservation of food by adding salt is called salting. The meat and fish are covered with salt to drain out water by osmosis. Whereas, curing involves adding some combination of salt, sugar, spices, vinegar, or sodium nitrate or nitrite to animal foods. Some common curing ingredients are:

A. Salt

It is a cheap and simple method of preservation. A salt concentration of 10 percent is sufficient to restrict the growth of *Clostridium botulinum*, but lower amounts used in conjunction with other additives or thermal processing can help control spoilage. Salt is predominantly used in the dry curing of bacon or as brine for wet curing.

Mode of action

(i) Salt (sodium chloride) kills and inhibits the growth of micro-organisms by drawing water out of the cells of both microbes and food alike through osmosis.

(ii) It replaces the moisture with salt thus prevent or retards the growth of spoilage organisms.

(iii) It slows down the action of proteolytic enzymes.

(iv) It causes dehydration of meat and aquatic foods.

(v) Chloride ion present in common salt directly acts on the microbial cells.

(vi) It is responsible for tenderness in meat during curing and also imparts flavour by interaction with fatty acids.

It produces harsh, hardening effects in meat and aquatic foods which is minimized by the use of sugar and dextrose in the brine solution. Salt is also having some relationship to hypertension and sodium is the key factor responsible for this act. To minimize the risk of hypertension consumers prefer a mixture of sodium chloride and potassium chloride in a ratio of 6:4 or 5:5.

B. Sugar

It is used in curing solution to impart flavour and to reduce the harsh, hardening effects of salt. High sugar levels are needed to inhibit the growth of yeasts and moulds.

Mode of action

(i) Sugar is effective in preservation because it reduces the amount of free water available for bacterial growth.

(ii) Sugar interacts with amino groups of proteins in the Maillard reaction (browning reaction).

(iii) It acts as a source of nitrate reducing bacteria in the curing or in cured meat colour development.

(iv) It also encourages the growth of beneficial bacteria such as those of the Lactobacillus genus.

(v) It produces an acidic environment (pH 4.5) through lactic acid production which inhibits the growth of other microbes and accounts for the tangy flavour of some cured products.

C. Nitrate and Nitrite

Nitrates and nitrites are not only kill bacteria but also produces characteristic flavour and give meat a pink or red colour. Nitrate (NO_{3^-}) supplied by sodium nitrate or potassium nitrate, is used as a source for nitrite (NO_{2^-}) production with the help of nitrate reducing bacteria. The nitrite further breaks down in the meat into nitric oxide

(NO) which then binds to the iron atom in the centre of myoglobin's heme group, reducing oxidation and causing a reddish-brown colour (nitroso myoglobin) when raw. After cooking it produces characteristic pink colour due to formation of nitrosohaemochromogen.

The flavour development with the use of nitrate and nitrite is due to the production of benzonitrite and phenylacetonitrite by the reaction of nitrite with fatty acids. However, the presence of nitrates and nitrites in food is controversial due to the development of nitrosamines when the food, primarily bacon, is cooked at high temperatures. The nitrate and nitrite compounds themselves are not harmful, however, and are among the antioxidants. To minimize the production of nitrosamine alpha-tocopherol cooked salts like ascorbates or erythrobates may be used. For this purpose 550 ppm sodium ascorbate alongwith 120 ppm sodium nitrite is most suitable combination. The concentration of nitrate and nitrite in finished products is limited to 500 ppm and 200 ppm or lower, respectively. Finally, they are irreplaceable in the prevention of botulinum poisoning from consumption of dry-cured sausages by preventing spore germination.

D. Phosphates

These are used in curing solution to enhance the water binding capacity and to reduce the rancidity development. The phosphate is generally used in form of pyrophosphates and diphosphates.

Mode of action

(i) It raises the pH.

(ii) It causes unfolding of muscle proteins thereby making more sites available for water binding.

(iii) The chelate trace metal ions present in phosphate retard the rancidity development.

E. Other curing ingredients

The various ingredients like sodium ascorbate, erythrobate, sodium sorbate, monosodium glutamate, sodium and potassium lactate are also added in curing solution. Among these compounds sodium ascorbate and erythrobate are used as a antioxidant to reduce the nitrosamine formation and to stabilise colour and flavour, potassium sorbate as *Clostridium botulinum* and mould inhibitor and monosodium glutamate as a flavour enhancer.

Curing Methods

(i) *Dry curing*: In this method crystalline salt, sugar and nitrite/nitrate is intimately mixed or rubbed into the dressed meat and fishes. Self brine formation occurs in this method by the exudation of water from the meat and fishes. In this method curing ingredients gets entry into the meat and fishes by diffusion. Example is bacon curing.

(ii) *Pickle curing*: In this method a pickle solution is prepared from salt, sugar, nitrite/nitrate etc. in a desired concentration in water. The cuts of meat and fish are then submerged in that pickle until the cured has completely enters the meat or fish. The examples of the products prepared by this method are corned beef.

(iii) *Artery pumping*: In this method a brine solution is pumped in the meat and fishes through artery or multiple needles in the muscular portion. The examples of the products prepared by this method are ham and picnic.

(iv) *Direct addition method*: In this method curing solution is directly added into the finally ground meat for better results. The examples of the products prepared by this method are communited meat products.

The chemical action of curing is highly complex with slow reactions of proteins and fats through autolysis and oxidation. These reactions can be driven by autooxidation alone through it is typically accompanied by enzymes in the curing food as well as beneficial fungi and bacteria. For better results curing should be maintained at 3-4°C for about 3-5 days depending upon product type.

5. *Thermal Processing*

Simple heat treatment of meat by boiling, cooking or roasting is an efficient meat preservation method for shorter periods, and can significantly reduce the microbial counts of fresh meat. Unfortunately, these products are subject to recontamination by micro-organisms brought in during subsequent product handling and from the environment, but it takes some time before the spoilage flora become critical again. Although these products are not safe from the microbiological point of view, experienced manufacturers and consumers have developed methods of coping with them. But to kill the spoilage micro-organisms in the meat and aquatic foods mainly two temperature regimes, pasteurization and sterilization are generally utilized.

Pasteurization of meat and aquatic products includes heating of the products at temperature in the thermal centre at the range of 58°C to 75°C for a sufficient period of time. While sterilization refers to a thermal shock of high temperature for a very short interval using a high temperature short time (HTST) technique to the meat and aquatic products at a temperature over 100° C for a time less than 15 seconds. The sterilized products can be stored under ambient temperatures for up to three or four years. The another specific method (Ultra high temperature sterilization) used for treating meat to obtain the results disclosed herein involve placing meat in a closed heat source, e.g., an electric oven, maintained at a temperature between 900° C and 1300° C for a time sufficient to denature surface proteins up to a depth of not more than 2 mm, i.e. typically between 5 and 30 seconds.

Terminology Used in Thermal Processing

i) *Decimal Reduction Value (D-Value):* It is a time usually in minutes to kill 90% of micro-organisms present in the food at a given temperature.

ii) *Z-Value*: It is a increase in °C or °F temperature to obtain ten fold increase in the death rate of the micro-organisms.

iii) *F-Value*: It is a time required in minutes at 121°C to destroy spores or vegetative cells of a specific micro-organisms.

iv) *Thermal Death time (TDT):* It is a time required to destroy given number of micro-organisms at a specified constant temperature.

6. Smoking

Smoking is an ancient technique for flavour development and preservation of meat and aquatic foods which is commonly used with curing. Smoking involves cooking meat or fish very slowly over a low wood fire. It preserves food by binding or removing water so that it is not available for the growth of micro-organisms and also inhibits fat oxidation. These methods impart a distinctive colour and flavour to foods. In emulsion type sausages it forms protective skin over the product. Some studies, however, show that smoked meats and fish may contain toxic and even carcinogenic compounds which they absorb from wood smoke such as sodium nitrite. It combine with other chemicals to form cancer-causing nitrosamines.

The smoke particles, after being absorbed by the product, inhibit bacterial growth on the surface of the product. The smoke particles also have a positive effect on the taste and colour of the product. The heat of the fire dries the fish or meat during the smoking process and if the temperature gets high enough, the flesh is cooked. This means that bacterial spoilage and spoilage due to enzyme activity is prevented. Drying and cooking of the flesh when being smoked play an important role in the preservation. If a product is well dried during smoking then it can be stored for a long time. There are three ways of smoking:

Cold smoke method: the temperature during the smoking is at most 30°C which means the product does not get cooked.

Hot smoke method: during this process the product does get cooked but not dried (temperature varies between 65 and ±100°C.

Smoke drying: during this process, the product is first hot smoked, so that it gets cooked, and then, with continued smoking the product is dried (temperatures vary between 45-85°C).

Composition of Smokes

The compounds produced in the smoke includes phenols, organic acids, alcohols, carbonyls, hydrocarbons and certain gases such as $CO_{2,}$ CO, $O_{2,}$ N_2 and N_2O. Among all these compounds phenol is a main ingredient and exerts their action by three ways:

(i) They act as antioxidant.

(ii) They impart typical smoky colour and flavour to the product.

(iii) They are having bacteriostatic properties and contribute in preservation.

Other compounds such as alcohol have minor bacteriostatic properties, organic acid coagulate the surface protein and has some preservative quality while carbonyls imparts colour, flavour and aroma to the product. The hydrocarbons present in the smoke is said to be carcinogenic.

Smoke Production

Smoke is generally produced in a specially constructed smoke house in which saw dust or hard wood and sometimes combination of both is used for combustion. The high temperature (about 300°C) is always preferred for smoke production because it reduces the chances of carcinogenic compounds development. During the combustion of wood or saw dust about 300 compounds are produced but among all phenol and aldehydes accounts about 50% of total compound.

Now a day's liquid smoke is preferred by the industrialist which is produced by the pyrolysis of hard wood or sawdust in which polycyclic hydrocarbons are removed by filtration. It is having some benefits over traditional smoke i.e. can be used directly in the products, little pollution, less chances of carcinogenic compounds production and faster application.

Smoke reduces some nutritional quality of animal products by the action of phenols and polyphenols on sulfhydryl group of proteins and carbonyl groups on amino groups. By this way smoke destruct lysine and thiamine but little effect on niacin and riboflavin is observed.

7. Canning

The canning process involves placing foods in cans or jars and heating them to a temperature that destroys micro-organisms that could be a health hazard or cause the food to spoil. Canning also inactivate enzymes that could cause the food to spoil. As the cans or jars are sealed hermetically, re-contamination from outside is prevented. In general, canned products can be stored for a long time without refrigeration. In this preservation technique some quality loss in form of taste, colour and amount of certain essential nutrients occurs. The time and the temperature required for heating depends on kind and form of micro-organisms, water content, pH, amount of salt, fat and types of cans or glass jars. In fish and meat the number of micro-organisms initially present may be large, the internal water content is high and the pH is close to neutral. It is therefore difficult to kill all micro-organisms present and to get a safe product. The only safe way to sterilize low acid products such as fish and meat is by prolonged heating in a pressure canner or sterilizer in which temperatures higher than 100°C (212°F) can be reached. The main reason pressure canning is necessary to avoid the hazard of the *Clostridium botulinum*, an indicator organism for canning. Though the bacterial cells are killed at boiling temperatures, they can form spores that can withstand these temperatures. The spores grow well in low acid foods, in the absence of air, such as in canned low acid foods. When the spores germinate and grow to high numbers, they produce the deadly botulinum toxins (poisons). The spores can be destroyed by canning the food at a temperature of 115-121°C (240-250°F) for the correct length of time. This temperature can only be reached in a pressure canner. As the canning of fish and meat requires a lot of energy, clean water and a large investment in equipment, usually it can only be done at a small-scale industrial level. It is less suited for household-level preservation.

Processing Technique

(i) Preparation of Fish or Meat

Fish with a high fat content (herring, mackerel, tuna, sardines etc.) have much firmer flesh and softer bones. These fish can retain their original shape during heat processing are suitable for canning. Another advantage of canning fatty kinds of fish is that the oxygen entrapped in the can will be consumed during sterilization and this will prevent fat oxidation and rancidness, which is not, achieved with simpler preservation methods such as drying etc. Small fish may be kept straight in flat oval cans (herring) while big fish have to be cut into smaller pieces to get them into small tin cans.

Bottling of meat at 100°C is not advisable but sterilizing it at 115-121°C is possible. For this purpose we generally use clean, fresh pieces of meat. Removal of bones, cutting of meat into smaller pieces (about 4 cm thick) and use of seasonings in desired quantity is required. Brown the meat by roasting or frying; big pieces should be partially cooked before frying. For small pieces in sauce, stock or brine, various sizes of tins and jars can be used. For bigger pieces, use flat tin cans. In general, almost all meat products are suitable for canning. Only products which are eaten raw such as raw dry-cured ham or dry sausage are not suitable.

(ii) Precooking (Roasting or Smoking) of Meat and Fish

Precooking of meat and fish reduces the volume, microbial load and makes the flesh firmer. For precooking of meat, fish and gravy we generally preferred 70°C temperature for about 15-20 minutes. By the precooking of fish flesh releases around 15-30% of the body water.

(iii) Filling of Cans with Fish or Meat and Filling Liquid (Gravy)

After initial preparation, the products, which are still warm or heated to the filling temperature, are put into tin cans or glass jars as quickly as possible. These are then filled with hot water, hot broth, hot salt solution or hot oil to about half a centimetre under the rim. This is called the headspace; it is needed to give the food inside the jar room to expand during heating and to create a vacuum in the jar after cooling. Take care that no air pockets are sealed in with the product.

(iv) Exhausting

Exhausting is a removal of excess air from the headspace of cans prior to seeming. It is an essential step for minimising the strain on the cans, reducing oxidation of fat and vitamins by reducing O_2, preserves vitamin-C and creates partial vacuum in the cans.

(v) Seaming

Seaming is a process of putting the air tight seal between the cover and body of the container to prevent the entry of micro-organisms. The double seamer machine is used for creation of hermetic double seam. Tin cans can be sealed after adding the liquid, as long as the middle of the product has reached the sealing temperature. Always measure the temperature in the middle of the tin can. The sealing temperature must not be lower than 60-80°C depending on the product and the size of the can. If it is lower, the cans must be quickly reheated in a shallow water bath until the temperature in the middle of the tin can is equal to or higher than the indicated temperature. This procedure ensures that the can will not deform at the sterilizing temperature and that a proper vacuum is created after cooling. The time between filling, sealing and sterilizing must be as short as possible. Never use damaged cans or jars.

(vi) Thermal Processing or Retorting

In this step of canning heat treatment (115-121°C) is applied on the cans for most fish and meat products. In low acid products spores of pathogenic micro-organisms, which are not killed at 100°C can grow and multiply. To kill those spores sterilization for 60 minutes or longer at 121°C may be necessary. At 115°C spores will be killed but it takes longer time while sterilization below 115°C is generally not safe. To sterilize at temperatures higher than 100°C, a pressure canner or autoclave is needed.

(vii) Cooling and Washing

After retorting, cans are cooled as rapidly as possible to about 35-40°C, to provides a shock to the thermophiles. This temperature of cooling is essential to retain the heat in the product which will facilitate the evaporation of water on the surface and make it dry. For cooling and washing of cans it is necessary to use bacteriologically safe water to prevent the exposure of spoilage and pathogenic bacteria.

(viii) Labelling of Cans

Labelling of cans should be done with the information of contents, sale information and other relevant information's.

(ix) Storage and Distribution

The storage temperature should preferably stay below 20 °C to prevent the quality degradation of meat and other aquatic foods. If we want to store the product for a longer period of time above 2 years in tropical conditions with higher temperatures (35°C or more) than a much more intensive heat treatment at 121 °C is necessary so that all micro-organism spores are inactivated. The store room should also be dry and kept at a constant temperature.

Terms Related to Canning

1. *Flash 18 Process*: It is a process of cans filling at 18 lbs air pressure in a room maintained at 225°F or 108^{0}C and holding at that temperature for sufficient period of time to achieve sterilization.
2. *D-Concept*: It is a time required in thermal processing to reduce the population of most resistant spores of *Clostridium botulinum* by 10-12 times at 250°F or 121°C.
3. *Aseptic Canning*: It is a process of obtaining aseptic conditions by sterilization of cans and product separately and then filling of the product into the cans in an aseptic atmosphere. For sterilization the temperature of 300°F or 149°C is continuously achieved.

8. Irradiation

Irradiation is a use of electromagnetic radiations (x or γ radiations) and accelerated electrons in the destruction or inactivation of many of the micro-organisms which causes meat and aquatic foods to spoil and cause food-borne illnesses. It is also known as cold sterilisation because in the process of microbial destruction by irradiation there is no significant increase in temperature. In this irradiation process DNA molecule of micro-organisms are fragmented and inherent water present in the micro-organisms are ionised into free radicles and hydrogen peroxide which leads to destruction of micro-organisms. The organisms responsible for spoilage of meat and aquatic foods by off odour, off flavour as well as the compounds that degrade foods are affected by irradiation. In fact, most spoilage bacteria as well as yeast and moulds are easily reduced by pasteurization doses. The complete sterilization does not occur because some organisms are spore formers which make them very resistant to the irradiation. However, commercially sterile meat products which are storable without refrigeration may be achieved by cooking, vacuum packaging, freezing to about -40°C and irradiated at 50kGy. But to achieve the little or no change in taste, smell and colour of meat, current FDA approved radiation doses that are 1 to 10 kGy in cold pasteurization are best suitable. In irradiation, production energy level should be in a limit that it should not produce radioactivity in the food being processed. Higher doses of ionizing radiation (approximately ten times the approved values) would cause reduction in polyunsaturated fatty acids, irradiation sensitive vitamins i.e. A, E, K, C and thiamine along with changes in colour, taste, and smell of meats. The doses requirements for different meat and meat products are:

Type of meat and meat products	Dose of irradiation
Fresh meat carcase or cuts	0.5-1.0 kGy
Packaged fresh meat	2.0-5.0 kGy
Processed meat	2.5-3.0 kGy
Poultry carcase	2.5 kGy

Types of Irradiations Generally used in the Preservation of Meat and Aquatic Foods

Ionising radiations are the main radiation used in preservation of meat and aquatic foods. Among the ionising radiations α and β rays are of very limited use due to their charged and X-rays are not good in conversion from electron beam particles while γ and accelerated electrons are of much value. Some non-ionizing radiations i.e. UV rays, infrared and microwaves are also lethal to micr-organisms and are of immense use in meat and aquatic foods preservation.

Gamma rays irradiation: These are electromagnetic radiations of a very short wavelength produced by the spontaneous disintegration of the atomic nucleus of certain radioactive nuclides such as ^{137}Cs or ^{60}Co. These are the cheapest form of radiations and among them ^{60}Co is the most common source of Gamma radiation. These rays are capable to penetrate the food products to a great depth exposing the pathogens in deep layers of irradiated products. This process is better than any means of pasteurization currently available. The upper dose limit for x or γ radiation is 5 MeV.

Electron accelerator irradiation: Electron accelerator produces high-energy electron beams thus produces very high level of energy in fractions of a second. These accelerated electrons produces electron beam which can kill about 99.9% pathogens in the meat but they have poor penetration power in layered food articles. This process is quicker than Gamma irradiation and can be switched off during off time. The upper dose rate for accelerated electrons is 10 MeV.

Ultraviolet rays (UV rays): UV rays are produced in the radiation wavelength of 100 and 3000 A^0 but it is most bactericidal at 2650 A^0. It causes mutation of cells of micro-organisms thus exert their action. These rays are not capable to penetrate in deeper parts of the foods so the use of UV rays is limited to surface sterilization of meat and aquatic foods only.

Microwaves: These are non-ionising radiations which lie between the infrared and radio frequency portion of the electromagnetic spectrum. These waves create oscillation in the products by rapidly changing alternating current field. The two frequencies of microwaves are in use 915 and 2450 MHz.

The irradiated foods should be labelled by the international symbol of irradiation that is known as Redura. This symbol is coloured green on white background and includes two leaves resting on the semicircle, with a green dot above it beneath a broken-lined semicircle.

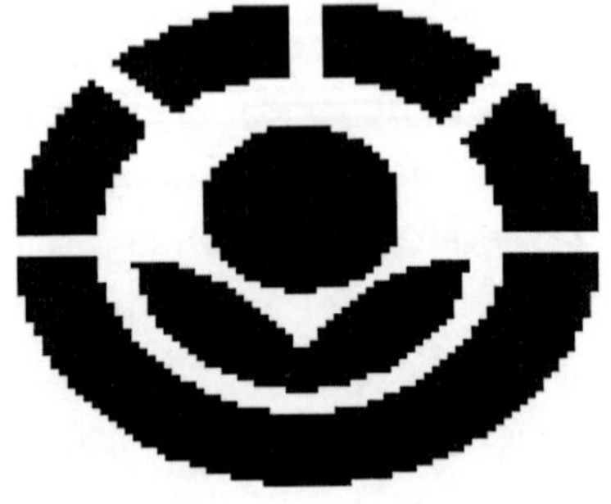

Treated by irradiation

Measurements and Terms Related to Irradiation

Rad : Radiation absorbed dose in conventional system. It is unit equivalent to the absorption of 100 ergs/gm of matter.
1 rad = 100(ergs/gm)

M rad : Megarad. It is equivalent to 1 million rad.
M. rad = 1million rad

Gy : Gray. It is a new unit of absorbed dose in SI system of unit and it is equivalent to 1 joule per kilogram of the irradiated product.
1 Gy = 1 joule/ kg or 100 rads

kGy : Kilo gray. It is equivalent to 100 Gy or 10^5 rads.
1 kGy = 100 Gy or 10^5 rads

MeV : It is equivalent to one million electron volts.

Radappertization: It is a type of irradiation sterilization or commercial sterilization in which higher doses of irradiation (30-40 kGy) is generally used. In this process all organisms associated with the meat and aquatic foods are killed but it also induces undesirable changes in flavour and texture of these products.

Radicidation: In this method 2.5 to 10 kGy dose of irradiation is generally used to kill all non spore forming pathogens other than viruses. This radicidation process is analogous to pasteurization.

Radurization: In this method of ionizing radiation a dose of 1 to 5 kGy is generally used to reduce the population of spoilage organisms. This redurization process is also considered equivalent to pasteurization in which food is exposed to ionizing radiation doses strong enough to reduce microbial or insect populations and thus, delay spoilage.

9. Chemical Preservation

The majority of food preservation operations used today also employ some kind of chemical additive to reduce spoilage. Of the many dozens of chemical additives available, all are designed either to kill or retard the growth of pathogens or to prevent or retard chemical reactions that result in the oxidation of foods. The most commonly used are the acids especially organic acids which are considered generally recognised as safe (GRAS) such as sorbic acid, benzoic acid and propionic acid. These acids checks mainly the growth of yeasts and moulds. World Health Organization (WHO) and Central Drug Research Institute (CDRI) at Lucknow have permitted only two chemicals for food preservation. These are sodium benzoate and Potassium metabisulphite. These are harmless and can be safely used in food items.

S.No	Name of chemical preservative	Dose	Mode of action
1.	Acids		
	a.) citric acid, propionic acid, benzoic acid, sorbic acid, acetic acid and their salts.	0.1 -0.2%	Yeast and mould inhibitors.
	b.) Acetic acid and lactic acid	0.1 -0.2%	Bacterial inhibitors.
2.	Sulphites (such as sulphur dioxide.	450 ppm	Insects and micro-organisms inhibitors.
3.	Nitrites (such as sodium nitrite)	200 ppm	Bacterial inhibitors.
4.	Sodium benzoate	0.1%	Bacterial inhibitor but not effective at normal pH of fish flesh.

10. Antioxidants Preservation

Antioxidants are compounds used in foods to prevent deterioration, rancidity or discolouration caused by oxidation. The most commonly used antioxidants are phenolic compounds such as butylated hydroxy anisole (BHA), butylated hydroxy toluene (BHT), tertiary butyl hydroquinone (TBHQ). Ascorbic acid and citric acid are also used to prevent the oxidative discolouration in meat caused by enzymatic oxidation. Whereas, sulphur dioxide is a compound serves dual purpose like preservation and antioxidant. The propyl gallate (PG) can be used as a animal fat stabiliser. Besides these traditional antioxidants some natural compounds such as extracts of rosemary and sage and compounds found in wood green tea may be used as antioxidants.

S.No.	Name of antioxidant	Doses in different meat products (in ppm)					
		In general use	In poultry products	In dry sausages	In fresh sausages & beef patties	In dried meat	In rendered animal fat
1.	BHA	200	100	30	100	100	100
2.	BHT	200	100	30	100	100	100
3.	TBHQ	200	100	30	100	100	100
4.	PG	200	100	30	100	100	100
5.	Tocopherols	300	300	-	-	-	300

11. Antibiotics Preservation

The use of antibiotics in food preservation is depend on the type of spoilage to be controlled, stability and suitability of antibiotics in a particular pH of food, stability to heat and lack of toxicity after consumption of food. Nisin and Natamycin are the most widely used antibiotics in the meat preservation while Aureomycin, Terramycin and Chloromycetin are the commonly used antibiotics in the fish preservation. Alongwith these antibiotics some others such as tetracycline, subtilin and tylosin are also used for this purpose.

S. No.	Name of antibiotics	Source of antibiotics	Favourable pH	Action
1.	Nisin	*Lactococcus lactis*	6.5 -6.8	Active against Gram+ve bacteria and inhibits growth of *Clostridium botulinum*.
2.	Natamycin	*Streptomyces natalensis*	5.0 -6.0	Effective against yeasts and mould but ineffective against bacteria.
3.	Lactic acid fermentation	*Lactbacillus, Lactococcus, Leuconostoc* and *Pediococcus*	-	It produces antimicrobial compounds i.e. hydrogen peroxide, diacetyl, bacteriocins and reuterin.

When natural or controlled microbiota or antimicrobials is used in food preservation and to extend the shelf life are sometimes referred as biopreservatives and technique of food preservation is termed as biopreservation. Lactic acid bacteria (LAB) are of special interest because they have antagonistic properties and their competence for nutrients, their metabolites. Nisin produced from LAB is an effective preservative.

In fish processing, biopreservation is achieved by adding antimicrobials or by increasing the acidity of the fish muscle. Certain types of plant extracts and essential oils as well as bacteriocins and bacteriophages are also used as the biopresrvation techniques.

The use of one or more than one preservation technique may be of immense use in the meat and aquatic food industry. It will also be helpful in reducing the cost in processing and the animal food will be available all time. The preservation technique may also impart colour, flavour and other sensory attributes besides prolonging the shelf life of animal tissues and aquatic foods. Now the recent innovations in meat and aquatic preservation are intelligent packaging, high pressure processing, pulse electric field, pulsed light, ultrasound technology, oscillating magnetic field, natural antimicrobials etc.

References

1. Egan, A.F. and Wills, P.A. (1985). The preservation of meats using irradiation. CSIRO Food Research Quarterly, 45:49-54.
2. Forrest, J.C., Aberle, E.D., Hedrick, H.B., Judge, M.D. and Merkel, R.A. (1969). Structure and Composition of Muscle and Associated tissues. In: Principles of Meat Science, W.H. Freeman and Company, San Francisco, pp 27-89.
3. Giese, J. (1994). Antimicrobials: assuring food safety. Food Technology, June Issue.
4. Gracey, J., Collins, D.S. and Huey, R. (1999). Anatomy, meat composition and quality. In: Meat Hygiene, 10th ed. W.B.Saunders Company Ltd. London, pp 57-65.
5. Hugo, W.B. (1991). A brief history of heat and chemical preservation and disinfection. Journal of Applied Bacteriology, 71:9-18.
6. Khurana, S. (2007). Meat Preservation. In: Universal Meat Hygiene in Public Health Care, International Book Distributing Co. Lucknow, pp 221-249.
7. Murano, E.A. (1995). Irradiation of fresh meats. Food Technology, Dec Issue: 52-54.
8. Panda, P.C. (1973). Formation, structure, food value and chemical composition of eggs. In: Text Book On Egg and Poultry Technology.Vikas Publishing House Pvt. Ltd., New Delhi, pp 9-46.
9. Sacharow, S. and Griffin, R.C. (1969). Basic food processes. In: Food Packaging, Richmand Virginea, pp 65-80.
10. Sharma, B.D. (1999). Structure, composition and nutritive value of meat tissues. In: Meat and Meat Products Technology (Including Poultry Products Technology), Japee Brothers Medical Publishers (P) Ltd, New Delhi. Pp 8-22.
11. Singh, V.P. (2008). Ageing of meat. In: Manual of Meat and Meat Products Technology (including poultry products technology), DUVASU, Mathura.
12. Wilson, W.G. (2005). Meat preservation and meat roducts. In: Wilson's Practical Meat Inspection, 7th ed. Blackwell Publishing, Oxford, pp 206-222.

□□□□

7 Ageing of Meat

Ageing of meat is also known as conditioning or tenderising or ripening or maturing and sometime resolution of rigor. It is a process of holding unprocessed meat above freezing point under controlled conditions. By this process we can make muscle soft and pliable thus meat becomes tender. When we keep the meat above freezing point at temperature between 0-3°C then all those changes occurs which are normally occurs at higher temperature i.e. atmospheric oxidation and enzymatic action of fat, bacterial action etc. When this temperature range becomes below freezing point then it inhibits completely the enzymatic action in the muscles. Ageing is required for marked increase in flavour, juiciness and tenderness of meat. In this process action of enzymes in meat plays key role while bacterial action is not of any importance. Meat tenderness and taste are definitely improved if carcasses or vacuum packed cuts are conditioned after slaughter but paradoxically beef is quite tender just two hours after slaughter and several days of conditioning are required to recover this degree of tenderness.

During the contraction of muscles, thick and thin filaments sliding to each other and decreases the length of sarcomeres. In turn, this decreases the length of fibrils, fibres and the whole muscle. If these muscles remain in contracted length when rigor develops, it causes massive overlap of thick and thin filaments leading to severe meat toughness. It is also necessary to avoid the cooling of meat too rapidly after slaughter, otherwise it cold-shortens and gets tough. If we avoid cold-shortening of muscles during conditioning, it will increase meat tenderness. But with too much conditioning, weight loss, surface spoilage and the cost of refrigerated storage increases.

Ageing of carcasses with little or no fat cover is not recommended by meat specialists. Because these carcasses loose moisture rapidly, loose weight excessively and discolour the meat surface rapidly. In addition, lean meat is also susceptible to deterioration through microbial growth, slime formation by bacteria and mould growth etc. Ageing is important for beef and buffalo meat while pork and lamb do not require ageing because they are slaughtered in the age where they are young and inherently tender. Additionally, the unsaturated fats found in pork fat oxidize during ageing causes rancidity and off flavour. Veal has very little protective fat covering and is high in moisture; thus it does not lend itself to ageing.

Factors Affecting Ageing

Ageing process of meat is determined by certain factors directly or indirectly and they may be either pre-slaughter or post slaughter.

Pre-Slaughter Factors

Breed, age, exercise and nutritional status of the meat animals prior to slaughter greatly affect ageing of meat post slaughter. Among the animals beef, buffalo meat, veal, rabbit meat have lesser rate of tenderization than lamb. Lamb has twice faster speed of conditioning than beef. Generally cross breeds of cattle have improved conditioning rate than indigenous breeds. And among muscles of an individual, longissmus muscle has greater conditioning rate during storage at 2°C.

Post-Slaughter Factors

The changes in meat during first 24 hrs of slaughter is utmost important for ageing. In this process myofibrils, connective tissue content surrounding myofibrils, amount of collagen and proteinous ground substance (proteoglycan) and action of calcium-activated proteases, calpins and lysosomal cystein proteases and cathepsins over myofibrils are the key factors responsible for ageing. The temperature of storage and degree of cooling the carcase also affects ageing process. If it is fast then meat gets cold shortening and if it is too slow then it destroys enzymes required for ageing. After onset of rigor mortis muscle temperature has largest effect on the rate of ageing. At 0-40°C rate of ageing increases by 2.5 fold for every 10°C rise in temperature while at temperature above 60°C rate of ageing drops rapidly due to enzyme denaturation. Storage temperature also has significant effect on rate of ageing as 80% of tenderization can be achieved in 10 days at 0°C while same effect can be obtained in 4 days at 10°C and within 1.5 days at 20°C.

Mechanism of Ageing

In early research, it was thought that increased tenderness might originate from the breakdown of rigor bonds between thick and thin filaments but now this appears unlikely because increased tenderness during conditioning still occurs when sarcomeres are at a stretched length that virtually eliminates any overlap of thick and thin filaments. Another factor that contributes to the increased tenderness of conditioned meat may be an increase in ionic strength that solubilizes myofibrillar proteins, particularly those of the thick filament.

Ageing is a process in which major changes takes place in muscle fibers but meat proteins are also affected by the action of different enzymes particularly proteolytic enzymes present in meat. Some of the enzymes (calcium-activated proteases, calpins and lysosomal cystein proteases and cathepsins) acts on muscle fibers especially on myofibrils and degradate Z-lines. In this process sarcomere is also separated. This action produces loosening of myofibrillor structure. And stretching at this point leads to fracture at Z-disc which is responsible for reduction of toughness of meat. But actomyosin bond remains intact as well as connective tissues surrounding myofibril is also less affected by enzymatic action.

Calcium-activated protease (Calpain) is an enzyme located in the cytosol. It slowly disrupts Z lines by releasing alpha actinin, a protein that holds the thin filaments into the Z line. This makes an important contribution to meat conditioning but many aspects of the calpain system still are unknown. Calpains occur in all vertebrate cells, where they are involved in general purpose enzymatic activity related to maintenance of cell shape and the response of cells to hormones. Also there are other enzymes inside the muscle fibre which might be involved in the conditioning effect. Cathepsin B and D occur in lysosomes (suicide bags to destroy unhappy cells) and parts of the sarcoplasmic reticulum. Acid phosphatase is another enzyme that has been found inside muscle fibres. Among these enzymes calpains and cathepsins are the main enzymes responsible for ageing in meat. Calpains becomes active at neutral pH and shortly after slaughter while cathepsins become active at acid pH after rigor. Calpains I is activated first at low calcium ion concentration normally at about 6.3 pH or about 6 hrs after slaughter. On the activation of calpains I, tenderization process started and gets sufficient pace after proper activation of this enzyme. After about 16 hrs of slaughter Calpains II gets activated due to appropriate concentration of calcium which causes further tenderization of meat. Approximately 50% of the tenderization occurs in first 24 hrs of slaughter, after which the rate of tenderization becomes exponential.

Muscle proteolytic enzymes which helps in ageing

Group of enzyme	Name of enzyme	pH required for proteolysis	Structurally important sites of enzymes during ageing
Lysosomal type	Cathepsin-B Cathepsin-D Cathepsin-H Cathepsin-L	3.0-6.0 2.5-4.5 5.0-7.0 3.0-6.0	Rapidly act on Troponin-T and I and C-protein. However, slowly act on myosin, actin, tropomyosin, α-actinin, nebulin and titin. It can also act on collagen at cross links of non helical telopeptides and mucopolysaccharides of ground substances.
Non-lysosomal type	Calcium activated sarcoplasmic factors (CASF) Calcium activated neutral proteinases (CANP) Trypsin like (Serine) proteinase Neutral (Thiol) proteinase Alkaline (Serine) proteinase	> 6.0 6.5-8.0 6.5-8.0 6.5-8.0 7.5-10.5	Troponin-T, Desmin (Z-line), Connectin (gap filament), M-line proteins and tropomyosin

Conditioning causes changes in a number of water-soluble compounds that affect meat taste including free amino acids, metabolites of ATP, organic acids and sugars. Free amino acids released by aminopeptidase activity are increased during the conditioning of pork, chicken and beef although the changes in beef are less than anticipated.

Effect of conditioning on red and white muscles

S.No.	White muscles	Red muscles
1.	Z-line in white muscles is more labile during conditioning	Z-line in red muscles are less labile
2.	Conditioning is more prone in rabbit and porcine muscles	Less prone in bovine muscles
3.	Semitendinosus muscle of bovine is more prone to degradation	Psoas muscle of bovine is less prone to degradation
4.	It has three times higher CASF activity than red muscle	It has three times lesser CASF activity
5.	Less susceptible to cold shortening	More susceptible to cold shortening
6.	During post mortem, isometric tension is less pronounced in red muscles	During post mortem, isometric tension is more pronounced in red muscles

Salient points of conditioning

- At the temperature of ageing (0-25^{0}C) collagen and elastin (connective tissue protein) do not denature. However, on the action of proteolytic enzyme collagen fibre swell during ageing.
- The extractability of myofibrillar proteins is greater at high ultimate pH.
- High temperature during post mortem hampers the extractability of myofibrillar proteins.
- Cold shortened muscles shows lower activity of μ-calpain and increased activity of calpastatin.
- During post mortem, sarcoplasic proteins are most labile proteins. Among all sarcoplasmic proteins, creatine kinase of beef, rabbit and pigs is most labile.
- Pigs affected by PSE conditions are supposed to be the higher temperature than normal pigs immediately post-mortem.

- The denaturation of protein leads to lower water holding capacity. The minimal water holding capacity of principal proteins in muscle is at isoelectric point (5.4-5.5).
- There is no increase in water soluble hydroxyproline containing derivatives even after storage in sterile fresh meat at 37ºC for a year.
- *Calpain*–L is a most important lysosomal proteinase for conditioning or ageing.

Methods of Ageing

For ageing of meat cooling of dressed carcase for 1-2 days at -0.5 to 3ºC and quarters, sides for 10-12 days at 2 to 3ºC is desirable. And for making retail cuts, carcase should be held for 24 hrs at 4.5 to 7ºC. In commercial practice of ageing carcase should be held for 2-6 weeks. However, good palatability can be achieved by ageing within 9 days by cutting the joints. On the basis of ageing temperature and condition of environment where ageing takes place, process of ageing can be classified into two broad categories:

Dry ageing: It is much more expensive and takes longer than wet aging. Meat which is dry aged is hung in a very clean, temperature and humidity controlled cooler for a period of two to four weeks. During this time, enzymes within the meat break down the muscle and connective tissue making it tender. Moisture is lost from the outer parts of the carcass causing an inedible crust to form which must be trimmed off and discarded. The carefully controlled environment, the time involved, and the loss of outer portions of the carcass make dry ageing a costly process.

Wet ageing: It occurs when meat and its own juices is vacuum packaged in plastic and boxed for distribution. Because the plastic packaging does not allow loss of moisture so the meat may absorb more moisture which results in an increase in juiciness and tenderness. Both methods of ageing work well and can create a better product. The difference is that dry ageing gives a more distinctive flavour while wet ageing is much less costly and rapid in dispensing and therefore a much longer shelf-life.

As we know ageing of meat is dependent on pre-slaughter factors as well as post-slaughter factors so we can induce the tenderness in meat by using pre-slaughter as well as post slaughter methods.

Pre-Slaughter Methods of Tenderization

Tenderization of meat by using certain enzymes at pre-slaughter living stage of animal is called Pro Ten Process which was introduced by Swift Company of Chicago, USA in late 1950s. In this method papain (obtained from papaya) solution is injected in jugular veins of animals. The dose rate varies from 300 to 500 ml depending upon breed, age, sex and weight of animals. For attaining maximum tenderness, animals must be slaughtered within 10-15 minutes of injection. The meat obtained after papain injection may contain about 4 ppm enzymes in raw meat which is activated when meat is subjected to cooking at 60-71°C. It is a method by which tenderness in meat can be achieved in low cost and under shorter period of time and also there is no weight loss due to shrinkage and trimmings. But it has not gains popularity due to animal welfare and ethical considerations, less acceptability of its texture and flavour, over tenderness of tongue, liver and kidneys of such animal and sometimes animal treated with these enzymes may get anaphylactic shocks, marked rigors and death.

Post-Slaughter Methods of Ageing

Post slaughter methods of ageing are more widely applicable. For this purpose various processes are applied but some of these may be summarized as:

1. Hanging and stretching of carcasses (Tender stretch method of hanging).
2. By severing certain bones and ligaments (Tender cut process).
3. Tenderizing meat by hammering and muscle stretching.
4. Quick freezing of carcase before sets of rigor-mortis.
5. Application of certain enzymes.
6. Infusion of calcium chloride.
7. Electrical stimulation.

1. Hanging and Stretching of Carcasses

It is a fact that shortening of muscles leads to toughness of meat. So stretching of muscles by hanging at certain points produces tender meat. In traditional method of hanging, a hook is placed behind the Achilles tendon. In another method of Texas A&M University aitch bone is used for hanging and hook is inserted in obturator foramen or pope's eye. By this way hind limb is relaxed. Hanging by aitch bone method is generally practiced for hot carcasses, sides and quarters within $1^{1}/_{2}$ hrs of slaughter while Achilles tendon method of hanging is applied in chillers after 24 hrs of slaughter.

In conventional method of hanging and stretching only five muscles of hind quarter becomes tender while other remains tough. The best example is tougher meat of psoas major muscle in conventional method, however, it is considered as most tender cut of beef and buffalo carcase. In this method rump, thick flank, striploin and scotch fillet becomes so tender and resembles like muscles of 3 weeks ageing at 2°C. Drawback in aitch bone hanging method is its slight alteration in appearance of muscles, however, flavour, juiciness and cutting qualities of carcasses remains same. Hanging and stretching method is most suitable for tougher cuts of beef and buffalo meat but can also be used for sheep, goat and other animal's carcasses.

2. Tender Cut Method

It is a process of making meat tender by cutting and splitting of certain bones and ligaments. In this process tenderization of meat is induced by alteration in tension on individual muscle in suspended carcase. For better results process should be carried out within 45 minutes of slaughter and carcase should be suspended by Achilles tendon.

3. Meat Tenderization by Hammering and Muscle Stretching

In this process pressure of hammer over meat is induced with stretching of muscles. In this way muscle fibers are brocken down which leads to decreas in toughness of muscles.

4. Quick Freezing of Carcase before Sets of Rigor-Mortis

In this process carcase is quick freezed before set of rigor mortis. Quick freezing produces small ice crystal in the meat which causes structural damage in the muscles. By this way it also releases enzymes responsible for ageing. Meat which is subjected to ageing prior to freezing is tenderer than that frozen within 1 or 2 days. The difference is also maintained in tenderness throughout its frozen storage for 9 months. Freezing rate affects the rate of tenderization after thawing but not the ultimate tenderness. Freezing at -10°C has double the rate of ageing than normal. The rate of tenderization is almost trebles when meat is frozen in liquid nitrogen (LN_2). The chances of cold shortening in muscles are more in this process and it also alters the colour and flavour of meat.

Cold shortening: If the muscle is chilled too rapidly before the metabolic changes takes place after slaughter then these may be chances of cold shortening. Cold shortening can cause the muscle fibre to contract and produces tough meat, affecting the colour, taste, tenderness, texture and eating quality. This is recognised by muscle pH which is still above 6.0 when the carcase has cooled to 12°C.

Heat shortening: Heat shortening condition observes in muscles when metabolic changes occurs after slaughter and before the muscle is chilled sufficiently. Heat shortening can cause the muscle fibre to contract and produces tough meat but toughness of meat is lesser than cold shortening. It will also affect the colour, taste, tenderness, texture and eating quality. Heat shortening occurs when a muscle pH is still below 6.0 and the carcase has cooled to 35°C.

5. Application of Certain Enzymes

It is method of artificial induction of tenderness in meat. In this method various enzymes obtained from fruits, bacteria and fungi are used. Some of the most commonly used enzymes are papain (proteolytic enzyme of *Carica papaya*, commonly known as papaya), ficin (a protease derived from figs), bromelin (proteolytic enzyme of pineapple) etc. These enzymes can be used separately or in combination, directly or in solution or powder form on cuts of carcasses. Some drawback of this method includes lack of uniformity in action of these enzymes, discolouration, mushiness and granulation of meat surfaces etc.

6. Infusion of Calcium Chloride

Infusion of calcium chloride is normally done in pre-rigor muscles on post mortem. It accelerate the tenderization process probably same as calcium-activated proteases and calpins. Marriott and Claus, 1994 reported that these compounds tenderizing the meat by breakdown of the myofibrillar proteins immediately post mortem but carcase should be hot with high pH.

7. Electrical Stimulation

Electrical stimulation is a application of electric current on carcase after slaughter. This process speed up the rigor mortis so on chilling of meat, possibility of cold shortening reduces. Method of electrical stimulation for tenderizing meat was suggested by Harsham and Deatherage of USA in 1951 but it was first time used in New Zealand for prevention of carcase from cold shortening. In large animals, two types of electrical stimulation is used i.e. higher voltage (500-1000 V, 5-6 ampears of current with 25 pulses per second for 2 seconds) and lower voltage (< 100V). Higher voltage electrical stimulation is normally applied after 30 minutes of slaughter while lower voltage within few minutes of slaughter and preferably during bleeding. The preferred site of electrical stimulation in the slaughter should be at dressing line between evisceration and carcase splitting points.

For electrical stimulation, two electrodes are used, one at carcase neck muscle or nose and another at hock. Its action is due to acceleration of rigor mortis. For electrical stimulation, current is applied immediately after slaughter which produces contraction in muscles and use up glycogen, ATP and creatine phosphate. In this process, rigor mortis is advances and pH about 6.0 is achieved within 2-3 hrs of slaughter. These conditions lead to increase in tenderness of meat and tender meat can be achieved in shorter period of time. The other benefits of electrical stimulation includes avoiding cold and thaw shortening, allows rapid chilling, produces better colour and flavour, retail cuts can be achieved rapidly.

8. Vacuum Packaging

When meat is stored in vacuum package in air free environment then it retards the growth of spoilage bacteria but ageing process continues. In this process maximum tenderness is achieved within 28 days of storage at -1°C. Optimum bloom and flavour can be obtained in this period. In vacuum packed meat ageing, slight sour or milky flavour appeared when we open the packed but it dissipate shortly and it can not affect flavour of meat afterwards.

Ageing is a process which is important for improvement in tenderness, flavour, water holding capacity and resolution of rigor mortis. It also plays an important role in processed meat by enhancement in flavour and textural development, in completion of curing reaction and drying as well as hardening of products. It causes tenderization of processed meat by the action of autolytic enzyme (cathepsin) which is found in meat.

References

1. Gracey, J., Collins, D.S. and Huey, R. (1999). Anatomy, meat composition and quality. In: Meat Hygiene. 10th ed. W.B. Saunders Company Ltd. London. 71-74.
2. Lawrie, R.A. and Ledward, D.A. (2006). The spoilage of meat by infecting organisms. In: Lawrie's Meat Science, 7th edn., CRC Press, Cambridge England. Pp 157-188.
3. Marriott, N.G. and Claus, J.R. (1994). Meat Focus Int., 372-375.
4. Ray, A.F. and Kaltenback, C.C. (1987). Aging Big Game. In: Bulletin 513R, Agricultural Experiment Station, University of Wyoming, Laramie, WY 82071.
5. Singh, V.P. (2008). Ageing of meat. In: Manual of Meat and Meat Products Technology (including poultry products technology), DUVASU, Mathura.
6. Stephen, J.J. and James, C. (2002). Meat refrigeration. In: Meat refrigeration. Woodhead Publishing Company, CRC Press, London.
7. Teye, G.A. and Okutu, I. (2009). Effect of ageing under tropical conditions on the eating qualities of beef. American Journal of food agriculture, nutrition and development. Vol. 9 (9).
8. Vaclavik, V.A. and Christian, E.W. (2003). Meat, Poultry, Fish and Dry Beans. In: Essentials of Food Science, 2nd ed. Springer (India) Pvt. Ltd. New Delhi, pp 172-173.

□□□□

8 Modern Processing Technologies of Meat and Meat Products

Meat processing is the set of methods and techniques used to bring substantial chemical and physical changes in the natural state of meat. These are the methods which are used for making meat and their products attractive, nutritious and marketable as well as for the prolongation of shelf-life. In processing techniques, grinding, chopping, addition of seasoning, alteration techniques for colour, heat treatments etc. are included but cutting, trimming and deboning are not included in processing operations.

History

Meat processing dates back to the prehistoric ages and probably the first processed meat product was sundried meat. Lator it turns to burning of meat over wood fire while salting and smoking of meat was practiced first time in the time of Homer, 850 B.C. In 63B.C.-14 A.D. at the reign of Augustus honey was tried for preservation of meat. Lator various types of cooking such as roasting, smoking, steaming and oven baking came in existance. Salt-preservation was especially common for foods including meat and meat products for warrior and sailor's diets, until the introduction of canning methods.

Modern food processing technology in the 19th and 20th century was largely developed to serve military needs. In 1809 Nicolus Appert invented a vacuum bottling technique that would supply food for French troops and this contributed to the development of tinning and then canning by Peter Durand in 1810. Although initially expensive and somewhat hazardous due to the lead used in cans. Canned goods would later become a staple around the world. Pasturization discovered by Louis Pasteur in 1862 was a significant advance in ensuring the micro-biological safety of food. In 20th century, food processing advances with the development of spray drying, freeze drying and the introduction of artificial sweeteners, colouring agents and preservatives such as sodium benzoate. In late 20th century ready to eat meat food products were introduced to cater the need of consumers.

Requirement of Modern Meat Processing Techniques

Modern meat processing technologies serves the purpose of convenience, variety, nutrition and reduced cost formulations alongwith other benefits like toxin removal, preservation, easy in marketing and distribution tasks and increasing food consistency. In addition, it enables transportation of delicate perishable meat foods across long distances and makes many kinds ofmeat and meat products safe to eat by de-activating spoilage and pathogenic micro-organisms. Modern meat processing techniques can also improves the quality of life for people with allergies, diabetics and other people who cannot consume some common food elements. It can also provide some of the extra nutrients required by human body such as vitamins, minerals, essential amino-acids and fatty acids. However, in another aspect these modern processing techniques can lower the nutritional value of foods and introduce hazards not encountered with naturally-occurring products. The use of additives lowers the nutritive value, chemicals used for preservation such as nitrites or sulphites may cause adverse health effects. The modern meat technologies also promote the development of junk foods with empty calories.

Basic Processing Techniques

1. Curing

Curing is a process of using salt, sugar, nitrate or nitrite, other colour fixing ingredients, phosphates and seasonings. In addition, various spices, baking soda, sodium erythorbate, hydrolyzed vegetable proteins and monosodium glutamate can also be used as curing ingredients.

Salt: Sodium chloride commonly known as salt is a basic ingredient used in curing. Its action is mainly due to dehydration and by altering the osmotic pressure.It slows down the action of proteolytic enzymes and chloride ions present in salt directly acts on micro-organisms.By this way it inhibits bacterial growth and susequent spoilage.Beside its preservative and antibacterial action, it also interact with fatty acids of meat thus enhances flavour and tenderness. Its recommended dose in meat products is 2-3% but it may increase or decrease depending upon the consumers preferences.Use of food grade salt is always recommended otherwise it may affect the colour and flavour of the product. The use of salt alone in meat and meat products is very limited (only in extremely fatty cuts) because it produces harsh hardening effects in products as well as it also produces dark undesirable colour which is not liked by most of the consumers. It is always used with sugar, nitrate or nitrite.

The use of salt in meat products is minimized due to its aderse effect on hypertension. For this purpose sodium chloride can be used alongwith potessium chloride because it is supposed that sodium elment of salt is mainly responsible for increase in hypertension in 20% of the human population. The ratio of potessium chloride in this mixture should not be more than 50% otherwise strong objectionable flavour in the product may develop. For optimum result, ratio of sodium chloride and potessium chloride should be 60:40 and by this ratio we can reduce about 34-35% of sodium content in the product. The replacement of sodium with potessium (due to increse in potessium content) reduces blood pressure even in normal individual. The later combination produces less salty taste as original by salt. It is paradoxical to note that potessium chloride has lower ionic strength and slightly higher water activity so the dose should be same as salt alone.

Sugar: The basic purpose of addition of sugar in curing solution is to minimize harsh hardening effect of salt, to enhance flavour and as a source of energy for nitrate reducing bacteria in curing solution. For flavour enhancement sugar interacts with amino groups of proteins and on cooking produces browning reaction. Most of the time 0.2-0.3% sugar is used in meat products by most of the processors but in ham it can be used upto 2%. Sometimes sugar produces excessive browning on cooking so there were several substitutes of sugars tried for the purpose. These substitutes may be corn syrup, molasses, honey and other natural sugar substitutes. Dextrose can also be tried but it is less sweet than sucrose and can be used for enhancement of water holding capacity of meat without altering flavour. Corn syrup can be used as the substitute of sugar because it is low in cost. Actually corn syrup is a mixture of sugars (dextrose, maltose, dextrins, polysaccharides and other higher sugars) obtaind by breackdown of starch but it is less sweet and soluble than sugar. Honey can also be used for this purpose particularly in hams and similar poultry products. It imparts sweet taste and some consumers like its taste but it is costly than other sugar substitutes.

Nitrate and Nitrite: For the supplementation of nitrate and nitrite mainly sodium nitrate and nitrite is used in meat products. The basic function of these compounds in meat and meat products is stablization of meat colour (pink red colour), contribution of characteristic cured meat flavour, inhibition of growth of poisioning and spoilage micro-organisms and to retard rancidity development. Initially nitrate was approved for fixation of cured meat colour but it is now a day outdated or used in very few meat products like country ham, lebanon bologna and canned meat products. However, use of both nitrate and nitrite is not recommended in baby canned meat products. Today nitrate is used only for the source of nitrite because nitrite acts quickly and required in less quantity. In addition, nitrite also prevent the growth of *clostridium botulinum* which is a heat resistant organism. In recent practice, many processors preferred to use the combination of both nitrate and nitrite because it gives additional nitric oxide and slow release of nitric oxide from nitrate gives additional safety factor. The recommended dose rate of nitrate and nitrite in most of the meat products is 500 ppm and 200 ppm respectively. If it is used in comination of nitrate and nitrite then it can be used at the rate of 200 ppm. A carcinogenic compound nitrosamine is formed in curing reaction by the interaction of nitrite with secondary amines. And it is believed that this nitrosamine is found in small quantity in nearly all cured meat product. To eliminate the formation of nitrosamine α-tocopherol coated salt can be used. It can also be reduced by the use of ascorbic acid and erythrobate in curing solution. Bacon is a produt in which elimination of nitrosamine is very difficult because it is produced by cooking at high temperature and nitrite interact with secondary amines in this product. To reduce the chances of nitrosamine formation 550 ppm sodium ascorbate alongwith 120 ppm sodium nitrite can be used. The colour reaction in nitrate and nitrite curing may be summerized as:

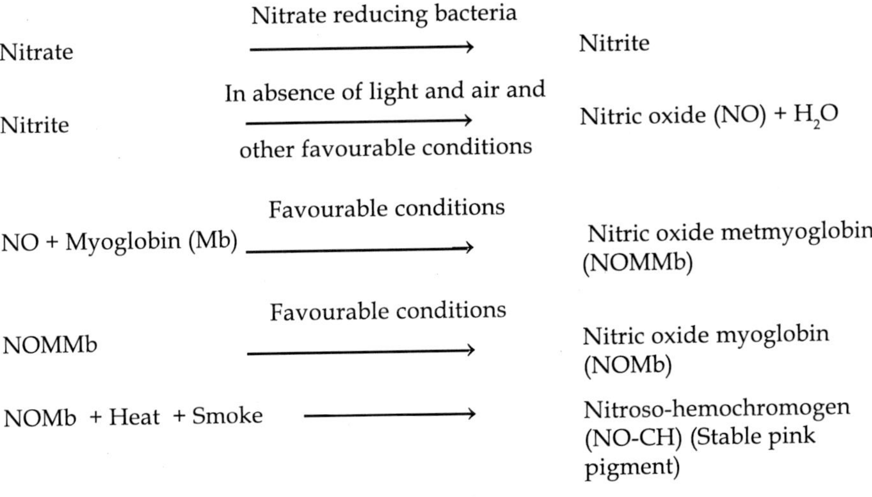

Cured meat flavour development in nitrate or nitrite curing is due to formation of benzonitrile and phenylacetonitrile compounds. These compounds are formed when sodium nitrite interact with fatty acids of meat and meat products.

Phosphates: Phosphate is used in meat in form of pyrophosphate and diphosphate but it is active only in form of diphosphate. Use of tetra-sodium pyrophosphate provides better binding but in curing brines a mixture of sodium tripolyphosphate and hexametaphosphate is used. The use of phosphate in meat enhances its water binding capacity by the unfolding of muscle proteins thus provides more sites for water binding. Due to enhancement in water binding capacity yield is also increased. Alkaline phosphate is mainly used for this purpose because it rises the pH and increases the water binding capacity while acid phosphate lowers the pH and produces more shrinkage resulted into less yield. For the balance of pH, both alkaline and acid phosphate may be used. Beside,the enhancement of meat product yield due to inceased water binding capacity and brine retention it also retards rancidity development by chelating the trace metal ions. The dose rate of phosphate in common meat products commonly ranges from 0.1-0.2%. Phosphates are corrosive in nature so the equipments used in phosphate cure must be of stainless steel. Phosphate is mainly used in cured solutions which are used by pumping especilly in ham, bacon, roast beef, cooked corned beef, pastrami and some poultry products. In these products phosphate produces certain effects i.e. cookout reduction, better slicebility, better juiciness and good flavour. In emulsion type products like sausages, phosphate produces all these effects alongwith better emulsification by improved protein extraction.

Ascorbate and erythorbate: Ascorbate and erythorbate commonly known as ascorbic acid and erythorbic acid. The salt of these similar isomers (sodium ascorbate and erythorbate) are generally used in meat products to stabilize the cured meat colour and also for reduction of nitrosamine formation. These compounds are when used in meat then accelerate the rate of curing, increases the yield of nitric oxide production. Ascorbate is also acts as an antioxidants thus stabilizes cured meat colour and flavour. In cured meat colour reaction ascorbate imparts in conversion of metmyoglobin to myoglobin thus accelerates the rate of curing. Ascorbate or erythorbate can be used in both intact meats and emulsion type meat products in a dose rate of 500 ppm. In emulsion type products particularly in sausages it greatly reduces the processing time. The use of ascorbate or erythorbate in processing of frankfurters can reduce about $1/3^{rd}$ time of total processing.

*Sorbate:*The use of sorbate in meat comes under the category of Generally Recognised As Safe (GRAS). Sorbate commonly known as sorbic acid is commonly used in fish, dairy and bakery products in form of potessium sorbate. The use of 2.5% potessium sorbate in meat products is approved only in dipping solution of stuffed dry sausages to inhibit the mould growth. It is a potent antibacterial agent and is also effective aginst mould growth. It is also able to inhibit the growth of *clostridium botulinum* when used with low levels of nitrite (0.26% potessium sorbate with 40 ppm sodium nitrite).

Monosodium Glutamate (MSG): It can be used in various meat products for enhancement in meat flavour.

Hydrolised vegetable proteins (HVP): It's use is limited to only meat sausages but it can be used in other meat products for enhancement of flavour and incorporation of vegetable proteins.

Lactate: Lactate is mainly used in form of sodium and potessium lactate to prolong the shelf life of the meat products because it prevents the spoilage in meat. It's 2.5 to 3.3% solution can be used in curing of various meat and meat products. Among sodium and potessium lactate, lator one is bitter in taste and is less preferred over sodium lactate.

Curing Methods

Curing is one of the oldest methods of preservation. Traditionally pork meat is subjected to curing. Cuts most commonly cured from pork are the ham, shoulders and belly while jowl and loin are sometimes cured. Most commonly cured beef cuts are briskets, strips of round or chuck and plates which can be cured as beef bacon. Sanitary conditions can affect the flavour of fresh or cured meats. Thus, it is essential to have clean equipment and facilities to produce the highest quality cured product. There are basically two methods of curing i.e. dry and pickle. Another method of curing is combination curing in which combination of both dry and pickle is used.

a. Dry curing involves the application of cure mix directly on the meat. Curing is done in the refrigerator. After curing, the meat is rinsed to remove the excess salt and then cooked. By the rubbing of dry curing ingredients on the meat makes brines by the extraction of moisture in form of meat juice and these ingredients then get entry into meat through diffusion process. Dry curing is used in curing hams and bacon as well as smaller cuts of meat. The dry salt curing method is mainly applied for fatty cuts and speciality products like dry cured bacon and country cured hams in which salt alone is rubbed on meat cuts. For the curing and storage of cured meat cuts wooden barrels or shelves were used. Now a day they are replaced with galvanized iron or stainless steel pressure boxes. Wooden and concrete vats can also used for this purpose. In this method curing time varies as per product i.e. ham and shoulders are cured for 2 to 2.5 days, bellies for 7 days and bacon for 10 to 14 days. Dry curing is used for relatively high priced speciality products, it enhances shelf-life due to dryness and firmness production and it imparts good flavour in meat products. It also has some draw backs such as high cost involvement in form of poor space utilization and amount of labour required, high inventory due to slowness of curing and production of harsh salty flavour of the final product.

b. Pickle or brine curing is also a popular method for curing meat. Brine curing involves mixing the curing salt with water to make a sweet pickle solution. The meat is cured with this brine by injecting the brine using a meat pump or by soaking the meat for a specific time. Curing takes place in the refrigerator and the meat is cooked after curing. Meat cuts intended for curing are submerged in the pickle until cure mix penetrates completely in the cuts. Pork shoulders are generally submerged in pickle in this method but it can also be used for making corned beef. Strength of the brine is expressed as degrees brine which is a measure of its density which can be determined by salanometer or salometer. Usually a pickle of 60-70° brine strength is commonly used and the ingredients used in pickle include salt, sugar, nitrite and/or nitrate etc. The curing time also depends on pickle strength and product type for example hams and shoulders are cured for 2 to 2.5 days in this pickle for optimum result. Some drawbacks of this method are poor utilization of space and slow turnover of meat inventories. Now a day a combination of methods, artery pumping and stitch pumping has restricted this technique but still it is popular technique for traditional meat products curing.

c. Injection curing is primarily used in hams, picnic shoulders (pork), briskets, round cuts and clods (beef). For farm curing, in which storage of meat product is done without refrigeration, sweet pickle of 75 to 85 degrees of strength is normally used. In this process meat is placed in a box or bin or on the shelves of a rack and cure for 7 days. However, for mild curing and subsequent storage under refrigeration, sweet pickle of 45 degree strength is normally preferred. Storage mode remains same but its storage time is 9 days. There are several methods of injection cure but some of these methods are spray, artery pumping and stitch pumping.

Artery pumping is basically limited to ham curing and to lesser extent to picnics. For artery pumping pickle of salt, sugar, nitrite/ nitrate and phosphate of the 65 to 80 degree strength is normally injected in the branch of femoral artery. It will facilitate the curing ingredient into the whole ham but some processor prefers to inject the pickle in each branch of this artery for more uniformity. In this method enough pickle solution is pumped to increase the weight of the cut by 8 to 15 percent. The time of curing normally remains 1-3 days but some processors directly exposed the product for smoking without holding. This system of curing gives better yield due to use of alkaline phosphate and it also reduce the time of curing subsequently. For example, in traditional system time of ham curing was about 7-14 days. Drawbacks of this system includes its use in limited products, due care during cutting and refrigeration is basically required.

Stitch pumping is a method of curing in which a needle of several openings or multiple needles are used to pump the cure in meat cuts. In single needle stitch pumping, pickle of 65 degree strength is used and it can be used upto 10% of the weight of cuts. It is a suitable method for curing picnics, shoulders, bellies and other miscellaneous cuts. In this method pickle is pumped into the meat with the help of needle having several openings. Drawback of this includes accumulation of pickle at the site of injection thus diffusion of pickle in meat cuts becomes delayed. To make diffusion of pickle more uniform in cuts, multiple needle stitch pumping system is adopted. In this system multiple needles are used for curing the pickle in meat cuts which gives more uniform distribution of pickle in the cuts. This method also reduces the labour cost and save the time of curing. It is a suitable method for bellies cure but can also be used in curing of hams.

d. In combination method of curing both dry rub cures with injection of sweet pickle solution are applied. It is a suitable method for curing hams. Combination method shortens the curing time and also reduces the chance of spoilage because the cure process takes place inside and outside the ham. Curing takes place in the refrigerator and the ham is cooked after curing.

e. Direct addition Curing or Sausage Curing is an entirely different method in which curing salt and spices are mixed with ground meat. Curing takes place in the refrigerator and the sausage is cooked after curing.

For curing of poultry, cover brine curing procedure and stitch using procedure is commonly used. In first system birds are put in curing vat and hold them under the brine with a clean board, stone, or container of water. Be sure the brine fills the body cavity. At the time of curing, brine temperature should be between 0-4^{0}C. And time of curing should be at least one week. In later system, stitching of brine is done with a 12-gauge needle and pumping of brine is done at numerous locations to insure uniform distribution into all parts of the carcass. The pickle solution can be used upto 11.8% of the carcase weight. Curing time normally remains 2 to 3 days.

In normal practice, curing takes place in refrigerated temperature. But to speed up the process hot or thermal cure process can also be adopted. In this method pickle of 70 degree strength is heated at 135-145°C. It can reduce the curing time from 3-5 days to 30 minutes to 1 hr. Hot curing also facilitate good yield, greater efficacy of smoke, more uniform curing, less pickle pockets and imparts good flavour in the products.

2. Smoking

Smoke is a very complex material containing more than 300 components such as alcohols, aldehydes, acids, ketones, phenolic compounds and various toxic elements and meat sometimes carcinogenic substances. The toxic substances inhibit the growth of microbes, phenolics retard fat oxidation and the whole complex imparts the characteristic flavour to meat and meat products. Among these compounds of smoke, phenol acts as bacteriostatic compound and formaldehyde as a bactericidal. In addition, smoke also produces surface dehydration, lower surface pH, bacteriostatic properties and antioxidant properties. Smoke at the point of generation is commonly exists in gaseous form but soon after it is converted into vapour and particle state. Among all three states, vapour phase is most desirable because it contains most of the volatile compounds which are mainly responsible for characteristic smoke flavour and aroma. Last state is very undesirable because it contains tars and polycyclic hydrocarbons which are considered as carcinogenic. The factors responsible for better action of smoke on meat cuts and products include smoke density, velocity, relative humidity and type of the product subjected to smoking.

Smoke Generation Process

Smoking of the meat products are normally done in specially constructed smoke houses. For the generation of smoke variety of woods can be used like apple, hickory, alder, maple (hardwood), sawdust or chips and some soft woods. But better results can be obtained from hardwood and sawdust and use of soft woods like pine is always avoided. Most of these woods consist of cellulose (40-60%), hemicellulose (20-30%) and lignin (20-30%). During combustion of wood it produces following compounds:

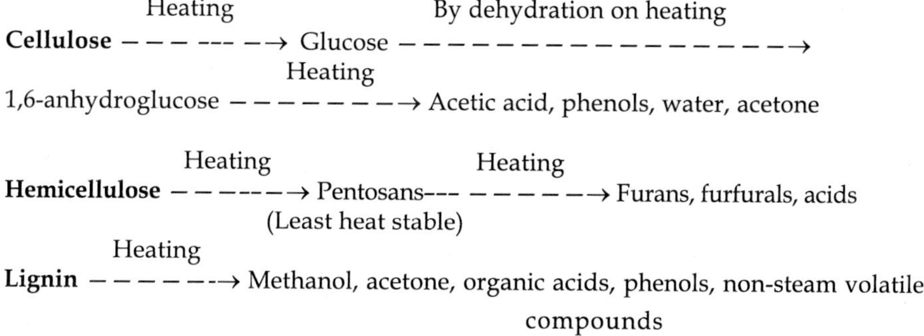

In smoke generation process combustion and oxidation occurs simultaneously. Most of the changes occur between the temperature range of 198.8°C and 398.8°C. The changes which take place at different temperature during smoke production may be summarized as:

Temperature	Yield products
100 °C	CO,CO_2, acetic acid
198.8 °C -260 °C	Gases , volatile acids
Between 260 °C -310 °C	Pyroligenous liquor, tar
310 °C-343.3 °C	Phenols and its derivatives
343.3 °C	Best quality smoke is produced as well as this temperature minimizes the production of carcinogens
398.8°C	Most desirable temperature for phenol production but also produces benazpyrene and other polycyclic hydrocarbons(carcinogenic compounds)

In most of the cases smoking and cooking takes place simultaneously which gives fully cooked and ready-to-eat meat. During the process of smoke generation humidity in the smokehouse should be maintained at 80–90% to minimize the weight loss and drying of the product. It can be achieved by dampening the sawdust or wood chips used for the smoke or by placing a pan of water near the heat source.

Compounds Produced during Smoking and their Mode of Action

Smoke contains about 300 compounds including chemicals and gases. The major chemicals are phenols, organic acids, alcohols, carbonyls, hydrocarbons and gases are carbon dioxide, carbon monoxide, oxygen, nitrogen and nitrous oxide etc.

Phenols: There are about 20 different phenolic compounds produced in smoke generation. Most of which are bacteriostatic in nature but bactericidal effect of phenol is a combined result of heating, drying and chemical components reaction. The main chemical responsible for bactericidal property of smoke is formaldehyde. Phenolic chemicals are also responsible for colour and flavour development especially in vapour phase, antioxidant property of smoke is mainly due to phenols of high boiling point. The colour development in smoked meat is mainly due to interaction of carbonyls in vapour phase with amino groups of meat. Phenols help in Maillard reaction and other factors assisting colour development are moisture (should be minimum 12-15% at surface) and relative humidity (should be more than 40%). The phenolic chemicals responsible for colour flavour and aroma developments are listed below:

Meat quality characteristics	Chemicals responsible
Smoked meat colour	Phenols of high boiling point such as 2,6-dimethoxyphenol, 2,6-dimethoxy-4-methyl phenol and 2,6-dimethoxy-4- ethyl phenol.
Smoked meat flavour	Guaiacol, 4-methyl–guaiacol, 2,6-dimethoxyphenol.
Smoked meat aroma	Syringol

Alcohols: Alcohol is a least important component of smoke because they are not playing any significant role in colour and flavour development except some bactericidal effect. The main role of alcohol in smoking is as a carrier of volatile components. There are many different alcohols are produced in smoke but the most important one is methanol or wood alcohol. It is obtained by destructive distillation of wood in smoking process.

Organic acids: The major role of organic acids is in skin formation in sausages and other similar products. They also have minor effect on preservation by increasing acidity on the surface of smoked meat but have no or insignificant effect on flavour and aroma. The organic acids found in smoke are of 1-10 carbons. Among them 1-4 carbon acids such as formic acid, acetic acid, propionic acid, butyric acid and isobutyric acid are main acids and mainly found vapour phase of smoke. Others (C 5-10) are of very less importance and mainly found in particle phase of smoke.

Carbonyls: More than 20 carbonyls are found in smoke which exits in steam-distillable and non-steam-distillable fractions. Major components belong to non-steam-distillable fraction but they are of not any use in meat smoking. The major contribution in smoked meat colour, flavour and aroma is of short-chain steam-distillable fraction carbonyls. The typical colour development in smoked meat is mainly due to carbonyls and in some extent due to phenols. The reaction of typical brown colour development in smoked meat products is due to Maillard or browning reaction. The steps in browning reactions are:

Aldol condensation (Aldose + Amines of meat) $\xrightarrow{-H_2O}$ Schiff's base ----→ Amadori rearrangement (N-substitute glycosylamine) $\xrightarrow{+2H}$ Strecker degradation (Enol) $\xrightarrow[-NH_2]{-CO_2}$ furfurals or hydroxymethyl furfurals formation (brown or black in colour)

Hydrocarbons: Smoke contains a number of polycyclic hydrocarbons which are not of any significance in preservation or organoleptic properties of smoked meat. Among them benzapyrene and dibenzanthracene are considered as carcinogenic. So the removal of these hydrocarbons in particulate phase of smoke is required. For this purpose liquid smoke can be used. These hydrocarbons can also be removed by combustion of hardwood or sawdust at a temperature of 300 °C.

Gases: Smoke constitutes number of gases particularly CO, CO_2, O_2 and N_2O. These are mainly related to the impartation of flavour but they may also contribute towards colour. CO_2 is suppose to react with the meat pigment myoglobin and forms carboxymyoglobin while CO produces carbonmonooxide myoglobin. O_2 when met with myoglobin then forms oxymyoglobin or metmyoglobin and gives muddy colour to the smoked meat. N_2O helps in formation of nitrosamine and nitrite which can be prevented by the use of ascarbates or erythorbates.

Methods of smoking: Smoke generation may be of natural air circulated type, forced air circulating or air conditioned type and continuous processing smokehouse type. Later method is more suitable for smoking of frankfurters.

Liquid Smoke Process

To facilitate the easy smoking, less production of carcinogens and faster smoking process now a day liquid smoke is used. In addition, liquid smoke has several other benefits i.e. no need of smoke unit installation, less atmospheric pollution, particulate phase of smoke can be removed which reduces the formation of carcinogens, smoking can be repeated several time with the faster rate.

Process of generation: Pyrolysis of hardwood sawdust ----→ smoke capture in water through absorption tower----→ recycling of smoke for generation of desired concentration----→ ageing ----→ filtration with cellulose filter to remove the hydrocarbons.

Application process: Liquid smoke either can be used directly over meat or it may be diluted with water or vinegar or citric acid. The use of citric acid or acetic acid may help in skin formation in frankfurters and related meat prodcuts. For better results, combination of liquid smoke (20-30 parts parts), citric acid or vinegar (5 parts) and water (65-75 part) may be tried. Application methods of liquid smokes includes direct addition, dipping, spraying, vapourizing, automizing etc.

3. Thermal Processing

The basic purpose of thermal processing is to produce palatable meat product with longer shelf life. The other benefits of thermal processing includes stabilization of colour, innactivation of autolytic enzymes, killing of pathogen and poisioning cusing micro-organisms, improvement in tenderness and enhancement of meat flavour. There are two temperature shedules are generally adopted in thermal processing, pasteurization and sterilization. Pasteurization is a moderate type of heat treatment in which meat and its products are exposed to a temperature of 58 -75°C. This temperature range kills spoilage organisms and inactivate other but it is not able to destroy spores of certain organisms. Pasteurized meat products require refrigeration storage. Sterilization is a method of severe heating of meat and meat products at the temperature above 100°C. At this temperature most of the organisms and their spores are destroyed or damaged beyond its repair but some nutrients are also lost in this process.

Commercial Sterility: It is a condition of meat product free from micro-organism capable of growing in the product at non-refrigerated condition (over 50°F or 10°C) at which the product is intended to be held during distribution and storage. This commercial sterility condition of product may be achieved by application of heat alone or in combination with other ingredients and/or treatments. These products are safe for eating because the pathogens of concern are destroyed or inactivated. Such product remains shelf-stable as long as the container is intact because any spoilage organism that favours the environmental conditions within the container (i.e., anaerobic) and normal storage temperatures (i.e., mesophilic bacteria) are also destroyed with the thermal process.

Principles of thermal processing: The basic principle behind the thermal processing and heat transfer to the meat product is by conduction or by conviction and/or by radiation. Conduction is a process of heat transfer in the meat products from one particle of meat to another without using any medium while in conviction a suitable medium such as water, air or steam is used to transfer heat to the meat product. Radiation is a process of heat transfer in meat products through space. These methods can be used separately or in combination depending upon the product nature and consumers choice.

Methods of thermal processing: In thermal processing of meat and meat products basically three methods are applied. The choice of method is entirely depends on nature of meat used and type of product is planning to made. These methods are dry heat processing, moist heat processing and microwave heat processing.

a. *Dry heat processing*: In dry heat processing hot air is commonly applied on the product for a sufficient period of time. This is a choice method for relatively tender cuts of meat. It is also a method of cooking in smoke houses of low relative humidity. The yield of finished meat product is relatively low in this method. The example of dry heat methods are roasting, broiling and frying. Now a day's hot air oven is good example of dry heat processing.

   Roasting is a method of using dry heat in which roast (meat cut) is exposed to hot air oven at 121.1 -176.6°C by using open roasting pan. In this process shelf-basting of meat cuts takes place. Cuts which are preferably cooked by this method are beef prime rib roast, beef sirloin, top round, veal leg, pork loin, pork shoulder, cured ham, lamb leg, lamb shoulder, lamb loin and racks.

   Broiling is a use of dry heat in tender cuts of meat. In this method meat hanged in iron wire grill and directly exposed to heat generated by electric or gas oven or charcoal oven. The continuous turning of meat is required in this method. This method of cooking is mainly applied in tender beef steaks, lamb chops, steaks from cured ham and the frozen meat products like patties and hamburgers.

Frying is suitable method for small tender cuts like fine sliced chops, steaks, bacon and small cuts of poultry. In this method cuts are emerged in fat in frying pan or in deep fat fryer and heat source is applied on this pan for a sufficient period of time.

b. *Moist heat processing*: It is a method of choice for tough meat cuts. In this method water or steam is used to cook the product. If water is used then it allows putting lid on the pan or product is cooked under pressure in pressure cooker. This is a fast method and gives better yield to the product and also conserves more nutrients than dry heat methods. Autoclaving and pressure cooking of the meat and its products comes under this category. The typical examples of moist heat cooking are stewing, braising, pot-roasting, simmering and pressure cooking.

Stewing is a method of use of moist heat in which small pieces of boneless meat are first browned (not always) in fat and then water is added in it and allow to cook at 71.1 -76.6°C in a covered pan. It is a suitable method for cooking of less tender and boneless cuts.

Braising is a combination of both dry and moist heat treatment in which meat is first browned in fat and then water is added in it and allows to cook in water vapour before boiling at a temperature of 71.1 -76.6°C. It is a suitable method for less tender cuts of meat such as beef roast and rump, lamb breast and shank, pork chop and steaks etc.

Pot-roasting is a similar method as braising but the addition of vegetables in meat cuts (as discussed in braising) at a desired time of cooking is an essential step.

Simmering is a method of using moist heat source in which meat cuts are filled in casings or plastic bags and then allow them to cook at the temperature below boiling (71.1 -76.6°C). This method can be used for cooking of certain beef cuts and sausages.

Pressure cooking is excellent method for tough cuts of meat. In this cooking method meat cuts are immersed in water and cooking takes place in pressure cooker. It rapidly gelatinizes the collagen of meat and makes the meat tender. But it also causes destruction of muscle structure and the texture of meat.

These methods (dry and moist) can be used alone or in combination. When they are used in combination then gives better texture, tenderness, flavour and overall palatability. Processed products are generally cooked by this combination method. The best example of this combination method is braising.

c. *Microwave heat processing*: Microwave heat processing is an excellent example of using electromagnetic spectrum in which heat is generated in magnetron vacuum tube inside the oven. For the generation of heat in microwave two frequencies (915 and 2450 MHz) are commonly utilized with the wavelength of 32.8 and 12.25 cm, respectively. Among these frequencies 915 MHz is better due to its double peak action, its first peak heat the food at surface and second peak at the center while 2450 MHz frequency heating is limited only to the surface. Heat generation through microwaves is known as volume heating due to its three dimensional heating process. In this process energy is converted into heat by intermolecular collisions. So the temperature of surrounding environment is not greatly changed during cooking of food. But use of metal pans in microwave cooking is always prohibited because microwaves are reflected from metals. For this purpose glass, pottery, wood and paper can be used. Microwave cooking gives uniform, rapid heating with less energy requirement. It also have some limitations such as lack of browning, requirement of proper and timely turning of the product and excessive exposure gives sogginess to the product.

4. Canning

Canning is the perfect way to preserve food with desirable flavour, texture and appearance for later use without the addition of chemicals and additives found in commercially preserved foods. Nearly all kinds of meat can be canned but lean meats or meat with the fat trimmed is ideal for canning.

Principles of canning: In canning process meat products filled in sealed containers are exposed to temperatures above 100°C in pressure cookers. Temperatures above 100°C, usually ranging from 110-121°C depending on the type of product, must be reached inside the product. Products are kept for a defined period of time at temperature levels required for the sterilization. The heat treatment in this process should be enough to kill or inactivate most heat resistant micro-organisms including the spores of Bacillus and Clostridium. Practically complete sterility is seldom achieved so the commercial sterility is the alternate in which all viable organisms are either destroyed or rendered dormant and the process also inactivate meat enzymes required for autolysis.

Types of containers used in canning: Containers used in canning must be hermetically sealed and airtight to avoid recontamination from environmental microflora. Most of them are metal containers (cans), glass jars or plastic or aluminium/plastic laminated pouches. Most cans or tins used in this process may be produced from tinplate. They are usually cylindrical but they may be of different shapes such as square, rectangular or pear-shaped or oblong. The interior of the cans is lined with a synthetic compound to prevent any chemical reaction of the tinplate with the enclosed meat food. Cans made up of aluminium are frequently used for smaller size, easy-to-open, better deep-drawing capability, low weight, resistance to corrosion, good thermal conductivity and easy recycability. Glass jars are sometimes used for meat products but are not common due to their fragility. Retortable pouches which are used in meat industry are made up of either of laminates of synthetic materials alone or laminates of aluminium foil with synthetic materials. Thermo-stabilized laminated food pouches have a seal layer which is usually made up of PP (polypropylene) or PP-PE (polyethylene) polymer and the outside layers are usually made of polyester (PETP) or nylon. Small can-shaped round containers are made from aluminium foil and polyethylene (PE) or polypropylene (PP) laminate are widely used for small portions particularly for sausage mix. One advantage of the retortable pouches or laminated containers is their good thermal conductivity which can considerably reduce the required heat treatment time and hence is beneficial for the sensory product quality.

Canning process: Red meats, poultry, game and sea foods are low-acid foods and must be processed in a pressure canner to assure their safety. The necessary steps in canning are preparation of meat and gravy, precooking, filling, exhausting, seaming, retorting, cooling, storage etc. The details description of these steps is given in chapter-6. Canning of the meat products are of three types i.e. pasteurized canned food, sterilized canned products and aseptic canning.

In this process different types of retorts are used such as nonagitating retort, continuous agitating retort and hydrostatic retort. But nonagitating retort is most common method in India for meat and fish products.

Establishing a Thermal Process in Canning

The combination of the factors such as how much heat and for how long is necessary to destroy micro-organisms in the food product and how fast does the product heat (in case of conventional canning) or how does the product flow (in case of aseptic processing) is used to establish the thermal process. As we know establishment of the thermal process is depend upon the method of processing (conventional canning or aseptic processing). In conventional canning, the product is filled into the container, the container is hermetically sealed and the container and product are thermally processed at a specified time and temperature to achieve commercial sterility. While in aseptic processing packages or packaging material and the food product are sterilized in separate systems. Product sterilization involves heating a pumpable product to a sterilizing temperature and holding it at that temperature for sufficient time to sterilize the product. The packaging materials are sterilized with heat, chemicals, radiation or a combination. The sterile package is then filled with sterile product, closed and hermetically sealed in a sterile chamber.

F-value of the Meat Product

By measuring the product temperature during thermal treatment through inserting a thermocouple into the critical thermal point (cold point) of the container (can), the summary F-value achieved can be determined. The temperature taken in the critical thermal point of the can/container each minute during sterilization corresponds to a partial F-value. All partial F-values obtained starting from the internal temperature of 100°C until the sterilization is ended and including the cooling phase until the product temperature falls below 100°C are added up. The sum of all partial F-values is the summary F-value achieved in

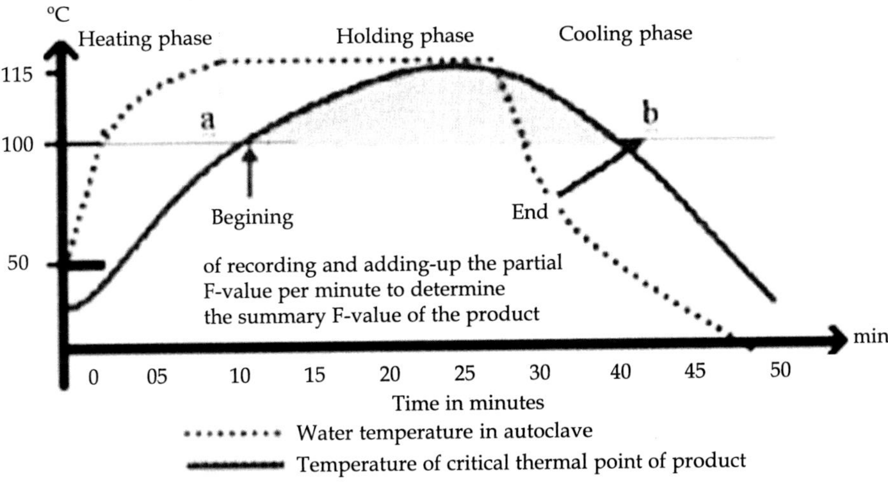

Fig.: F-value calculations during heating, holding and cooling phase (*Source*: FAO/WHO, 1993)

(In the figure temperature value starting from +100°C during the heating phase (a) – measured in the critical thermal point of the product – the F-values (per minute) are added up until a temperature below +100°C is reached during the cooling phase (b). The partial F-values associated with temperatures below 100°C are very small and hence do not contribute significantly to the overall amount of heat treatment or summary F-value of the product. Partial F-values below 100°C can therefore be neglected in the summary F-value calculation for meat product sterilization.)

the product. It is noticeable point that partial F-values associated with temperatures below 100°C are very small and hence do not contribute significantly to the overall amount of heat treatment or summary F-value of the product. Partial F-values below 100°C can therefore be neglected in the summary F-value calculation for meat product sterilization.

For the calculation of the *Cl. botulinum*–based partial F-values (F-value per minutes) the following additional parameters apply:

D-value: Decimal reduction time of *Cl. botulinum,* which is the time at a given temperature needed to reduce the microbial population to 10%, of its original numbers (e.g. at 121°C approximately 12 seconds)

Z-value: It indicates the necessary increase in temperature (°C), which is needed to decrease the decimal reduction time (in the above example 12 seconds) to 10% (=1,2 seconds in the example). For Cl. botulinum this z-value is 10°C (is different for all other microorganisms).

This fact of the Z-value being 10 for the reference microorganism *Cl. botulinum* facilitates F-value calculations. The rule is that temperature increases/decreases by 10°C will change partial F-values by the factor 10 (decimal increase/decrease)

Time/temperature effect for Z-value

Temperature	F-value (minutes)	Minutes at 121°C to achieve F-value 1
101°C	1	100
111°C	1	10
121°C	1	1
131°C	10	0.1

12 - D - Concept

Knowledge of the decimal reduction rate of *Cl. botulinum* enables the calculation of the safe elimination of this micro-organism. It is assumed that a batch of cans is contaminated with one spore of *Cl. botulinum* per can. It is required that the sterilization be such that there is a likelihood of only one spore surviving in a trillion (10^{12}) cans, or in other words a 12-fold decimal reduction (down to 10^{-12}). Mathematically the complete elimination to zero micro-organisms cannot be established.

The decimal reduction time of *Cl. botulinum* at 121°C is 0.21 min., and for the 12-fold effect the result is 12 x 0.21 min. = 2.5 min. The period of 2.5 min. at 121°C is equivalent with F-value 2.5. This F-value of 2.5 is also called "botulinum cook" or "12-D-concept" and signifies the elimination of *Cl. botulinum* under practical conditions. When applying the above decimal increase/decrease rule at 111°C (10°C lower than 121°C), the "botulinum cook" would be achieved only after the ten-fold time = 25 min. instead of 2.5 min. at 121°C.

Thermal death time (TDT) test: It is a test based on the amount of heat required for destruction of micro-organisms in food products. TDT retorts, tubes, and/or cans; three-neck flask, oil baths, sealed plastic pouches, and/or capillary tubes. The equipment and instrumentation used will depend on the type of product being tested – whether it is low-acid, acidified, thick puree, solid or a liquid. In TDT tests heating of a known amount of micro-organisms are done in a buffer solution or food at several temperatures and for several time intervals at each temperature. The results from the TDT tests are used to calculate D- and Z-values. These values are used to define the heat resistance of concern micro-organisms.

Thermal establishment for fully sterilized canned products: In the food industry the most heat resistant pathogens are *Clostridium botulinum* spores for which a minimum F-value of 2.52 needed. The most heat resistant spores for spoilage are the *Clostridium sporogenes* spores which require minimum F-values of 2.58. Based on these microbiological considerations and including a sufficient safety margin, sterilized canned products should be produced with F-values of 4.0-5.5. The retort temperatures to be used may vary between 117°C and 130°C depending on the heat sensitivity of the individual products. A shelf life of up to four years at storage temperatures of 25°C or below can be achieved for canned products. In tropical countries, where the storage temperatures may exceed 25°C, specific canned products for tropical conditions are manufactured. In these cases the summary F-values have to be increased to F-value 12-15, which permits safe storage of the finished products under storage temperatures up to 40°C.

Thermal establishment for commercially sterile products: F-values of 4 and above as required for fully sterilized canned products are often detrimental for the quality of certain canned foods. Thus technologies have been developed, which use a sterilization pattern of slightly less than F-value 4, which means that under certain circumstances some spores may survive. In order to tackle this risk, other hurdles can be employed to curb microbiological growth. In this connection first step is curing substance with nitrite. It inhibits the growth of spores and lowers water activity (a_W) due to reduced water content or a_W reducing ingredients such as fat, non-meat proteins and salts.

5. Drying

Drying is an oldest method of meat preservation in which natural temperatures, humidity and circulation of the air, including direct influence of sun rays is used. It consists of a gradual dehydration of pieces of meat cut to a specific uniform shape that permits the equal and simultaneous drying of whole batches of meat. Intensity and duration of the drying process depend on air temperature, humidity and air circulation for example drying will be faster under high temperatures, low humidity and intensive air circulation. Reduced moisture content of the meat is achieved by evaporation of water from the peripheral zone of the meat to the surrounding air and the continuous migration of water from the deeper meat layers to the peripheral zone. There is a relatively high evaporation of water out of the meat during the first day of drying after which it decreases continuously. After drying for three or four days weight losses in meat upto 60–70 percent may be observed that is equivalent to the amount of water evaporated. Consequently, moisture losses can be monitored by controlling the weight of a batch during drying. Continuous evaporation and weight losses during drying cause changes in the shape of the meat through shrinkage of the muscle and connective tissues. The meat pieces become smaller, thinner and to some degree wrinkled. The consistency also changes from soft to firm to hard. In addition to these physical changes, there are also certain specific biochemical reactions with a strong impact on the organoleptic characteristics of the product.

Meat drying is a complex process with many important steps, starting from the slaughtering of the animal, carcass trimming and selection of the raw material, proper cutting and pre-treatment of the pieces to be dried and proper arrangement of drying facilities. In addition, the influence of unfavourable weather conditions must also be considered to avoid quality problems or production losses. The secret of correct meat drying lies in maintaining a balance between water evaporation on the meat surface and migration of water from the deeper layers.

Meat suitable for drying: As a general rule only lean meat is suitable for drying. Dry meat is generally manufactured from bovine meat although meat from sheep, goats and venison can also be dried. The meat best suited for drying is the meat of a medium-aged animal. Meat from animals with poor nutritional condition can also be used for drying but the higher amount of connective tissue is likely to increase toughness.

Drying Process

Carcase cutting into sides and quarters and
hanging with Achilles tendon

↓

Trimming

↓

Deboning
(There should be least possible damage to the muscles)

↓

Cutting of meat for drying
(Muscles should be splitted exactly along the muscle fibres and
strips must be cut uniformly and smoothly as possible.
The diameter of strip must remain same throughout the length)

↓

Primary treatment (pre-salting) of meat strips before drying

↓

Suspension of meat for drying
(Meat strips should be suspended individually from one end for

proper drying with free air circulation along the whole length of the pieces for uniform drying. Suspension methods are metal hook and clip suspension, metal or wood sun dryer.)

↓

Meat drying should be done for atleat four to five days, till the development of wrinkle free uniform appearance, uniform dark red colour with a mild salty taste

↓

Packaging and storage
(Plastic bags or card board packages are most appropriate and vacuum packaging is a most suitable method)

Dried Meat Preparation for Consumption and Various Dried Meat Products

Dried meat is normally rehydrated provide the resemblance same as fresh meat.Rehydrated dried meat has almost the same nutritive value as fresh meat.Rehydration is in most cases combined with cooking. The addition of other additives in meat is entirely dependent on consumer's choice. Though dried meat is not common in India but they are very specific in African and American countries.

Dried meat product	Countries in which it is popular	Type of meat used	Preparation method and Speciality
Odka	Somalia and East African countries	Lean beef	Drying of meat is done in similar manner as described above but meat strips for drying are bigger and dry salting is used. After six hours of drying strips are cut into smaller pieces and cooked in oil. Its shelf-life is more than one year.
Qwanta	Ethiopia and East African countries	Lean beef muscles	Long strips of 20 to 40 cm are primarily coated with sauce (sauce mixture of salt 25%, hot pepper or chilli 50% and seasonings 25%) are allowed to dry in kitchen by hanging on wire for about 24 to 36 hrs. After that meat pieces are exposed to wood smoke and then fried in butter fat and dried again.
Kilishi	Nigeria and West Africa	Lean muscles of beef, goat and lamb	These muscles are dried in sun or tray-drying in a warm air oven. Muscles are trimmed for connective

Contd.

Dried meat product	Countries in which it is popular	Type of meat used	Preparation method and Speciality
			tissue and adhering fats and sliced into a strips of 0.5cm thickness,15 cm length and 6 cm width. These meat strips reduces 40-50% moisture in 2 to 6 hrs then they are infused in defatted wet groundnut cake paste or soybean flour and it is then added with water, garlic, bouillon cubes, salt, pepper, ginger and onion and allowed for sun drying and roasting. When packaged in hermetically sealed, low density plastic bags then they can store for one year.
Biltong	Southern African countries	Meat of beef and antelope, particularly from sirloin strips	Meat strips (1-2 cm thick) are cured in brine for about 12 hrs (sugar, coriander, aniseed, garlic, spices, 0.1 percent potassium sorbate can also be added) and then dipped in a mixture of hot water and vinegar (10:1) and then sun dried for one day. Then strips are shifted in shades for further drying. Some times they smoked (not always). Final biltong is soft inside, moist and red in colour with a hard brown outer layer are most liked by the consumers. In airtight packages the product can store well for more than one year.
Pastirma	Turkey, Egypt and Armenia	Meat of beef and camel	50 to 60 cm long meat strips with less then 5 cm in diameter is rubbed and covered with salt and nitrate. These strips are arranged in piles for 1 m high and kept for one day at room temperature. They are turned, salted and stored in piles for another day. After washing these strips are air-dried for two to three days in summer and for 15 to 20 days in winter. Then again piled up to a height of 30 cm and pressed with heavy weights for 12 hours. For next two to three days the meat pieces are again pressed for 12 hours and air dried for 5 to 10 days. After that entire surface of meat is covered with 3 to 5 mm thick layer of

Contd.

Dried meat product	Countries in which it is popular	Type of meat used	Preparation method and Speciality
			a cemen paste made up of ground garlic and trefoil seed, red paprika, mustard and water. These strips are again stored in piles for one day and then dried for 5 to 12 days in a room with good air ventilation. After that pastirma will be ready for sale.
Charque	Brazil and South American countries	Beef	Large pieces (5 cm thick) are dipped in saturated salt solution for about one hour and then allowed to drain. It can also be salted by dry salting method. Then meat pieces are passed through a pair of wooden rollers or a special press to squeeze out some surplus moisture and flatten the meat slabs. These slabs are then spread out on bamboo slats or loosely woven fibre mats in a shed. For industrial production it can be exposed to the sun on wooden rails. Initial drying directly in the sun (at 40°C) is limited to a maximum period of four to six hours then it is dried in shade or a dim sun light.

Modern ingredients used in meat industry

In modern era when consumers are more concern about their health and quality of meat so the traditional ingredients used in the meat processing is now replacing fully or partially in the products. It is essential to make the daunting demand of today's consumers with the health benefits. There are some ingredients which are now the part of many meat products are listed below with their significance in the meat products:

Category of ingredients	Examples	Functionality	Replacement rate
1. Fat replacers a. Fat mimetic	• Whey, egg proteins based fat mimetic like Simplesse, Dairylo etc.	They are protein and carbohy drates in nature and maintain the physical and sensorial characteristics of triglycerides.	Not able to replace as 1:1of fat but acts as a good source for reduced calorie for products.
b. Fat substitutes	• Oat based mimetic i.e. Qatrim etc. From vegetable oils examples are Olestra, Saltrim, Caprenin etc.	Reduced cholesterol, improves PUFA/SFA and n-6/n-3, prevents saturation of fatty acids and trans fatty acid formation.	Replaced as 1:1 of fat and resembles with triglycerides
2. Dietary fibre enhancer	Oat fibre, sorghum, wheat fibre, carrot, sugarbeet, citrus fibre extract, pea and gram hull, apple pulp, bottle gourd, inulin, chitosan etc.	They are plants and carbohyd rates analogous, not digested by human intestine and produces health benefits. They reduce cooking loss due to high water and fat bindings and helps in improvement of product texture.	Up to 10% of the product formulation.
3. Salt replacers	• Various combinations of sodium chloride, potassium chloride and calcium chloride. • Combination of sodium citrate, corboxy methyl cellulose and carrageenan. • Combination of potassium chloride, tartaric acid, citric acid and sucrose.	Used to replace the sodium in meat products because it is believe that it is harmful to the hearts. But need is to maintain the beneficial effects of salt.	These combinations can be used to replace 40% sodium chloride.

Contd.

Contd.

Category of ingredients	Examples	Functionality	Replacement rate
4. Fatty acid profile replacers	• Linseed oil as a source of linoleic acid and omega -3-fatty acids. • Fish oil as the source of omega-3-fatty acids. • Vegetable oil as a source of CLA.	Used to enhance the amount of beneficial fatty acids in meat based human foods.	-
5. Antioxidants	• Naturally occurring antioxidants like aloevera, mustard, rosemary, sage, fenugreek, soya protein, tea catechins, whey protein concentrates, chitosan, lycopene etc. • Others may be BHA, BHT, TBHQ, PG, Tocopherol, sodium ascorbates etc.		-
6. Enzymes as a texture modifier etc.	• Papain, bromelin, ficin Used to suppress the lipid oxidation in meat products. • Pronase E and fungal extract • Transglutaminase, tyrosinase, laccase etc .	For Protein degradation and tenderization.For flavour and texture enhancer.To enhance the firmness of meat products.	-

Modern Processing Techniques

1. *Preblanding*: Preblanding is a process of mixing and grinding of curing ingredients partly or fully in the ground meat in desired proportion. The basic aim of preblanding is better extraction of meat proteins for stable emulsion preparation, to reduce the chances of oxidation of meat and spoilage. Preblading serves the purpose of compositional analysis of the meat mixture and guide the processor for adjustment of fat contents in products at mixture level. The another greater imporatnce of preblanding is the mixing of ingredients at hot bonned meat level or in the state of prerigor meat which provides better protein extraction and stable emulsion. Preblanding facilitates the mixing of cures in different meat blocks separatly and also helps in least cost formulation. It is prerequisite in preblanding that ingredients should be of sound quality and practices of cleanliness and sanitation must be adopted.

2. *Restructuring*: Meat restructuring technology enables the production of value-added meat products from low quality cuts and trimmings from whole of the carcase. In addition, this technology can improve products characteristics such as texture, fat content, binding strength and shape; meanwhile, it can also satisfy the increasing demand for convenience and variety. The factors affecting the quality of restructured meat products includes appearance, comminution and formation, particle size, mixing time, meat type and fat content. The basic method in this technology are chunking and forming, flaking and forming, tearing and forming. These methods can be used separately or in combination for production of restructured meat.

   Chunking and forming is a process step of restructing meat in which meat is passed through grinder or dicer to make the chunks of size not more than 1.5 inches cubes. Ingredients such as salt, phosphate and seasonings are added to extract the protein and non-meat binders are also used at this stage to bind the meat chunks. These chunks are then mixed or tumbled for forming and then pressed to form meat logs. These logs are then freeze stored till further processing. Restructuring technology conserves the structural and textural properties of natural meat but expose the meat for autooxidation.

Flaking and forming is a process of slicing or flaking of meat log with the help of fine slicer or flaking machine. After that it is treated with salt and phosphate to provide tacky structure to the meat flakes. The next step is tempering of these slices or flakes by putting them into plastic bags under vacuum and stored under frozen condition. The desired configuration then can be achieved by hydraulic pressing. After that it is stored under freezer till further use. This process step of restructuring provides fine and uniform meat for better processing with texturally similar meat to steaks, chops or roast. But the problem of autooxidation and cost involvement is there.

Tearing and forming is not well recognised method due to lack of facilities for tearing the meat fibers. In this process meat has more structural integrity, less membrane damage and less chances of autooxidation. It also provides similar texture of meat as in intact meat cuts.

3. *Sectioning and forming:* Sectioning and forming of meat is a process of making single fused piece of meat from different pieces or chunks of meat. In this process meat pieces or chunks are adhered to make a product with the resemblence of intact cut in its appearnce and consistency. Sectioning and forming of meat facilitates easy slicing, lower cooking losses, readily molding or shaping, lower priced cuts are converted into higher value cuts with uniform colour, curing and have better process control. The drawbacks are involvement of higher cost on equipment and labour and lack of marketability.Proces of sectioning or forming has three main steps such as creation of protein matrix, plibility improvement and shaping of product and stabilization of bond by heating. By this process we can produce the meat products like turkey rolls, sectioned and formed ham, beef roles etc. There are three main steps in sectioning and forming product preparation.

Creation of protein matrix is an important step in production of sectioned and formed meat. Protein matrix is created either by extraction salt soluble proteins (myofibrillar proteins) through tumbling or massaging of meat pieces or chunks or by addition of nonmeat proteins at surface. The nature of protein matrix at surface decides the bond strength on heating. Other factors contributing towards bond strength on heating are fragmentation of fibers, contents of myosin whereas, actin and sarcoplasmic proteins (water soluble proteins) play a minor role in this process. The nonmeat proteins used in creation of protein matrix are egg white, dried egg albumin, dried skim milk, sodium caseinate, soy protein concentrates and isolates etc. These proteins are not capable to produce strong bond as through protein extraction from meat but these are low in price and increses protein in bulk.

Plibility improvement and shaping of product is a second important step in producing sectioned and formed meat. In this process physical manipulation of product is done by tumbling and massaging to make the meat soft and plible. This physical manipulation facilitates easy availability of proteins for shaping the product. The shaping of product is mainly done by pressing the protein matrix in casings or by tying with string and sometimes forcing into metal containers before heating.

Stabilization of bond by heating is a final step in production of sectioned and formed meat. For getting good bond strength in these products it is heated to an internal temperature of 57.2°C to 68.3°C and then cooled properly. Normally at this temperature all major myofibrillar proteins such as myosin and actin are denatured. Sometimes product is smoked alongwith heating for better prduct quality but not always.

Equipments used in sectioning and forming of meat are mainly mixers, tumblers, massagers and ultrasonics. Mixers are simply a machine used for mixing ingredients like salt and polyphosphates in meat. Tumblers are stainless steel drums arranged either in side-loaded impact or multiple batch tumblers. In this equipment meat is drops from apex of the tumbler for pressure and strong blow.

Now a day vacuum processing tumblers are also available. The massagers are slow mixers designed to gently stir or agitate the chunks of meat. Use of low frequency ultrasounds (ultrasonics) in meat causes disruption of meat tissues which leads to softness and pliability of these tissues.

4. *Communition*: Communition is a process of subdividing raw meat into a meat pieces of uniform size. Communition is mainly used for formation of sausages and degree of communition gives variety of products. Coarsely communited meat products are salami, pork sausages and summer sausages while fine sudividing of meat into viscous mass leads to a formation of emulsified sausages such as frankfurters and bologna. The products which are communited but not comes under the category of sausages such as hamburger, ground beef, meat burgers, meat patties etc. Equipments commonly used in communition are meat mincer and bowl chopper.

5. *Emulsification*: Emulsification is a process of mixing of two or more immiscible compounds or materials together by mechanical means. The basic aim of emulsification is to produce meat product with optimum emulsification stability. Meat emulsion is a two phase system, dispersed phase; consisting of either solid or liquid fat particles and the continuous phase having water containing salts and dissolved, gelled and suspended proteins. Thus they can be classified as oil-in-water emulsion. Meat emulsion is not a true emulsion since the two phases involved are not liquids and the fat droplets in a emulsion are larger than 50 μ in diameter. The continuous phase mainly consists of water, water soluble proteins and salt soluble proteins. The dispersed phase or discontinuous phase consists of fat droplets. In this process meat protein is extracted by chopping the meat with salt and ice water. Ice water is used to prevent the rise of temperature during chopping. In chopping and mixing process fat globules are coated with myofibrillar proteins especially myosin. For making good and stable emulsion ingredients used in emulsion making should be of good quality and uniform in size. The formation of fat pockets

should always be avoided. This emulsion can be used in different forms for preparation of different products but most common products are sausages, others are meat balls, meat patties, meat kofta, meat samosa etc.

6. *Meat extension*: To enhance the bulk and reduce the cost of preparation of certain meat products, several types of non-meat ingredients are incorporated. These are generally termed as extenders or binders but less frequently as fillers, emulsifiers or stabilizers. Some of these are having very good functional properties. The permissible amount of these extenders in meat products should not be more than 3.5% as per USDA meat regulations. Besides, lower the cost of formulation and yield of the product, they can also improve meat sliciability, flavour, protein contents as well as emulsion stability and fat binding. For the meat extension starch of potato and flours of wheat, rice, corn, peas etc can be used as filler (for cost reduction), skim milk powder, whey powder and sodium caseinate as a binder while sodium alginate, carrageenan and arabic gum can be used as stabilizers or emulsifiers.

7. *Intermediate moisture meat processing*: Intermediate moisture meat is considered as dry meat with respect to its bacterial spoilage resistance but its moisture content in the range of 20 to 30%. These meat products are relatively soft, easily masticated and moist feeling in mouth but they are microbiologically stable at room temperature even some products are also resistant to mycotic infections. The basic principle behind the production of intermediate moisture meat is reduction in water activity (aw). The examples intermediate moisture meat are country style cured ham, jerky, pepperoni and dry sausages.

8. *Hot processing*: Hot processing of meat is a practice of utilizing meat just after slaughter when it has ATP intact in some extent. It gives better emulsion stability due to better meat protein extraction and save the energy used for chilling the meat. In India, it is a routine practice but it is a new thing for developed countries because they are habitual to process chilled meat for various product preparations.

9. *Hurdle technology*: The term hurdle was coined by Leistner and Rodel in 1976. Hurdle technology is a combined control of certain parameters like chilling, heating, pH, water activity, redox potential, use of preservative and competitive microflora in meat industry. So we can say it is a use of two or more factors for control of microbial growth in the meat and meat products thus helps in extension of products shelf life. In addition, it also improves products texture, taste, juiciness, tenderness and safety. These parameters may be applied at any stage right from animal slaughtering to meat processing and also in final product development. So it is an overall check up system of the industry.

10. *High pressure processing*: The high pressure technology is a recent innovation in meat industry in which high pressure upto 400 MPa is generally applied either in fresh meat after initial treatments or in fully cooked meat products. This treatment enhances solubility of myofibrillar proteins, improves water retention and textural qualities of the products. It is an important technology to produce the healthy and functional meat products. It also acts as a preservative method because high pressure damages the cell membrane of micro-organisms responsible for meat or meat products spoilage and contamination.

11. *High Intensity Pulsed Electric Field*: In this technique high intensity pulsed electric field is applied to cause the disruption and structural changes in cell membrane of the harmful micro-organisms. It is a process of non-thermal inactivation of micro-organisms so it is beneficial process to obtain the good quality meat products. However, the authentication of the process and product quality is needs to be elucidated. The factors decide the effectiveness of the technology is strength and exposure time of electric field, food type, pH, a_W etc.

In connection of above discussion we can say that there are hundreds of processing methods exiting locally in different countries and are more confined to these countries or in the regions of a particular country. For example different states of India are having their particular and popular meat dish with their peculiar recipe and method of formulation. Like

Yakini and Gustaba in Kashmir, Rapka in Arunachal Pradesh, Pork pickle in Himachal Pradesh and Nihari in Delhi.

References

1. Anjaneyulu, A.S.R., Gadekar,Y.P. and Patil, G.S. (2013). Development in ingredient and processing systems for meat products. In: 5th Convention of Indian Meat Science Association and National Symposium on Emerging Technologies Changes to Meet the Demand of Domestic and Export Meat Sector, Feb 7-9: 49-56.
2. Barbut, S. (2004). Other poultry preservation techniques. In: Poultry Meat Processing and Quality by G.C. Mead, Woodhead Publishing Limited (CRC), Cambridge, England. Pp 187-209.
3. Elton D., John A.,C. Forrest, F. E., Gerrard, E. W., Mills H. B., Hedrick M. D., Robert A.J., and Merkel (2009). Principles of Meat Science. In: Wikipedia
4. Forrest, J.C., Aberle, E.D., Hedrick, H.B., Judge, M.D. and Merkel, R.A. (1969). Structure and Composition of Muscle and Associated tissues. In: Principles of Meat Science, W.H. Freeman and Company, San Francisco, pp 27-89.
5. Joint FAO/WHO Food Standards Programme CODEX ALIMENTARIUS COMMISSION Recommended International Code of Hygienic Practice for Low Acid Canned Foods, 1993
6. Pearson, A.M., and Gillett, T.A. (1997). In: Processed Meats. 3rd ed. CBS Publishers & Distributors, New Delhi. Sun X. D. (2009). Utilization of restructuring technology in the production of meat products: a review. Informa World, 7 (2): 153 - 162.
7. Sacharow, S. and Griffin, R.C. (1969). Basic food processes. In: Food Packaging, Richmand Virginea,pp 65-80.
8. Sachdev, A.K., Verma,S.S. and Gopal R. (1998). Technologies for value- added poultry products. Indian Food Industry,17(1): 25-28.
9. Sharma, B.D. (1999). Structure, composition and nutritive value of meat tissues. In: Meat and Meat Products Technology (Including Poultry Products Technology), Jaypee Brothers Medical Publishers (P) Ltd, New Delhi. pp 8-22.

□□□□

9 Packaging of Meat and Meat Products

Food packaging is an essential technique for preserving food quality and minimizing food wastage. It is a scientific technique of containing food against physical, chemical and microbiological contaminants. In addition package also display the product in most appropriate manner and provide product information to the consumers while at the same time allowing convenient handling and efficient distribution. The packaging of meat and meat products are particularly important because meat is highly nutritious food and provides good medium for the growth of micro-organisms. Meat and meat products are also susceptible to bacterial growth due to their high water activity. Exposure of meat and meat products on atmospheric temperature and sunlight leads to various types of deteriorative changes. For example when cut meat surfaces exposed to ambient air provide excellent breeding grounds for most bacteria. Minced meat is even more at risk due to the large exposed surface area. Packaging provides protection of food against external and internal factors but once food gets deteriorated it can not be controlled by packaging. For this reason rigorous hygiene in all processing and pre-packaging steps is vital for packaging of perishable food items like meat and meat products.

Functions of Package

For the quality preservation and protection of meat and meat products good quality package has great importance. These package may be classified into primary package (main package that holds the food that is being processed), secondary package (which combines the primary packages into one box) and tertiary packaging (which combines all of the secondary packages into one pallet). The package used for meat and meat products packaging provides following functions:

1. *Physical protection*: Package provides protection of meat and meat products against physical forces like shock, vibration, compression, temperature etc.
2. *Barrier protection*: Package provides barrier to meat and meat products against light, oxygen, water vapour, undesired gases, dust, dirt, vermin etc.
3. *Contaminants protection*: Package gives protection to the food products against external contaminants such as microbes etc.
4. *Information transmission*: Package and label communicate about product use, their mode of transport, storage, disposal of package etc. It also provides information about ingredients used, their quantity, batch number, date of expiry, price etc.
5. *Marketing*: Package provides convenient means for dispatching the product in desired quantities whether bulk or retail. It's labelling and decoration on exterior makes products attractive and appealing to the consumers.
6. *Security*: Package provides security risk during transportation or shipment. It also protects the food product against pilferage losses, thefts and tempering. Authentication and other security measures can easily be adopted through package.
7. *Convenience:* Packages provides convenience in distribution, handling, stacking, display, sale, opening, reclosing, use and reuse.
8. *Portion control:* Single serving packages serves precise amount of contents for control usage. Bulk commodities can be divided into packages that are more suitable size for individual households.

Packaging Materials

A wide variety of polymers and materials are used in production of package. Among them plastic packaging materials are more common. Selection of packaging materials for a particular food depends not only on its technical suitability (i.e. how well the package protects a food for the required shelf life), but also on the availability and cost in a particular area and any marketing considerations that favour choosing a certain type of package.These packaging materials are broadly classified into traditional packaging materials and modern packaging materials. The modern packaging materials are again classified into cellulose, metal, glass, plastics and mixed materials.

Traditional Packaging Materials

These materials have been used since the earliest time for domestic storage and local sale of foods. However, with the exception of glazed pottery, they have poor barrier properties and are only used to contain foods and keep them clean. They are also unsuited to the needs of commercial production processes and are considered by many customers to be less attractive than the newer 'industrial' materials described below. The main types of traditional materials are leaves, vegetable fibers, textiles, wood, leather and pottery. Leaves are cheap and readily available and are used as wrappers for products such as cooked foods. For this purpose Banana or plantain leaves were using since ancient time. Other leaves which can be used are maize leaves, pan leaves, green coconut palm, papyrus leaves and bamboo leaves. Rattan fibres was also using for carrying meat in many parts of the world. Fibres from kenaf and sisal plants can be used to make net bags to transport the food. The examples of textile containers are woven jute sacks which are used to transport a wide variety of bulk foods including grain, flour, sugar and salt. Plant fibre sacks are flexible, lightweight and resistant to tearing. They have good durability and may be chemically treated to prevent them from rotting. Muslin and cheesecloth are open-mesh and can be used for packaging of processed meat like smoked ham etc. Wooden containers protect foods against crushing, have good stacking characteristics and a good weight-to-strength ratio. Wooden boxes, trays and crates have traditionally been used as shipping containers for a wide variety of solid foods. Leather containers made from camel, pig or kid goat hides have traditionally been used as flexible, lightweight, non-breakable containers for water, milk and wine. Pottery is still used domestically for storage of liquid and solid foods such as yoghurt, beer, dried foods, honey, etc. If they are glazed and well sealed they prevent oxygen, moisture and light from entering the food and they are therefore suitable for storing oils and wines. They also restrict contamination by micro-organisms, insects and rodents. Glass or plastic containers have largely replaced pottery because of its high weight, fragility, variability in volume when hand-made, and the difficulty of adequately cleaning pottery containers for re-use.

Modern Packaging Materials or Industrial Materials

These materials have been developed over the last 200-300 years and are the main types of packaging used by small-scale food processors. The availability of glass, metal or plastic containers varies considerably in different countries, and this, together with the relative cost of different materials, determines their uptake by local processing industries. Where these materials have to be imported, large minimum order sizes can be a significant constraint on the development of a processing sector.

A. Cellulose, Paper and Cardboard Package

Plain cellulose is a glossy transparent film which is odourless, tasteless and biodegradable. It is tough and puncture resistant, although it tears easily. However, it is not heat sealable and the dimensions and permeability of the film vary with changes in humidity. It is used for foods that do not require a complete moisture or gas barrier.

Among the paper and cardboard, moulded paperboard trays are used for packaging of eggs, meat or fish. Corrugated cartons are used as shipping containers for bottled, canned or plastic-packaged foods. Wet foods may be packed by lining the corrugated board with polyethylene or a laminate of wax-coated greaseproof paper and polyethylene these materials are used for chilled bulk meat, dairy products and frozen foods.

A natural polymer of cellulose known as cellophane is widely used for packaging of fresh meat when it is coated with nitrocellulose on one side.In this process uncoated side remains in contact of meat. These films are cheap, good in mechanibility and dimensional stability.

B. Metal Containers

There are two basic types of metal cans: those that are sealed using a 'double seam' and are used to make canned foods and those that have push-on lids or screw-caps that are used to pack dried foods. Double-seamed cans are made from tinplated steel or aluminium and are lined with specific lacquers for different types of food.

Metal Cans: Metal cans are mainly used for canning the meat products. They have a number of advantages over other types of container. As on sealing they provide total protection of the contents. In addition they are tamperproof, provides wide range of shapes and sizes and are convenient at ambient storage and presentation. However, the high cost of metal and the high manufacturing costs make cans expensive compared to other containers. They are heavier than plastic containers and therefore have higher transport costs.

Aluminium: Other types of metal containers include aluminium foil cups and trays, laminated foil pouches as alternatives to cans or jars, collapsible aluminium tubes for pastes and aluminium barrels. Aluminium foil is commonly known as 'Alu foil'. The thickness of 0.025 mm to 0.15 mm is generally used for the packaging of food products.The advantages of aluminium are that it is impermeable to moisture, odours, light and micro-organisms, and is an excellent barrier to gases. It has a good weight-strength ratio and a high quality surface for decorating or printing. They can easily recycle.

Steel: Steel is a widely used packaging material for food, paint and beverage as well as aerosols. Recycling steel brings significant resource and energy savings. The current recycling rate for steel cans is 62%.

C. Glass

The use of glass jars are only limited to meat pickle. Although, glass bottles and jars have some of the advantages over metal cans and packages. As they are impervious to micro-organisms, pests, moisture, oxygen and odours. They do not react foods or have chemicals that migrate into foods and can be heat processed, recyclable and re-useable, rigid and are suitable for stacking without damage. Unlike metal cans they are transparent to display the contents.

The main disadvantages of glass are the higher weight than most other types of packaging which incurs higher transport costs. Additionally containers are easily broken, especially when transported over rough roads. They have more variable dimensions than metal or plastic containers and have potentially serious hazards from glass splinters or fragments that can contaminate foods.

D. Plastic

Plastic is widely used packaging material due to its several advantages over other packaging materials like sturdiness and low weight.

i. *Polyethylene:* Polyethylene is most widely used flexible packaging material. It is cheap, easily available and can carry anywhere but it is non biodegradable.

   Low-density polyethylene (LDPE): LDPE is prepared by exposing ethyline to a very high pressure (1200 atmospheric pressure) and temperature range of about 150-200°C. Normally LDPE of 0.91-0.925 density is used for food packaging. It is heat sealable, inert, odour free and shrinks when heated. It is a good moisture barrier but has relatively high gas permeability, sensitivity to oils and poor odour resistance. It is more flexible and less expensive than most films and is therefore widely used. LDPE is also used for shrink or stretch-wrapping. Stretch-wrapping uses thinner LDPE (25-38 mm) than shrink-wrapping (45-75 mm) or alternatively, linear low-density polyethylene is used at thicknesses of 17-24 mm. The cling properties of both LDPE and HDPE are adjusted to increase adhesion between layers of the film and to reduce adhesion between adjacent packages.

   High-density polyethylene (HDPE): HDPE is stronger, thicker, less flexible and more brittle than low-density polyethylene and has lower permeability to gases and moisture. It is produced at 40 psi atmospheric pressure and 60-150°C temperature. Normally 0.941 to 0.965 density HDPE is used. It has higher softening temperature (121°C) and can therefore be heat sterilised. Sacks made from 0.03-0.15 mm high-density polyethylene has a high tear strength, penetration resistance and seal strength. They are waterproof and chemically resistant and are used instead of paper sacks.

ii. *Polypropylene (PP):* Polypropylene is a clear glossy film with a high strength and is puncture resistance. It is prepared by polymerization of propylene and has resistance against oil and grease. It has moderate permeability to moisture, gases and odours which is not affected by changes in humidity. Its stretching ability is although less than polyethylene. Its applicability is almost same as LDPE. Oriented polypropylene is a clear glossy film with good optical properties and a high tensile strength and puncture resistance. It has moderate permeability to gases, odours and a good barrier to water vapour and it is not affected by changes in humidity. It is widely used to pack snackfoods and dried foods.

iii. *Polyvenyl chloride (PVC):* PVC is generally produced by polymerization of venyl chloride in the presence of suitable catalase. The common use of PVC is in pickle packaging.

iv. *Polyvinylidene chloride (PVDC):* PVDC is very strong and is therefore used in thin films. It has very low gas and water vapour permeability and is heat shrinkable and heat sealable. However, it has a brown tint which limits its use in some applications.

v. *Nylon or polyamides*: These are clear films with good mechanical properties. These are heat resistant and suitable in a wide temperature range (from 60 to 200°C). However, the films are expensive to produce and require high temperatures to form a heat seal. These films have low permeability to gases and are greaseproof and permeability changes at different storage humidities. They are used with other polymers to make them heat sealable at lower temperatures and to improve the barrier properties and are used to pack meats. Nylon 6, 11 and 12 are used for packaging of fresh and processed (bacon) meat.

vi. *Polyester*: Polyester is a condensation product of polyalcohol with diacids. It is unbreakable, very light in weight and is excellent gas barrier.

vii. Polystyrene is a brittle clear sparkling film which has high gas permeability.

E. Mixed Materials or Films

Package made with mixed materials serves the specific functions and are more energy efficient than single material packaging. But it creates difficulty in recycling because it is hindered by the lack of facilities and technology necessary to separate materials and to avoid contamination. Mixed materials packaging can be reprocessed into other products such as floor coverings, shoe soles and car mats, incinerated to produce energy, or landfilled.

i. Flexible plastic films

Flexible plastic films have relatively low cost and good moisture and gases barrier. They are heat sealable to prevent leakage of contents. These films are light in weight and fit closely to the shape of the food, thereby wasting little space during storage and distribution. These films have good wet and dry strength and are easy to handle and convenient for the manufacturer, retailer and consumer. The main disadvantages of these films are its production from non-renewable oil reserves and non biodegradability. For this purpose 'bioplastics' are used which are derived from renewable sources and are biodegradable. However, these materials are not yet available commercially in developing countries.

There are very wide range of plastic films which are produced from different types of plastic polymers. Each one has their specific range of mechanical, optical, thermal and moisture/gas barrier properties. These are produced by variations in film thickness and the amount and type of additives that are used in their production. Some films like polyester, polyethylene, polypropylene may be oriented by stretching the material to align the molecules in either one direction (uniaxial orientation) or two (biaxial orientation) to increase their strength, clarity, flexibility and moisture/gas barrier properties.

ii. Coated films

Coated films are those which are coated with other polymers or aluminium to improve the barrier properties or to impart heat sealability. For example, nitrocellulose is coated on one side of cellulose film to provide a moisture barrier but to retain oxygen permeability. A nitrocellulose coating on both sides of the film improves the barrier to oxygen, moisture and odours and enables the film to be heat sealed when broad seals are used. A coating of vinyl chloride or vinyl acetate gives a stiffer film which has intermediate permeability. Sleeves of this material are tough, stretchable and permeable to air, smoke and moisture. These films are used for packaging meats before smoking and cooking. Packs made from cellulose that has a coating of vinyl acetate are tough, stretchable and permeable to air, smoke and moisture. A thin coating of aluminium is termed as metallisation and produces a very good barrier to oils, gases, moisture, odours and light. This metallised film is less expensive and more flexible than plastic/aluminium foil laminates.

iii. Laminated films

Lamination of two or more films improves the appearance, barrier properties or mechanical strength of a package. The examples of some laminated films are given in table:

Laminated film	Typical food applications
Polyvinylidene chloride coated polypropylene (two layered)	Crisps, snack foods, confectionery, ice cream, biscuits, chocolate
Polyvinylidene chloride coated polypropylene-polyethylene	Bakery products, cheeses, confectionery, dried fruit, frozen vegetables
Cellulose-polyethylene-cellulose	Pies, crusty bread, bacon, coffee, cooked meats, cheeses
Cellulose acetate-paper-foil-polyethylene	Dried soups
Metallised polyester-polyethylene	Coffee, dried milk
Polyethylene-aluminium-paper	Dried soup, dried vegetables, chocolate

iv. Coextruded films

Coextruded films are produced from simultaneous extrusion of two or more layers of different polymers. These films have threefold advantage over other films such as very high barrier properties (similar to laminates) but produced at a lower cost (thinner than laminates) and are therefore easier to use on filling equipment. These layers of coextruded films do not separate. For the manufacture of these films mainly three groups of polymers are coextruded such as low-density and high-density polyethylene, polypropylene, polystyrene, acrylonitrile-butadiene-styrene and polyvinyl chloride. In three layered coextrusion films, outside layer has a high gloss and printability, middle bulk layer provides stiffness and strength and an inner layer is suitable for heat sealing. These films are used for packaging of confectionery, snack-foods, cereals and dried foods. For thicker coextrusions (75-3000 μm), pots, tubs or trays are used.

F. Biobased Packaging Materials

These are recent developments in packaging industry. As per the definition "Biobased food packaging materials are materials derived from renewable sources. These materials can be used for food applications". Biobased polymers may be divided into three main categories based on their origin and production:

1. Polymers directly extracted/removed from biomass. Examples are polysaccharides such as starch and cellulose and proteins like casein and gluten.
2. Polymers produced by classical chemical synthesis using renewable biobased monomers. A good example is polylactic acid, a biopolyester polymerised from lactic acid monomers. The monomers themselves may be produced via fermentation of carbohydrate feedstock.
3. Polymers produced by microorganisms or genetically modified bacteria. To date, this group of biobased polymers consists mainly of the polyhydroxyalkonoates but developments with bacterial cellulose are in progress.

Fresh Meat Packaging

Package for fresh meat packaging should be permeable to oxygen for the development of meat bloom. The package should also have the capability to prevent moisture loss during storage, prevents microbial contaimination, prevent meat from pick up of foreign odour and to prevent lipid oxidation.

Techniques used in Fresh Meat Packaging

i. *Overwrap packaging*: For packaging of primal and subprimal cuts of fresh meat thermoplastic films with good optical properties are used. The packaging materials commonly used is LDPE of 100 gauge and other options for packaging are rubber hydrochloride, 6, 11 nylon, highly plasticized PVC films of 70 gauge etc. Cellophane coated with nitrocellulose on one side is also a good option but meat should be kept in contact of uncoated side. Cellophane coated with PE provides good option for irregular cuts of fresh meat. In this method cuts are overwraped with these packaging films to protect it from moisture losses.

ii. *Tray with overwrap packaging*: This type of packaging includes a polystyrene foam or clearplastic tray which is sized for receiving a piece of fresh meat of predetermined cut. The tray is then overwrapped with a web of clear plastic wrapping material like thermoplastic film. The overwrapped tray is ventilated to ensure gas communication between enclosed regions of the overwrapped tray and the outside ambient without blockage due to run off juices from the meat product or shifting of the meat product within the tray during transport. For soaking of meat juice absorbant cotton can be used. A number of similarly ventilated overwrapped trays are then placed within an outer barrier bag which is first evacuated at normal atmosphere and then flushed with a preservation-enhancing gas. The outer barrier bag is then sealed. Upon opening of the outer barrier bag, exposure to oxygen causes the packaged meat products to bloom to a desired fiery red color. Upon removal from the outer barrier bag, the ventilated overwrapped trays are ready for retail case-ready display without the need for repackaging or cosmetic repair. Fresh meat can be stored for about a week under refrigeration.

iii. *Shrink film overwrap packaging*: Shrink film overwrap is commonly used for wrapping of large and uneven cuts of fresh meat. These films are having qualities of holding in streching condition at normal ambient temperature and gives good shrink on heating. These are suitable materials in carcase packaging for forzen storage. These films have good water vapour barrier, high structural strength, neat appearance, capacity for contour tight packaging etc. Packaging materials most preferably used are PP, PE and PVDC. It is suitable packaging method for giving appearance same as the cut packaged in it.

iv. *Vacuum packaging*: It is a technique used for long term storage of primal and sub primal cuts of beef and cara beef. In this technique meat cuts are placed in a gas-impermeable form of plastic like Alu foil/ PE, nylon/ PE, polyester /PE or PVDC/ polyester/ PE laminated bags at 2-4°C and a pH of 5.5 to 5.8. Vacuum packaging provides shelf life of most of the meat products for more than 2 to 3 months at refrigeration temperature except lamb and pork. The shelf life of lamb is about 21 days and pork is about 15 days. The reason of lower shelf life of lamb meat might be due to higher pH and in pork due to higher initial microbial load. For vacuum packaging mainly two methods are adopted. One is cryovac method, in which air is sucked out and then passed through either a waterdip or hot air tunnel. Second is drawing a vacuum without heat shrinkage. Among them, cryovac technique is better due to less drip production, oxygen cunsumption by tissues , accumulation of CO_2. In this technique vacuum is created inside the package which inhibit the microbial growth in the product. Draw back of this system is development of bluish colour during storage though it subside on reexposure on air and again produces normal red colour.

v. *Modified atmosphere packaging*: It is also known as Equilibrium modified atmosphere packaging (EMAP) or Modified atmosphere/ modified humidity packaging. It is a technique of modifying the composition of internal atmosphere of package in order to improve the product shelf life without interfering product colour, flavour and other quality and quantity parameters. It is done by using the gases alone or in mixture of gases usually oxygen, carbon dioxide,carbon monooxide and nitrogen. In other meats replacement of oxygen from 20% to 0% is desirable. It is replaced with nitrogen because it is a inert gas. It can also be replaced with CO_2 which can lower the pH or inhibit the growth of bacteria. CO can be used for keeping the red color of meat. In this packaging technique different meats have different requirements like red meat requires oxygen for oxidation of the myoglobin. To preserve the red colour of the meat (beef and buffalo meat), package should have high concentrations of oxygen (60% - 80%). Pork requires less oxygen due to high fat content. With the right mixtures, the shelf-life of consumer-packaged meats can be extended from 2-4 days to 5-8 days at +4°C. If master packs are used in distribution, high carbon dioxide levels can be used to increase shelf-life. Poultry is very susceptible to bacterial spoilage, evaporation loss, off-odour, discolouration and biochemical deterioration. The sterile poultry tissue becomes contaminated during the evisceration process. The practical shelf-life of gas-packed poultry is somewhere between 16 and 21 days. The spoilage of raw poultry is mainly caused by microbial growth, fuelled by the *Pseudomonas* and *Achromobacter* genera in particular. These aerobic bacteria are effectively inhibited by carbon dioxide in MAP. Levels of carbon dioxide in excess of 20% are required to significantly extend the shelf-life of poultry.

To avoid problems associated with collapsed packaging and excessive dripping with raw poultry, the gas/product ratio should be increased if higher levels of carbon dioxide are used. Where package collapse is not an issue (e.g. bulk or master bags), 100% carbon dioxide is recommended. In both retail and bulk modified atmosphere packs, nitrogen is used as an inert filler gas.

There are two techniques used in the industry to pack vegetables namely gas flushing and compensated vacuum or passively by designing "breathable" films known as equilibrium modified atmosphere packaging (EMAP). For its cheapness the gas-flushing is more widely used. In gas-flushing the package is flushed with a desired gas mixture, as in compensated vacuum the air is removed totally and the desired gas mixture then inserted.

Traditionally used packaging films like LDPE, PVC, EVA (ethylene-vinyl acetate) and OPP (oriented polypropylene) are not permeable enough for highly respiring products like fresh-cut produces. The films called barrier films are designed to prevent the exchange of gases and are mainly used with non-respiring products like meat and fish.

Frozen Meat Packaging

For the packaging of frozen meats like frozen pork chops, solid block of frozen turkey, frozen ground beef etc. LDPE of 0.035 to 0.05 mm thickness, moisture proof cellophane, PE coated polyester and polyamide coated PE and heat shrinkable films are most widely used. These packaging materials protect frozen meat texture and flavour. Frozen meat also requires protection from moisture vapour and oxygen transmission to avoid freezer burn. In addition, package should also have good durability at freezer temperature. It should have very high wet strength and should be impermeable to odour and flavour.

Cured Meat Packaging

Cured meat products such as ham, bacon, luncheon meat, frankfurters etc. require proper packaging to prevent deterioration of meat. The package used for these meat products should be able to prevent further growth of bacteria, yeast, moulds etc. These packages should be of good oxygen and water vapour barrier and should be capable of lamination or coextrision and hermetically sealing. Package should also be capable from protecting the product against light and grease. There are various methods for cured meat packaging, some of them are summarized as:

1. One of the most suitable method is *overwrapping* in PE films, PVC, PVDC and rubber hydrochloride.
2. Another method is the use of *laminates* such as cellophane/ PE and aluminium foil/paper laminate.
3. *Shrink packaging:* It is most suitable method for packaging of ham and other large uneven cuts of cured meat. The packages used are polyester/PVDC/PE copolymers etc.
4. *Vacuum and gas packaging*: These are the choice methods for long term storage of sliced bacon, luncheon meat etc. The packages generally used are laminated pouches of polyester/PVDC/PE or polyamide/ PVDC/ PE or metabolised polyamides/ ethylene venyl lactate etc.

The method of choice for cured meat packaging is vacuum packaging at commercial level. When Vacuum packaging combined with refrigeration, it produces great impact of prolonging the shelf. By this method we can slow down the bacterial growth in cooked meat and also reduced its decay. By removing the surrounding air around the cooked meat helps in slow down and in some cases prevent the spread of bacteria that require oxygen to grow and multiply which are ultimately spoils food. In addition, it prevents evaporation and possible contamination from other products. However, it is not a substitute of refrigeration but can be combined with refrigeration to greatly increase the shelf life of most products. The main requirement of cured meat packaging is its protection against evaporation losses or to prevent meat from becoming tough and dry.

Pre-cooked Frozen Meat Products Packaging

The packaging of precooked frozen meat products such as meat stews, roast, boiled sliced meat, hamburger, hot dog etc. requires special packaging to conserve their quality during storage. The requirements for these products includes protection from moisture loss and excessive air exposure. For this purpose package should be capable to withstand on boiling for about 20 minutes and it should also be good in sealability. There are various methods for packaging of precooked frozen meat products but some of them are as under:

1. *Use of boilable bags*: These bags are made up of polyester/ medium density polyethylene laminates. These are ideal packaging materials for meat stews, roast and boiled sliced meats.
2. *HDPE laminates*: For short term storage of precooked frozen meat products HDPE can also be used.
3. *Glassine bags*: These are the suitable packaging materials for hamburgers, hot dog. These bags can withstand and can be used in microwave heating of the products.
4. *Stout bags*: These bags are made up of Kraft and PE laminates and can serves the purpose of master container for packaging of all these products.

Packaging of Dehydrated Meat Products

Packaging of dehydrated meat products requires protection from oxidation and rancidity, light and foreign odour contamination and package should be impermeable to moisture and oxygen. There are number of packaging techniques are in use some of these are:

1. *Metal foil plastic laminates:* These packaging materials are widely used for dehydrated meat products packaging.
2. Outer paper/Alu foil/PE laminate and inner cellophane wrap can be used for compressed bars of dehydrated minced meat.
3. *Vacuum packaging technique:* It is a best packaging technique for dehydrated meat products. In this technique vacuum is sealed in PE coated polyesters.

Dried or dehydrated meats like biltong and beef jerky need a package which may not absorb ambient moisture because this extra moisture is responsible for spoiling the original characteristics of these meats. Many other meat products like pork pies, scotch eggs and cooked sausages may be stored for a longer period of time under vacuum. The principle behind vacuum packaging is quite simple i.e. by removing the oxygen to prevent and slowdown the growth of bacteria which intern brakes down enzymes and ultimately spoils the food. In this technique contamination from other food products is eliminated and in some cases smell is contained.

Recent innovations in packaging of meat and meat products including aquatic foods

1. *Active packaging:* Active packaging is a type of packaging which can change the atmosphere of the package to enhance the shelf life of the product without compromising the product quality. The active packages may serve the purposes of oxygen absorber as well as the absorbers of moisture, carbon dioxide, flavour/odour etc. Active packaging is also capable to release the carbon dioxide, ethylene antimicrobials, off flavours, antioxidants etc. These agents are adhered with the package which serves the purpose when required by the foods. The active ingredients which serves various functions in this package may be summarized as:

S. No.	Active function	Name of the ingredient that play the active role	Purpose
1.	Oxygen scavengers	Iron powder oxidation, ascorbic acid oxidation, photosensitive dye oxidation, enzymatic oxidation (glucose oxidase and alcohol oxidase), unsaturated fatty acids (oleic or linoleic acid), rice extract, immobilized yeast etc.	To absorb the residual oxygen which is essential maintain the quality of oxygen sensitive foods like pork and poultry products
2.	Carbon dioxide scavengers and emitters	These packages serve purpose of both CO_2 scavengers and emitters. These sachets may contain calcium hydroxide and sodium hydroxide or potassium hydroxide, calcium oxide, silica gel etc.	To maintain and enhance the organoleptic quality of carbon dioxide loving foods such as aquatic foods, fresh and processed meat products. It may also serve the purpose of bacteriostate.
3.	Moisture absorbers	The moisture absorbers may contain super absorbent polymer placed in-between two layers of polyvinyl acetate blanket.	To absorb the moisture and reduce the water activity. Thus reduce the microbial growth.
4.	Chlorine dioxide generators	Microsphere powder is able to release chlorine dioxide (1-100 ppm) for a day to 6 weeks.	To act against the broad spectrum micro-organisms and spores.
5.	Antimicrobial agents in package	Acid anhydrate, bacteriocins, enzymes, alcohols, organic acids, polysaccharides, cheleters etc.	These agents are used to extend the lag phase and retard the log phase of microbial growth to enhance the shelf life.

6.	Flavour/odour absorbers	Cellulose triacetate, citric acid, activated carbon etc.	Used to remove the undesired odour of fish and poultry products.

2. *Intelligent packaging*: Intelligent packaging is also known as smart packaging because it tells about the changes in the products quality, chemical nature and microbial deterioration etc through the changes in the indicators, sensors, tags etc. These indicators include time –temperature indicators, ripeness indicators, toxin indicators, biosensors, radio frequency identifications etc. The identification marks which tells about the product change well in time may be classified as given in next table.

3 *Edible and bio-based packaging*: Edible packaging material is an integral part of the food and placed on or between the foods and eaten alongwih the food. Now biodegradable biopolymers are used to make the edible coating. However, certain qualities are required for edible packaging like acceptability in terms of colour, flavour, taste and texture. The materials used for edible packaging must be generally recognized as safe (GRAS). In addition they must have the optical property, mechanical property as well as anti-browning and antibacterial properties.

S.No.	Name of identification mark	Type of identification mark	Purpose	Examples
1.	Indicators	Time-temperature indicators	These indicators are visual colour changers or radio frequency identification tags.	They are basically based on enzymatic reactions, polymerization, chemical diffusion etc.
		Freshness indicators	They perceive the indication of metabolites generation by microbial or chemical changes takes place in the food.	They may be classified as: a. Organic acids: n-butyrate, L-lactic acid, D-lactate, acetic acid etc. b. Biogenic amines: histamine, tyramine, putrescine, cadaverine etc. c. Carbon dioxide, hydrogen sulphides are indicative of spoilage and offflavour.
2.	Sensors	Gas sensors	They indicate the change through gas production in foods through the generation of translucent materials.	Amperometric oxygen sensors, organic conducting polymers, potentiometric carbon dioxide sensors, metal oxide semiconductor field effect transistors, piezoelectric crystal sensors etc.

Contd.

Contd.

S.No.	Name of identification mark	Type of identification mark	Purpose	Examples
		Oxygen sensors based on flouroscence	The oxygen level in the head space of package is measured and higher level can be monitored by the sensors.	It generally consists of long delay fluorescent or phosphorescent dye encapsulated in a solid polymer matrix.
		Biosensors	It is mainly based on the pathogen detection principle and related to the food safety.	Toxin Guard and Food sentinel system.
3.	Radio-frequency identification tags	Tag system	It works on the radio frequency waves passed through material to microchips and changes can be monitored on the computer monitor.	Radio-frequency identification tags containing minuscule microchips.

Biomolecules used in edible packaging

Biomolecules	Examples	Functions
Polysaccharides	Starch and its derivatives, cellulose derivatives, alginates, carrageenan, plant and microbial gums, chitosan, pectinates, red sea weed agar	They are biodegradable, edible and hydrophilic in nature and acts as good barrier to carbon dioxide and oxygen but poor barrier to water vapour. Some bio-molecules such as agar can easily be used with antibiotics and bcateriocins nisin in meat and fish products.
Lipids	Paraffin wax	They are hydrophobic in nature so generally used with polysaccharides to reduce hydrophilicity and water vapour barrier property. Antibiotics, antifungal, antioxidants etc. can easily be incorporated in these bio-molecules for meat and fish products.
Proteins	Collagen, edible gelatin, corn zein, cotton seed, egg white, wheat gluten, pea protein, soya protein, fish myofibrillar proteins, chitosan, casein, whey protein etc.	They must be insoluble on heating to maintain film and food integrity, protein must have cross links, some materials provides colourless, odourless and flavourless coating to the foods such as whey protein.
Composite film	Gelatinized starch/hydrophobic co-polymer/polyethylene or improved starch alongwith pectin film is recommended for red meat packaging	They must have the properties of all bio-molecules like lipid layer exert moisture barrier property, protein layer provide structural matrix and polysaccharides provides good Co_2 and O_2 barriers.

Packaging is a scientific and smart approach to protect, preserve, conserve, transport, display and to make meat products salable and marketable. It is not only important to all above reasons but also provides comfort and choice to the consumers to bye particular type of product. Various types of products require different types of package and also needs different types of techniques. Some package provides us food as fresh as naturally fresh and as nutritious as natural. The recent innovations in the field of packaging provide the biodegradability, selectivity, edibility, sensibility etc alongwith the traditional functions of packages.

References

1. Battcock, M., Azam-Ali, S., Axtell, B. and Fellows, P. (1998). Training in Food Proessing: Successful Approach. IT Publication.
2. Church, I.J. and Parsons, A.L. (1995). Modified Atmosphere Packaging Technology: A Review, Journal of Food Science & Agriculture, 67:143-152.
3. Day, B.P.F. (1996). A perspective of modified atmosphere packaging of fresh produce In Western Europe, Food Science and Technology Today, 4:215-221.
4. Fellows, P., Franco, E. and Rios, W. (1996). Starting a small food processing Enterprise. IT Publications/ACP-EU.
5. Fellows P., Hampton, A. (1992).Small Scale Food Processing: A Guide to Appropriate Equipment. IT Publications/ CTA.
6. Parry, R.T. (1993). Principles and applications of MAP of foods. Blackie Academic & Professional, England, 1-132.
7. Peter Fellows, P. and Axtell, B. (1993). Appropriate Food Packaging. ILO/TOOL.
8. Phillips, C.A. (1996). Review: Modified Atmosphere Packaging and its effects on the microbial quality and safety of produce, International Journal of Food Science and Tech, 31: 463-479.
9. Sharma, B.D. and Kumar, R. R. (2013). Optimizing shelf life of meat and meat products using innovative packaging solutions. In: 5th convention of Indian Meat Science Association and National Symposium on Emerging Technologies Changes to Meet the Demand of Domestic and Export Meat Sector, Feb 7-9: 59-71.
10. Singh, V.P. (2008). Ageing of meat. In: Manual of Meat and Meat Products Technology (including poultry products technology), DUVASU, Mathura.
11. Zagory, D. & Kader, A.A. (1988). Modified atmosphere packaging of fresh produce, Food Technology, 42(9):70-77.

□□□□

10 Formulation and Development of Meat and Sea Foods

Formulation of meat and sea food products requires various ingredients which are commonly known as food additives. Food additives are those non-meat ingredients which are used to enhance colour, flavour, aroma and texture of the meat and sea food products. These food products can fulfil the demand of modern consumers. As per the definition of Food and Drug Administration (FDA) food additives are those substance which are used to provide a technical effect in foods. The use of food additives has become more prominent in recent years, due to the increased production of prepared, processed, and convenience foods. Additives are used for flavour and appeal, food preparation and processing, freshness, and safety. These additives can be classified as curing ingredients, extenders and binders, flavour enhancers and other additives. For the formulation of different products both raw materials and ingredients should be of food grade and sound hygienic strength. In the starting of this chapter we will discuss about ingredients used then the specific formulations will be discussed for better understanding of meat and sea food processing.

Curing Ingredients

Curing agents such as salt, phosphate, sugars, nitrite and nitrate, sodium ascorbate and erythorbate etc. have traditionally been used in various meat formulations from long back. The details of these ingredients have already been discussed in chapter-8 of this book. So we will try to discuss other ingredients which are relevant for meat and sea food products other than these ingredients. Cure accelerators such as ascorbates and erythorbates are used to speed the curing process. They also stabilize the colour of the final product. The examples are ascorbic acid, erythorbic acid, sodium erythorbate, citric acid, sodium citrate, sodium acid pyrophosphate, glucono delta lactone (GDL) etc. Glucono-delta-lactone (GDL) acts as a curing accelerator in meat and meat products. It is permissible up to 1% in sausages and up to this level it lowers the pH about 0.5 thus inhibits the growth of spoilage micro-organisms. GDL also facilitate the cured colour development.

Binders and Extenders

A number of non-meat ingredients are used in meat and sea foods to provide variety in the products and lower the cost of meat and sea food products are termed as binders and extenders. These ingredients are also used to enhance product yield, flavour, sliciability and protein contents improvement alongwith emulsion stability, fat and water binding in the emulsion. Number of ingredients comes under this category such as flours and starches, non-meat proteins, colloid and gums etc. These binders and extenders are further can be classified into various categories i.e. fillers, binders, emulsifiers or stabilizers based on its purpose of use in meat products.

1. *Fillers*: Fillers are mainly used in meat products to reduce the cost of formulations. The examples are mainly flours of wheat, rice, pea, corn and starches of soya and potato. Starches are long chains of glucose molecules which hold water. Most unmodified starches needs heat to become thick however, some modified and natural starches may become thick at room temperature. These products work well in marinates to help in coating of the products. Starches are not however, allowed in hams or roast beef but can be used in non-standard products. Starches are allowed in cured pork products at a level not to exceed 2%. It is also noticeable point that starches can not be used in conjunction with any other binder. The flours are mainly made up of cereal grains rich in carbohydrates and can not ferment without enzymatic action. By the addition of water these flours becomes sticky and facilitates

the adhering of meat particles with each other. Flours can be utilized in variety of meat products but the most wide use is in low fat ground beef.

2. *Binders*: Binders are mostly non-meat proteins used for proper binding of the meat ingredients for better emulsion stability. The examples are soy proteins, milk proteins, yeast proteins and egg proteins. Soy proteins and deheated mustard flour are used as protein sources to allow for further extension and as binders for added water. Protein binders cannot be used in products called ham but are allowed in highly extended ham loaves or poultry rolls. The typical usage level is between 0.5% and 5.0%. Levels used depend on the protein form whether isolate or flour. For example soy isolate can bind between seven and ten times its weight in water while soy concentrate binds less water (approximately five times its weight) and imparted more beany flavour.

   Soy proteins are relatively low in cost and have excellent power to maintain traditional product characteristics. But the use of higher level of soy proteins gives poor taste and texture otherwise it imparts good flavour and texture. Actually soy proteins cover a wide range of products derived from the soybean such as soy flours, soy protein concentrates or isolated soy proteins.

Composition of Soy Protein Products

Soy protein type	Protein (%)	Carbohydrates (%)
Soy Flour	50	38
Soy Protein Concentrate	70	24
Isolated Soy Protein	90	Less Than 3

Soy proteins are available in many different sizes and shapes like powder, granule, flake, chunk, fibrous and hydrated. Powdered soy proteins work best in products where no visible soy protein is desired in the finished product like frankfurters and luncheon leaves. Soy proteins are also performing excellently in coarse ground fresh products and have the ability to impart texture to the finished product. A lot of low cost hamburger patties are manufactured containing either textured flours or textured concentrates. Soy proteins are available either coloured or uncoloured. Uncoloured textured products are used in fresh meat products such as beef or pork patties while coloured products are effectively used in cooked products such as pizza toppings, chilli and burritos but they have light caramel appearance. The basic function of soy protein in meat products are water binding and fat absorption.

Milk proteins are generally used in meat products for better binding at higher temperature because milk proteins are more heat stable than meat proteins. Commonly used milk proteins are non-fat dried milk (NFDM), calcium reduced non-fat dried milk, dried whey powder, whey protein concentrates, sodium caseinate, skim milk powder (SMP), butter milk powder etc.

Composition of milk proteins (Source: Processed meat by Pearson and Gillett, 1997)

Ingredients	Moisture(%)	Fat(%)	Protein(%)	Lactose(%)	Ash(%)
NFDM	3.0	0.8	35.9	52.3	8.0
Calcium reduced NFDM	3.0	0.8	36-39	52.3	4-7
Dried whey powder	4.5	1.1	12.0	73.5	8.0
Whey protein concentrate	2.0	2-9	20-60	18-60	3-18
Sodium caseinate	4.0	0.8	92.0	-	1.5
SMP	4.0	1.5	83.0	1.0	10.0
Butter milk powder	2.8	5.3	34.4	50.0	7.6

NFDM is mainly used in meat products for better binding of water and fat and it is cheaper than meat proteins. In addition, it can also improve the texture and flavour of the products especially in emulsion type sausages. The legal limit for its use is 3.5%. Calcium reduced NFDM acts similarly as the normal NFDM but due to reduction in calcium ion up to 20 to 70%, it has better solubility than normal NFDM. Dried whey or whey protein concentrates are the by-products of cheese industry and the principle protein found in whey is lactalbumin. They act mainly as binders and thickeners besides incorporating protein in the meat products. The legal limit is 3.5 to 8.0% in different meat products. Sodium caseinate is used as a water and fat binder but it is not a good fat emulsifier at normal pH. Some other milk products like skim milk co- precipitates and whole milk powder may also be used in meat and meat products but they are not of very commonly used.

Yeast proteins are very good emulsifying agents and rich in protein as well as vitamin-B complex. They are mainly used in form of dried yeasts or yeast extracts but extract form is commonly used in meat products due to better flavour imparting characteristics. Dried yeasts has 45-52% proteins and mostly used in meat pizza and sausages rolls while yeast extracts are used in almost all types of meat products and has 38-54% proteins.

Egg proteins are mainly used in meat products to enhance the binding ability but it also imparts certain sensory attributes. It is also provides better emulsion stability. For improving the functional properties and maintaining the nutritional value of low value meat, egg proteins serves as a good source of protein and binders in low cost. It can be used in form of whole egg liquid, whole egg powder, albumin powder and sometimes with yolk incorporation. But whole egg liquid and powder are the main forms of interest for meat processors.

Hydrolyzed vegetable proteins (HVP / HPP) are mainly used to enhance the meat flavour in product. Meat aroma is produced from amino acids in the presence of sugar. The process of production of different meat flavours are as follows:

Fructose or maltose or sucrose

Glycine------------------------------------→ Beef broth aroma

Glucose or fructose

Glutamic acid ----------------------------→ Chicken like aroma

Maltose

Glycine-------------------------------------→ Baked ham aroma

Sucrose

Lysine---------------------------------------→ Boiled meat aroma

3. *Emulsifiers or stabilizers*: Emulsifiers or stabilizers are mainly used in low fat products for better texture and juiciness. Under this group gums are the main ingredients and the examples of important gums are carrageenan and sodium alginate. Carageenans and xanthan gum are thickening and gelling agents be used in cured pork products at a level of 1.5% but if used in combination with xanthan gum or locust bean gum then the amount can not exceed 0.5% of the product formulation. It is extracted from red seaweed and is found in three basic types i.e. kappa, iota and lambda. The ability of carageenan to form a gel in meat products leads to increasing yield, consistency, sliceability, spreadability, cohesiveness and decreasing purge, fat content and slicing loss. Carageenan can be incorporated into the meat as part of a marinade or it can be added directly to meat as a dry powder. Salt makes carageenan insoluble in water and therefore causes carageenan to be dispersed in the system only (not thickening the solution but only dispersed). Carageenan should therefore be added after addition of salt so it does not bind water (swell) before it is incorporated in the meat product. In some cases it is necessary to disperse carageenan without salt. For this purpose there are special coated carageenans dispersible in pure water. The use of carageenan as a dry powder almost never causes any trouble. Immediately after incorporation carageenan has no function but as the temperature rises and the carageenan starts to swell, the viscosity increases and water retained in meat. Cooking to 68-72°C in the center ensures complete dissolution of carageenan. During the subsequent cooling process the carageenan at a temperature of approximately 50-60°C, sets to a firm and cohesive gel. Therefore, it is of utmost importance that the product is cooled as quickly as possible.

Sodium alginates are mainly used in restructured fresh meat products but the role of alginate in processed meat products is not well known. For the initiation of gelling and binding properties it requires calcium carbonate. Other gums used for this purpose are locust bean gum from *Ceratonia siliqua*, guar gum, gellan gum from carbohydrate fermentation by *Pseudomonas elodea* and xanthan gum by fermentation of carbohydrates with *Xanthomonas campestris.*

Spices, Seasonings and Flavouring

Spices, seasonings and flavourings are used to add flavour to the products and also affect the consistency of the ground sausage mixture. The wide range of spices, seasonings and flavourings are available for use in meat and meat products. The type, amount and qualities of the ingredients produces variety in meat products as per the choice of local consumers in a particular area. Spices are defined as any aromatic vegetable substance that is intended to function as flavour contributer in foods instead of contributing the nutritional substance of the food. The active aromatic or pungent properties of spices that contribute the most to the flavouring effect is mostly present in volatile oils, resins or oleoresins of the spices. These properties are present in the whole spice or in extracts of the active components. The use of spice extracts has some advantages over whole spices such as controlled intensity of the flavour, diminishes microbial contamination, facilitate easier storage and less conspicuous visual appearance compared with spice particles.

Flavourings are substances that are extracted from a food such as fruits, herbs, roots, meats, seafood etc. Adding various flavorings and spices to cured meat products is becoming increasingly popular. Originally few spices such as pepper, allspice, etc. can be rubbed on the surface of dry cured hams. These probably do not penetrate too far into the ham itself and their flavour effect is primarily confined to the surface. With the advent of brine curing, however, flavourings could be introduced directly into the meat. Seasonings are another general term that refers to any substance which is used to impart flavour to the food product. Some examples of common spices and seasonings includes all spices, pepper, cardamom, caraway, coriander, cumin, garlic, sage, mustard, nutmeg, paprika, rosemary, thyme, and turmeric. Spice extracts are used in the flavouring of cured meat products with the combination of dextrose to make them more soluble in water.

Traditional Spices and Flavourings

Coriander has a sweet, aromatic, rose-like flavour and is mostly obtained from dried ripe fruit or seed of a parsley herb. The flavour produces by coriander is sweeter, aromatic and rose flower like. It can be used in frankfurters and bologna as an alternative of nutmeg. It gives taste on middle side of tongue.

Mustard is a number-one spice used in meat industry. It is slightly bitter in flavour though oriental mustard has a very pungent flavour. The compound responsible for typical oriental mustard pungency, sharp odour and acrid flavour is allyl isothiocyanate. However, de-heated mustard has no flavour and contains about 29% protein. It can be used at the rate of 1% in frankfurters or bologna emulsion. In sausages it contributes little or non for flavour.

Fennel has a sweet licorice or warm anise like flavour. It is obtained from fennel seed (*Foeniculum vulgare*) and mostly found in India and Argentina. It is most commonly used in Italian sausage, pepperoni and other Italian-flavoured meats.

Cumin has a strong, musty flavour which is sometimes termed as dirty socks smell. A heavy and possibly objectionable flavour associated with Texas or Mexican meat products, chili and curry powder. It is a flavouring ingredient and also has inhibitory effects against fungi. It is obtained from cumin seed of parsley plant.

Sage has a bitter, aromatic and warm bitter flavour similar to the flavour of Vicks Vapo-rub. It is produced from leaves of *Salvia officinalis L.*, belongs to mint family. It is a suitable spice for bitter taste development in fresh pork sausage, pork pizza and poultry dressings.

Paprika has a sweet flavour and mostly imparts red colour of capsanthin in meat products especially in sausages. It is an important spice obtained from annuum species of capsicum family and contains number of carotinoids. It is a choice spice for low fat meat products due to requirement for colour development in such products. It has little to no flavour development in processed meat products with the exception of capicola.

Chili pepper has a sweet, pungent, slightly burnt flavour and also gives cooked taste. Chili is cooked to darken but gives cooked or burnt flavour in Texas and Mexican meat products.

Red pepper has a pungent, biting hot flavour, which is not detected in front of mouth but gives hot throat sensation after use. Its small quantity imparts more flavour in seasoned products and commonly used in crushed form to aid visual appearance. It is a product of frutescens species of capsicum family.

Black pepper has a hot, pungent or piney flavour used in summer sausages. It gives taste on the tip of tongue. Black and white pepper both are obtained from berry of vine *Piper nigrum* and together accounts about 35% of total spice market globally.

White pepper has a less pungent flavour than black pepper. The origin of both black and white pepper is same but white pepper is prepared by removing the pericorp before or after the drying of berries. It is mostly used in meat products not required black specs on it.

Nutmeg belongs to the pear shaped tropical fruit of Mytistacease tree and its mace is thin, lacy, bright red aril which surrounds the nutmeg. It produces sweet and pungent flavour and mostly used in frankfurters and bologna. Mace has a stronger flavour and lighter colour than nutmeg. It also gives typical spice flavour in most hot dogs and bologna. Its taste can be judged on front side of tongue.

Mace has a sweet, pungent flavour which is sweeter than nutmeg. It also gives lighter colour than nutmeg and mace comes from scarlet membrane of nutmeg kernel.

Garlic has a strongly adored, pungent flavour which is obtained from dried bulb of *Allium sativum L.* It produces hearty flavour in beef frankfurters, Polish and Italian sausage. Its taste can feel in mouth. It has some antibiotic property alongwith taste incorporation

Onion provides compliments garlic flavour with sweetness in meat products. It has antibacterial action in meat products and belongs to same genera *Allium*.

Ginger induces bitter taste in meat products alongwith antioxidant properties. Taste of ginger may be perceived on middle side of tongue.

Other Additives

Some additives are used for specific purposes in meat products which comes under this group. Examples are antioxidants, bacterial cultures, compounds used for flavour enhancement, synthetic fat replacers, fat mimics, maltodextrins, oat bran and oat fiber, animal proteins (gelatine and serum proteins) etc.

Antioxidants are the compounds used to retard oxidation of fat they may be either naturally occurring or produced synthetically. Naturally occurring antioxidants are mainly tocopherols or vitamin-E. Whereas, synthetic antioxidants are of two types depending on their solubility such as fat soluble and water soluble. Fat soluble antioxidants include butylated hydroxyanisole (BHA), butylated hydroxytoluene (BHT), catechin, quercetin and 2, 6-dimethoxyphenol (DMP) while water soluble is ascorbic acid, citric acid, phosphoric acid and nitrite.

Bacterial cultures of different bacteria are used to ferment the meat products. It makes the product palatable and also reduces the chances of nitrosamine formation. The pure cultures used for this purpose may be obtained from *Pediococci, Lactobacilli, Micrococci* and one subtype of *Streptococci* etc. Among them *Micrococci* and *Streptococci* are good for flavour and aroma production while *Pediococci* and *Lactobacilli* are good for acid production. *Streptococci* are not commonly used due to the threat of food poisoning.

Monosodium glutamate (MSG), Ionosine monophosphate (IMP), Guanosine monophosphate (GMP) are the compounds used for enhancing the meat flavour. These compounds are mainly used in meat loaves, soups, stews, hash and canned ham. In general these additives are very useful in the products having little meat protein contents.

Synthetic fat replacers are non-calorie additives have all the functions of fat but not metabolized by enzymes. The use of these compounds is not yet approved by the authorities for use in meat products. The known examples are olestra, esterified propoxylated glycerols, dialkyl dihexadecyl malonate and trialkoxy citrate etc.

Fat mimics are the group of compounds used for thickening, bulking and microparticulates. These compounds are used together in a meat product to give a desired texture. Examples of thickeners (provides lubrication) are gums, starches and hemicelluloses while bulking agents (controls absorption) are polydextrose, low viscosity hydrocolloids and polyols. Micro-particulates are used for smoothening the fat replacing system which includes microcrystalline cellulose and microparticulated proteins.

Maltodextrins are generally used in low fat meat products. These are easy in use, low in cost and excellent in water holding. The permissible limit is 3% in different products like sausages. These are actually cleavage products of amylase and amylopectin with the help of beta amylase. Examples are corn and oat maltodextrins.

Oat bran and oat fiber are generally used to improve texture of low fat meat products. Oat bran can be used with spices and flavourings for improvement in mouth feel while oat fiber has ability to lower the blood cholesterol when used in meat products.

Animal proteins such as gelatine, milk proteins and serum proteins can be used satisfactorily in meat products. *Gelatin* is a hydrocolloid extracted from pork skin by acid treatment or from beef bones or calf skin by alkali treatment. They have good binding with water and makes meat products softer because gelatin swell in cold water. On dessolution in hot water it forms gel at 20°C which melts below mouth temperature (<30°C). Another animal protein is *serum protein* particularly serum albumin and fibrinogen. These proteins impart flavour, increases water holding capacity and provide good binding in low fat meat products.

Different Types of Meat Products

1. Kabab

Kabab is a baked or charcoal-grilled or pan fried piece of meat with necessary ingredients. It is a very popular meat product in India and came in existence during the times of Changez Khan. At his horse back riders would kill an animal, clean it, cut it into pieces, thread the pieces over the daggers or swords and cook over open fire. That was the first Kabab, a piece of meat threaded on a dagger and cooked over open fire. In United States, Kabab refers to Turkish definition of Shish Kabab.

In Turkey, Shish kabab means skewer with grilled meat. With time, the Kabab has evolved from whole muscle meats to minced meats and even non-meats. The latest in the evolution is Tikka masala originating in United Kingdom.

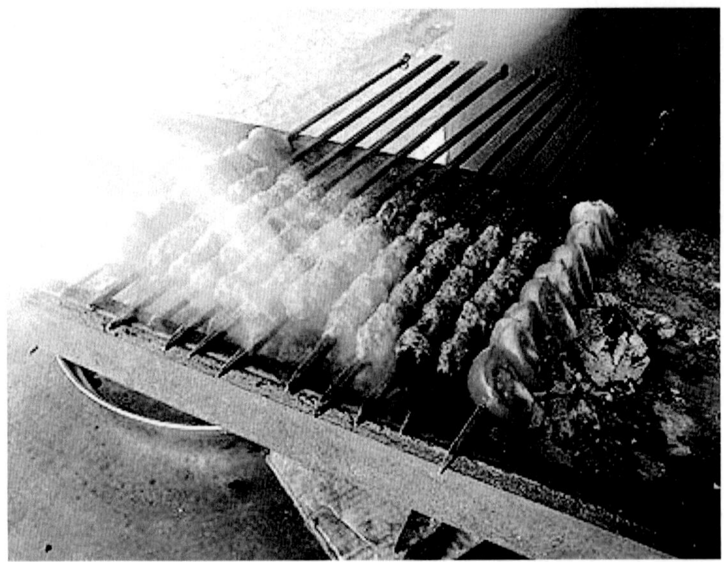

Kabab preparation (*Source:* wikipedia.org)

Kabab is a wide variety of meat dishes originating in southwest and south Asia and now found worldwide. In English, kabab with no qualification generally refers more specifically to shish kabab or doner kabab served wrapped in bread with a salad and a dressing. But in southwest and south Asia, kabab includes grilled, roasted, and stewed dishes of large or small cuts of meat, or even ground meat; it may be served on plates, in sandwiches, or in bowls. The traditional meat for kabab is lamb but depending on local tastes and taboos it may now be beef, goat, chicken, pork, fish and sea food or even vegetarian foods like tofu. Like other ethnic foods brought by immigrants and travellers, the kabab has become part of everyday cuisine in multicultural countries around the globe. Meat kababs are mainly of two types whole muscle meat kabab and minced meat kabab.

Whole Muscle Meat Kabab

The whole muscle meat is cut in to convenient pieces that are either threaded over the skewers or cooked over charcoal grill. The meats are either tenderized with Papaya or Yogurt mixture. The examples of whole muscle meat kababs are lamb boti kabab, chapli kabab, chicken tikka kabab, pather kabab, reshmi chicken kabab and tabak Maaz.

Minced Meat Kabab

In North India, minced meat kababs are popular in which meat is first minced with necessary ingredients and then given a shape of kabab. The minced meat is tenderized with either yogurt or Papaya and then almost pulverized by the heel of the palm. The examples of minced meat kababs are galawati kabab, kakori kabab, seekh kabab, shami kabab and shikampur kabab.

Recipe and Procedures of Some Indian Kababs

i. Seekh Kabab Recipe- Popular in North India

Ingredients

½ kg ground lamb or ground turkey meat or meat of choice

Spices

1 Small finely chopped onion

½ Small finely chopped tomato

2 tablespoon fresh finely chopped coriander

2 teaspoon ginger paste

1 teaspoon garlic paste

½ teaspoon garam masala

Salt as required

Garnish

1 circular shape sliced onion

1 circular shape sliced capsicum

1 circular shape sliced tomato

1 circular shape sliced lemon

Procedure

1. Ground meat is mixed with spices.
2. Ideally, kababs should be cooked in a tandoor for about 10 minutes but grill or oven can also be used in absence of tandoor.
3. Tightly pack meat on skewer and sliced garnish are arranged in between meat. Grilling is done for about 12 to 15 minutes at 300°F or 148.8°C.
4. Pre-heated oven maintained at 300°F or 187.7°C can be used. On it tightly pack meat on skewer is arranged as sliced garnish placed between meat. It is then placed on a baking tray coated vegetable oil and allow to Cook for 12 to 15 minutes. Turn periodically once in a 6-7 minutes.
5. After proper cooking kabab is removed from heat and can be served hot with the onion and lime slices.

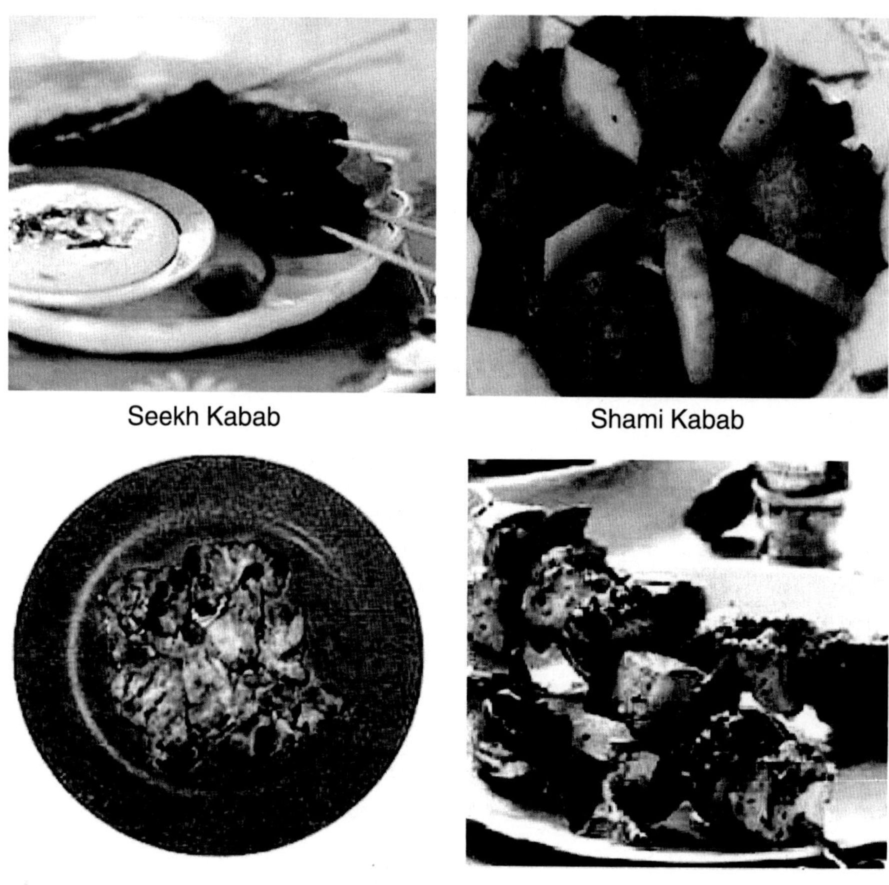

Seekh Kabab Shami Kabab

Boti Kabab Hussaini Kabab

Different types of kababs (*Source:* Indian food co.com)

ii. Shami Kabab Recipe

Popular in U.P. and Bihar.

Ingredients

750 g finely minced lamb meat or meat of choice

1 medium finely chopped onion

3 tablespoons mattar dhal (yellow split peas) or masoor dhal (red lentils)

Spices

1 teaspoon finely grated fresh ginger

1½ teaspoons finely chopped garlic

Salt as desired

2 cups water

½ teaspoon garam masala

1 tablespoon yoghurt or thick cream

1 small beaten egg

Ghee or oil for shallow frying

Filling mixture

1 fresh seeded and finely chopped green chilli

1 tablespoon finely chopped fresh cilantro

I spring onion with green leaves

½ teaspoon finely grated fresh ginger

Procedure

1. Lamb meat or meat of choice, onion, dhal, ginger, garlic, salt and water are put into a heavy saucepan and bring to the boil with stirring.
2. Cover and mok over low heat until meat, lentils and onions are soft (about 45 minutes).
3. Uncover and cook with stirring till all the liquid has been absorbed (for about 1 hour).
4. Allow to cool and then mix garam masala and yoghurt or cream.
5. Add one tablespoon of beaten egg and mix well till mixture will become completely smooth.
6. Divide it into eight portions and make them in flat circle form.
7. Filling mixture (about 14 teaspoon) is added in middle of the mixture, close the meat mixture around it, pinching edges together. Flatten gently to form a small round patty.

8. Shallow fry on a heavy griddle or frying pan with ghee or oil.
9. Product is generally utilized as hot because it is a cocktail snacks available in a bite-size.

iii. Tikka Kabab Recipe (also called Boti Kabab in Punjab, India)

Ingredients

0.25 kg boneless mutton or chicken in a form of cubes

2 teaspoon ginger-garlic paste

2 teaspoon cumin powder

1 teaspoon roasted cumin powder

¼ teaspoon black pepper powder

½ cup curd

1 teaspoon vinegar

½ teaspoon red chilli powder

1 teaspoon garam masala

Salt as desired

2 teaspoon ghee

6 black pepper

5 coarsely ground green cardamom

Juice of 2 lemons

Procedure

1. Mix ginger and garlic and spices in yogurt and marinate the meat.
2. Dip the meat in ghee and arrange the pieces on skewers.
3. Roast or grill or bake them for 15-20 minutes with timely turning to prevent burning.
4. Paste with lime juice and sprinkle black pepper and cardamom powder and roast for another five minutes.

iv. Hussaini Kabab Recipe (also known as Skewered Barbecued Lamb)

Ingredients

2 kg boned lamb leg

Spices

1 teaspoon crushed garlic

1½ teaspoons finely grated fresh ginger

1 teaspoon freshly ground black pepper

2 tablespoons finely ground almonds

2 tablespoons yoghurt

1 teaspoon ground coriander

1 teaspoon ground cummin

Salt as desired

2 tablespoons sesame oil

1 tablespoon lemon juice

Procedure

1. Lamb leg is prepared by trimming of excess fat. Then lean meat is make into 2.5 cm cubes and put into a large howl.
2. Mix all the ingredients, cover and leave for 2 or 3 hours or refrigerate and leave for about 4 days.
3. 4 or 5 pieces of meat are now threaden on each skewer and barbecue over glowing coals or under a preheated griller until crisp and brown all over. Periodic turning is required to ensure proper cooking of lamb.

2. Sausages

The word sausage originally comes from the Latin word *salsus* which means salted or minced meat preserved by salting. In sausage preparation highly seasoned minced meat usually pork or beef traditionally stuffed in casings of prepared animal intestine. Sausage has been known since ancient times and some of its varieties came to be known by their city of origin: the frankfurter from Frankfurt am Main, bologna from Bologna, the wiener from Vienna (Wien). Sausage meat may be eaten fresh, smoked, dried, or pickled. It may be mixed with other meats and additives such as cereals, vegetable starch, soy flour, preservatives, artificial colourings, salt, various herbs and spices. Casings may be intestine, paraffin-treated fabric bags or synthetic sleeves of plastic or reconstituted collagen. All sausages require refrigerated storage but special attention to be given to dry cured sausages. Cooked and dry sausages are ready to eat while fresh and frozen sausages must be cooked before eating.

The process of sausage manufacturing originated from the necessity to increase the uses of remnants of meat, fat of clearness meat parts and less noble cuts, adding value to these products. There are many different types of sausages. The differences between them are related with the type of meat, the size of meat grinder disk, the seasonings, the casing diameter, the buds length and the presence or not of smoking.

History of Sausage

In the ancient time when there was no refrigeration facility to preserve the meat and so making sausage was a way of overcoming this problem. Dry sausage was born as a result of the discovery of new spices which helped to enhance, flavour and preserve the meat. Different countries and different cities within those countries started producing their own distinctive types of sausage both fresh and dry. These different types of sausage were mostly influenced by the availability of ingredients as well as the climate. Some parts of the world with periods of cold climate such as Northern Europe were able to keep their fresh sausage without refrigeration, during the cold months. They also developed a process of smoking the sausage to preserve the meat during the warmer months. The hotter climates in the south of Europe developed dry sausage, which did not need refrigeration at all. Basically people living in particular areas developed their own types of sausage and that sausage became associated with the area. For example Bologna originated in the town of Bologna in Northern Italy, Lyons sausage from Lyons in France and Berliner sausage from Berlin in Germany.

Types of Sausages

Sausages may be of various types depending on its composition and its method of preparation.

Basis of sausages classification	Sausage type
1. On the basis of degree of chopping	i. Coarsely ground e.g. fresh pork sausage. ii. Emulsion or finely chopped e.g. frankfurters.
2. On the basis of amount of cooking	i. Uncooked e.g fresh smoked pork sausages. ii. Cooked e.g. salami, frankfurters, bologna etc.
3. On the basis of amount of smoking	i. Unsmoked e.g. breakfast sausages ii. Smoked e.g. fresh smoked pork sausages , fresh smoked kielbasa
4. On the basis of amount of water added	i. Without added water e.g. Italian pork sausage ii. Added water e.g. emulsion type sausage
5. On the basis of amount of curing	i. Uncured e.g. bockwurst. ii. Cured e.g. frankfurters
6. On the basis of amount of fermentation	i. Unfermented e.g. fresh beef and pork sausages ii. Fermented e.g salami, pepperoni, thuringer
7. On the basis of amount of moisture in final product	i. Fresh e.g. fresh beef and pork sausages ii. Smoked e.g. fresh smoked pork sausages. iii. Cooked e.g. frankfurters, bologna, knockwurst. iv. Cured e.g. frankfurters v. Meat loaves and speciality products vi. Dry and semi dry e.g. salami and cerevelat, thuringer or summer sausage
8. On the basis of USDA meat inspection system	i. Fresh e.g. fresh beef and pork sausages

Contd.

Basis of sausages classification	Sausage type
	ii. Uncooked smoked e.g. fresh smoked pork sausages, fresh smoked kielbasa iii. Cooked smoked e.g. bologna , pepperoni iv. Cooked e.g. frankfurters, bologna, knockwurst. v. Dry and semi dry e.g. salami and cerevelat, thuringer or summer sausage vi. Luncheon meat, loaves and Jellied products

Fresh Sausage

For making of fresh meat sausage, fresh meats that have not been previously cured are commonly used. The quality characteristics (colour, texture, taste, tenderness etc.) of these sausages are directly related to ratio of fat to lean. These sausages must be refrigerated and thoroughly cooked before eating. Examples include Boerewors, Italian Pork sausage, Fresh pork sausages, Breakfast sausages, whole hog sausages and Fresh Beef sausage.

Fresh Smoked Sausage

These are fresh sausage which are smoked for development of colour and flavour. After smoking, the sausage can then be refrigerated and cooked thoroughly before eating. Examples include fresh smoked pork sausages, fresh smoked Kielbasa, Mettwurst and Roumanian sausage.

Cooked Sausage

These sausages are made up of fresh meats comminution and then fully cooked. The sausage is either eaten immediately after cooking or must be refrigerated and is usually reheated before eating. Examples are Braunschweiger, Veal sausage and Liver sausage.

Cooked Smoked Sausage

These are same as cooked sausage but they are cooked and smoked, or smoke-cooked. They can be eaten hot or cold but needs refrigeration storage. Examples are Wieners, Kielbasa and Bologna.

Dry and Semi Dry Sausage

These are the most complicated of all sausages to make, as the drying process has to be carefully controlled. These sausages are produced by fermentation. The fermentation is usually done by natural process(back slopping) or by addition of lactic acid culture. Dry sausages are lightly smoked, firmer, high in price but low in yield (60-70%). Whereas semidry sausages are usually fully cooked, semi soft and high in product yield (70-80%). These sausages can be readily eaten and can be kept for very long periods under refrigeration. Examples of dry sausages are Salamis and Cervelats while semidried sausages include Thuringer or Summer sausage.

Luncheon Meat, Loaves and Jellied Products

In this category of sausage Luncheon meat, meat loaves, Scrapple and Bockwurst are the main products. Luncheon meat is a cured cooked product prepared from comminution of mechanically deboned meat. Meat loaf is a comminuted meat product obtained from mechanically deboned meat. The permissible limit for addition of ice-water is up to 3% in both the products. Scrapple contains 40% meat along with other cereal ingredients like soy flour or meal. Bockwurst is a product of mainly pork or beef that is uncured, comminuted, cooked or uncooked. The meat content in this product must be above 70% and other ingredients include milk or water, eggs and vegetables.

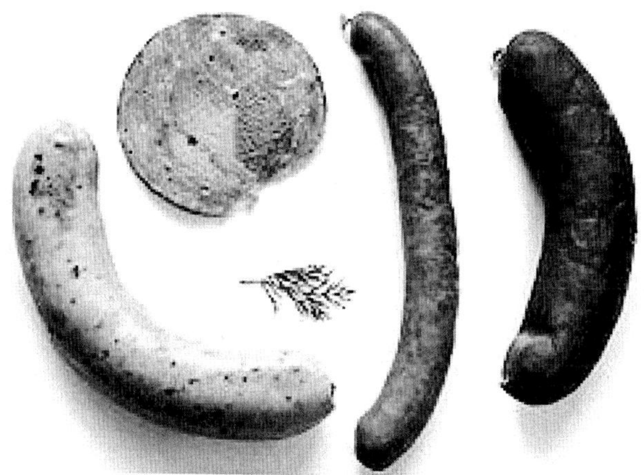

Meat sausages (*Source:* sausage wikipedia)

Requirements for Sausages Preparation

Grinder, Mixer, Bowl Chopper and Stuffer

For the grinding of meat, grinder is important equipment that has different cutting plates for grinding of meat to the correct consistency. Cutting plates are mostly available in four sizes: 3/4 inch coarse grind, 3/8 inch Medium-course grind, 3/16 inch Medium grind and 1/8 inch Fine grind. Grinder may be of manually operated or an electric grinder. This grinder should also have sausage stuffing attachment with different size stuffing horns. This attachment is required to stuff different size sausage casings. For commercial purpose electric grinder and a separate sausage stuffing device is required. Electric grinder is normally powered by a 220V motor and then has a separate sausage stuffer. In some of the sausage production especially for emulsion type sausages, mixer and bubble chopper are the important equipments.

Casings

Casings are of variety of sizes and are usually sold by the hank, bundle, cap or ounce. It is always difficult to know about the casing requirement for a particular quantity of meat. For this purpose some thumb rules can be used. One kg of meat requires about 2 feet (32-35 mm) of medium-size hog casing or about 4 feet (20-22 mm) of medium-size lamb casing.

Types of Casings

Casings	Characteristics
Lamb and Sheep Casing	These casings are very tender and used for making breakfast sausage, frankfurters, and fresh pork sausage.
Hog Casing	Undoubtedly the most popular casing which can actually be used for almost any sausage.
Beef Bungs, Rounds, and Casing	For sausages that require a very thick casing such as bologna and salami.
Collagen Casing	This casing is made from the gelatinous substance found in the connective tissue, bones and cartilage of all mammals. The substance is harvested from the animals and reconstructed in the form of a casing. Most sausages in USA is stuffed into this casing.
Fibrous Casing	This casing is used to make dry and semi-dry sausage. The fibrous casing is extremely strong and is used to stuff sausage that is very tightly packed, as it will not break. The inside of this casing is coated with protein that allows it to shrink with the meat as it dries out.
Muslin Casing	This casing is made of muslin and is used for sausages such as liverwurst, blood sausage, salami's and bologna's.
Cellulosic Casing	This is an artificial casing made from solubilized cotton linters. It is very uniform, strong and less susceptible to bacteria as other types of casings. Skinless hotdogs are made with cellulosic casings.
Synthetic Casing	This casing is made from alginates and requires no refrigeration. It is used by mass producers and can be made in different colours. Red for bologna, clear for some salami's and white for liverwurst. Much like the cellulosic casing it is uniform and strong.

Generally natural casings are preferred over artificial due to development of best flavour and appearance to the final product. In addition, natural casings also enhance and complement the natural juices and quality of the meat and spices and permits deep smoke penetration during smoking.

Method of emulsion preparation: the procedure for production of stable meat emulsion may have following steps:

1. *Grinding*: The lean meat chunks of variable size and shape along with fat contents are screw feed in the barrel of grinder. The meat is then pressed into holes of grinder plate after cutting with rotating blades into uniform size. The diameter of meat pieces is determined by the size of holes.
2. *Mixing*: The pieces of fat and lean are then feed into a mixer for uniform mixing of fat and lean particles. Mixing also facilitates extraction and coating of fat particles with salt soluble proteins.
3. *Emulsifying*: Meat mix is now passed in a bowl chopper and then salt is added @4.5% of lean meat weight. Chopping of meat with salt is done for a couple of minutes. Then ice, sodium nitrite and ascorbate or erythorbate and other ingredients are added. The basic purpose of adding ice is to reduce emulsion temperature after chopping of 5-10 minutes (desired temperature at this stage is 11°C-12°C). After chopping all extenders, seasonings and sweeteners are added and again chop these ingredients for about 5-10 minutes.
4. *Stuffing*: The emulsion dough or batter is now transferred to sausage stuffer for extruding into casings. Commonly air pressure of 125 psi is used for stuffing the batter into casings.
5. *Linking and Tying*: After stuffing of emulsion and casings, the encased mass is tied with thread or metal clips on a definite distance. In small sausages twisting may also be done.
6. *Smoking and Cooking*: The prepared sausages are placed in a smoke house for smoking and cooking at a temperature of 68.3 -71.1°C. The rate of cooking is greatly affected by air velocity in a smoke house. But humidity in the smoke house plays very minor role in cooking. However, 35-40% humidity is required to transfer smoke in the sausages. Sausages should not touch the surface of smoke house.
7. *Chilling*: For chilling, sausages are first showered with cold water and then placed in refrigeration for further use.

8. *Peeling and Packaging*: After chilling of sausages at internal temperature of 1.6 to 4.4°C, these are taken out. This process is known as peeling. These peeled sausages are then packed in a suitable package.

Formulations for Some Common Meat Sausages

i. Fresh Pork Sausages

These are coarse ground type sausages which are very popular for breakfast in Europe and America. This kind of sausage consists only of ground seasoned pork and its manufacture involves only a few operational steps. Seasoning formulae vary widely with particular market and regional preferences, but generally speaking, there are two seasoning extremes: a sage and sugar flavour and, on the other hand, a hot seasoning.

Ingredients: The ingredients required for production of 100 kg fresh pork sausages are 90 kg fresh pork trimmings with 60 to 70% lean and 10 kg fresh pork back fat. The seasonings required for this purpose are 1800 g salt, 150 g ground white pepper, 100 g mace, 200 g sage, 100 g sugar, 40 g savoury, 150 g ginger, 200 g chilli and 2000 g monosodium glutamate. The preferred casings are narrow (under 28 mm) pig rounds. In some formulations pork side and lean can also be used in a ratio of 3:2.

Procedure: Seasoning mixture is sprinkled over pork before grinding. The pork trimmings are primarily passed through 13 mm plate and then through 5 mm plate grinder and seasoning are added and mixed. The mixture is stuffed into previously soaked casings. It is considered that a highly acceptable fresh pork sausage can be produced by formulating the product to 35 percent fat level.

ii. Fresh Beef Sausages

These sausages are common in Arab countries. These are coarse ground type and do not necessarily use cereal binders. Rusk or other binders are added in the mixer or cutter either in a dry or pre-soaked state.

Ingredients: The ingredients required for 100 kg of fresh beef sausages are 85 to 90 kg lean beef or lean beef trimmings. 10 to 15 kg selected beef or mutton fat, 0.5 to 3.0 kg rusk is sometimes added to improve binding and 2 to 3 kg salted water may also be added to facilitate stuffing. In this product about one-third beef may be substituted by mutton, if desired. The seasonings are 2000 g salt, 50 to 100 g red pepper, 1 to 2 g chilli, 20 to 60 g cardamom, 20 g ginger, 10 to 50 g fenugreek and 20 to 60 g sugar. The preferred casings are sheep or goat casings of different diameter i.e. wide (22 to 24 mm), medium (20 to 22 mm), narrow medium (18 to 22 mm) and narrow (16 to 18 mm).

Procedure: The meat and fat are run separately through the coarse plates of the grinder (meat through 6 to 8 mm plate and fat through 5 to 6 mm plate). Both are then mixed and kept for few minutes and added with seasonings. The mixture is then regrinded through 5 mm plate and finally stuffed into pre-soaked salted goat or sheep casings. The stuffed casings are generally divided in units by twisting. The length of sausage units or links varies widely but short links of 5 to 7 cm and long links of 10 to 15 cm are common lengths. These sausages can be stored for about two days at refrigeration temperature.

iii. Sausage-Burger (Hamburger)

Technologically hamburgers are typical fresh beef sausages that are not stuffed in casings. However, stuffing hamburgers into appropriate casings may be advantageous for small scale manufacturers. Hamburgers are made up of ground seasoned beef without addition of others meats. Prerigor meat is an excellent raw material for hamburgers and it should be removed as soon as possible from the carcass and coarse ground through a plate having holes of 12 mm or even larger. Mixing with salt gives a product of high water binding capacity.

iv. Cooked or Summer Sausages

These sausages can be produced from beef and sometimes with the combination of both in equal proportion. The other ingredients used are fat, salt, dextrose, coarse ground black pepper, whole mustard seed, ground nutmeg, ground coriander, ground spice, sodium nitrite, garlic powder, lactic acid starter culture for fermentation at 37.7°C or 100°F.

Procedure: Ground beef and/or pork are passed through 1/8 inch. plate. The temperature of grinder should be maintained at 1.1°C or 30°F or less. Salt, sugar, spices, and cures are then blended with meat. After that starter culture is added and temperature is adjusted below 2.2°C. This mixture is then stuffed in appropriate dry sausage casings. The preferred casing used in this product is beef middles. For the fermentation of sausages temperature 35°C to 37.7° C, Relative Humidity in between 90 to 95% and pH of 4.8 to 4.9 is provided. For cooking of products in smokehouse, temperature should be around 62.7°C to 65.5°C and R.H. around 60% to 70%. After reaching the temperature around 145°F or 62.7°C product is taken out from smokehouse and allows cooling slightly at room temperature before shifting it to chill coolers.

v. Thuringer cervelat

These are coarse ground, fermented, semi dry sausages.

Ingredients: For the preparation of thuringer cervelat beef meat (12.5 kg) with 15% fat and pork trimmings (7.5 kg or 2.5 kg) with 20% to 50% fat and some organs like beef heart (2.5kg) is optional in this formulation. Other ingredients are 700g salt, 250 g dextrose, 250 g sugar, 115 g coarse ground black pepper, 75 g whole black pepper, 30 g mustard coriander, 15 g ground nutmeg, 15 g ground spices, 7.5 g sodium nitrite and 60 g Acid starter culture.

Procedure: Beef meat and pork trimmings are first grinded through 1/8 inch plate but temperature must be maintained at 1.1°C or below. Then salt, sugars, spices and cures are blended in it. After blending starter culture is added for fermentation. At this stage low temperatures (below 2.2°C) must be maintained. For stuffing traditionally double walled sewed bungs are used as a casing. For optimum production of colour and flavour smoke house should be adjusted at 15.5° C with 85% to 95% Relative Humidity at 4.6 pH. When internal temperature of the sausages reaches to 48.8°C then sausages are taken out from smoke house and allow cooling at room temperature for 4 to 6 hours before shifting to chill cooler.

vi. Pepperoni

For making the pepperoni beef bone less meat (7.5 kg), plates (3.5 kg), cheeks (5 kg), pork bone less meat (8.0 kg) is used. Other ingredients include 750 g salt, 250 g dextrose, 15 g pepperoni spices, 7.5 g sodium nitrite, 1.5 g sodium erythorbate and lactic acid starter culture.

Procedure: For grinding of pork and beef 3/16 inches plate is used while for other meats 1/8 inch plate is commonly utilized. After that meat mixture is added with salt, dextrose, spices, cure and erythorbate. Then starter culture is added in it for fermentation and mix is stuffed in suitable casings. For optimum production temperature should be around 21.1°C to 26.6°C with 80 - 90% Relative Humidity to a pH of 4.7. Light smoking of the product is desirable.

vii. Genova Salami

This is a product obtained from pork trimmings (25 kg) of 25% fat along with other ingredients like 750 g salt,250 g dextrose, 115 g ground black pepper, 100 g whole black pepper, 25 g garlic powder, 5 g sodium nitrite and Lactic acid starter culture.

Procedure: Grinding of pork through 3/16 inch plate at 1.1°C or less is the first step. Then mix it with salt, cure, and spices. Addition of starter culture and then filling it into suitable casings is a last step. For obtaining optimal quality characteristics product should be fermented at 23.8°C to 26.6°C with 85 - 90% R.H at pH of 4.8 to 4.9.

viii. Thuringer Blood Sausages

Ingredients: For the production of thuringer blood sausages 12.5 kg picnics (cured and cooked), 5 kg jowls (cured and cooked), 1.25 kg pork liver added with 6 gm 6.25% nitrite and 14 gm salt, 2.5 kg blood (cured with 156 ppm nitrite), 2.5 kg pork rinds (cured and cooked), 115 g ground black pepper, 115 g ground marjoram, 20 g ground spices, 15 g ground cloves and 30 g fresh onions or onion powder is used.

Procedure: Cured and cooked picnics and jowls are grinded with 1/2 inch plate while cooked pork rinds are grinded through 1/8 inch plate with liver. This mixture is mixed with warm blood. Spices and other ingredients are mixed with rinds, liver and blood. For filling of this material casings are used. Then product is water or steam cooked at 68.3 °C to 73.8 ° C internal temperatures and allows cooling in cold water.

ix. Non Specific Loaf

For the preparation of non-specific loaf, beef or pork with 40% fat is commonly used. Its 25 kg is added with 12 kg water or ice, 3 kg whey or other milk protein, 1.1 kg soy isolate, 0.8 kg salt, 0.5 kg dextrose, 75 g sodium nitrite, 15 g sodium erythorbate, 75 g ground white pepper, 15 g ground mace, 15 g ground coriander, 15 g ground cardamom, 15 g ground ginger and 75 g paprika.

Procedure: Lean meat is chopped with salt and ice or water at 4.4°C. Then it is added with soy, milk proteins, meat fat and other ingredients and again chops it at 15.5° C. After that blending is done with pickles, olives etc. for desired red coloured loaf. Fibrous casings are used for making non-specific loaf.

x. Bologna

These are comminuted semi solid emulsion type sausages commonly prepared from one or more kinds of meat of older animals. These sausages should not contain more than 35% fat and 10% added water but also contains milk powder. The procedure and other ingredients used are similar to cooked sausages.

xi. Hot Dog

These are fairly spicy sausages usually prepared in broader casings like weasand. Generally, hot dogs, unless kosher, are a combination of finely ground pork and beef combined with salt and spices. The flavour of most hot dogs is black pepper and nutmeg. Other hot dogs have a garlic flavour as a secondary flavour. Many chicken hot dogs have onion like secondary flavour. Smoke is another important flavour of hot dogs.

xii. Mortadella

These are dry, fermented, smoked or cooked sausages usually prepared from bladder of cattle or from artificial broader casings. The meat of beef, pork, turkey, chicken, chevon and mutton can be used for this purpose. Other ingredients used are ice, salt, sugar, black ground pepper, sodium nitrite and sodium ascorbate.

xiii. Liver Sausages and Braunschweiger

These are emulsion type water cooked sometimes lightly smoked sausages. In its formulation pork livers and jowls are used in a ratio of 1:1 along with other ingredients like salt, ground white pepper, coriander, nutmeg and sodium nitrite.

xiv. Frankfurters

These are cured emulsion type sausages commonly produced from beef and pork trimmings. The other ingredients used in its preparation are ice, salt, white pepper, nutmeg, cardamom, ginger powder, MSG, sodium nitrite and sodium ascorbate.

Meat Balls

Meat balls are also known as meat kofta in India. It is an emulsion type product in which ground meat, fat, bread powder, salt, condiments and spices are used for making stable emulsion.

Ingredients

65% lean meat

15% fat

2% table salt

10% bread powder

6.5% condiments

1.5% spices

Procedure

1. Lean meat is minced once through 9 mm plate and twice through 4 mm plate in meat grinder.
2. Mince the fat once through 4 mm plate in meat grinder.
3. Mix all the ingredients along with fat and minced meat and mix them thoroughly.
4. 15-20 g portion of this dough is now rolled into balls manually or mechanically
5. These balls are either deep fat fried in refined vegetable oil at 135°C for 2-3 minutes to get brown colour and fried flavour or these balls are cooked in hot water at 80°C for 10 minutes and then light frying for development of golden brown colour.
6. Packaging in LDPE pouches and can be stored for a week at refrigeration temperature.

Meat Patties

Meat patties are very popular product in India and mainly used as a filling in burger roll or sandwiches. These products can also be used separately with chutney or sauces. These products are emulsion based and contain less than 30% fat.

Ingredients

1kg	Lean meat
100g	Gram dal
200g	Fat
50 ml	Egg liquid
25g	Table salt
100g	Green curry stuff
20g	Spices

Procedure

1. Mince deboned lean meat once through 9 mm plate and then twice through 4 mm plate in meat grinder.
2. Mince fat twice through 4 mm plate in meat grinder.
3. Mince boiled gram dal through 4 mm plate in grinder.
4. Mix all the ingredients in meat mixer and make dough.
5. 100 g of dough is moulded into 70-80 mm diameter and 15-20 mm thick patties.
6. These raw patties may be frozen for further use or they can bake in an oven maintained at 200°C for 10-20 minutes. Internal temperature of patties must reach to 72°C.
7. Alternatively these patties may be deep fat fried for commercial purpose.
8. Packaged and stored under refrigeration for future use.

Tandoori Chicken

Tandoori chicken is a very popular chicken product in India. It is a delicious, nutritious and tender meat product. For making tandoori chicken normally broilers of six weeks of age are used because they have tender meat which can very well sustain during roasting.

Ingredients

Basic ingredients

500g	Chicken

Rubbing Ingredients

1 teaspoon	Table salt
2 dessertspoon	Lemon juice

Marinade Ingredients

6g	Cloves
10g	Ginger
1teaspoon	Coriander seed
½ teaspoon	Table salt
1 dessertspoon	Lemon juice
7g	Green papaya
½ teaspoon	Black cumin seed
½ teaspoon	Red pepper
2 table spoon	Curd

Sprinkling Ingredients

½ teaspoon	Ground powdered dried green mango (amchur)
½ teaspoon	Roasted ground black cumin
¼ teaspoon	Table salt
1 dessert spoon	Lemon juice
½ teaspoon	Ground fenugreek seeds
1 teaspoon	Ghee

Procedure

1. Chicken washing and patting with a piece of clean cloth.
2. Lightly pierce the entire surface of chicken with fork.
3. Apply ½ teaspoon salt and 2 dessert spoon lemon juice on the surface and in the body cavity of chicken and leave it for 30 minutes.
4. Fine paste of marinade is rubbing all over the surface and inside the body cavity and keep for 12 hours in refrigeration.
5. Bake the chicken in tandoor maintained at 190.5°C for 15-20 minutes. Turn chicken periodically during baking and paste ghee and remaining marinade 2-3 times.

6. Take out chicken from tandoor and sprinkle the sprinkling ingredients over baked chicken.

Soups

In soup preparation, soup stock and its quality is utmost important. This soup stock includes juices and soluble portions of meat or fish, bones and vegetables which have been extracted by long and slow cooking. The basis of stock may be beef, veal, mutton, fish, poultry, game birds or animal's meat and vegetables. Proportions used in soup should be 2/3 meat, 1/3 bone and 1 part water. All waste portions of meat and bone and bits of cold cooked meats that have not been charred in cooking can be utilized in making stock.

Ingredients for Soup Stock

Vegetables and Seasonings

Soup vegetables include carrot, turnips, onions, tomato and seasoning used in soup are bay leaf, cloves, peppercorns, salt, and pepper.

Stock Preparation Procedure

1. Cut the meat in fine pieces and put it in cold water for ½ to 1 hour.
2. Heat to boiling point and then simmer slowly for 5 to 7 hours.
3. No starchy substance is added at this stage. After completion of cooking, strain and cool it quickly and leave the stock uncovered until cold.
4. The fat should not be removed from stock or broths during cooling as during cooling of stock, thin covering over the stock excluding air and preventing decomposition. But it should be entirely removed before reheating stock or broth with the help of cloth or by using tissue paper or a piece of bread.
5. The meat which remains after straining the stock may be used in any recipe.

Brown soup stock is prepared from beef, and the best results are obtained by browning a portion of the meat or by using cold cooked meat that is browned. It is usually seasoned with vegetables, spices, and herbs. While *white Soup stock* is prepared from veal, turkey, chicken or rabbit and delicately seasoned. Soup stock which is prepared from mutton is used only in special recipes and should not be combined with other meats.

Meat Soup

Ingredients

8-12 cups of water

½ kg meat (pork, beef, lamb, chicken etc.)

Table salt as desired

3-5 cups of herbs and spices

Procedure

1. Place the meat in kettle and pour water over the meat and after covering put the kettle on the fire. Kettle should be turned in every 5-10 minutes for uniform heating.
2. After boiling, it should be cooked for about one hour but meat should always be covered with water.
3. Wash and chop the herbs and spices and put it in soup when it is ready.
4. When meat becomes tender it is sliced to a spoon size and again put it to the soup.
5. Desired amount of salt is added at last. It can be served with bread pieces.

Fish Soup

Ingredients

½ kg trout, salmon, cod or another fish

10-12 cups of water

Table salt as desired

One cup of whipped cream

3-5 cups of herb and spices

Procedure

1. Clean and wash the fish and cut into small pieces.
2. Cook these pieces of fish till development of tenderness (20-30 minutes).
3. Debone the fish and again put them in the soup.
4. Add the whipped cream and chopped herbs and spices in soup.
5. Cook the soup for about 20-30 minutes.
6. Add desired quantity of salt and can be served with bread pieces.

Spinach and Minced Meat Soup

Spinach and Minced Meat Soup is a delicious and nutritious food. It is delicately flavoured with cumin and ginger and can be used as appetizer. When it is added with crusty bread or plain boiled rice then it serves as whole meal.

Ingredients

500g	Spinach
500g	Minced meat
2 teaspoon	Oil
2 teaspoon	Cumin seed
1 teaspoon	Grated ginger
2 large	Chopped fine onions
2 large	Chopped fine tomatoes
1 teaspoon	Chilli powder
1 teaspoon	Freshly ground black pepper
1 litre	Meat stock
2 teaspoon	Lime juice

Salt as desired

Procedure

1. Wash and drain the spinach and keep aside.
2. Put the oil in pressure cooker over flame and add cumin seed. When cumin seed splutter then add grated ginger and sauté for a minute.
3. Add onion and sauté till its softness and then add tomatoes, chilli powder, pepper and minced meat.
4. Stir and allow the meat to become brown.
5. Now add spinach and meat stock and cover the pressure cooker and increase the speed of flame.
6. When meat turns to brown then slow the speed of flame to facilitate simmering.
7. Now soup becomes ready to serve along with lime squeezing.

Pickles

Pickle is a shelf stable meat product and can be stored for years together at room temperature without preservation. It's a convenient, nutritious and delicious meat product. Its production technique is very simple and requires no special equipments. These products can be prepared from any type of meat and non tender meat can also be utilized in this product. It can be prepared either by pressure cooking the meat or by simple roasting the meat and with or without preservative like butylated hydroxy anisol (BHA) and butylated hydroxy toluene (BHT). Several naturally occurring acids can also be utilized in this product depending on consumers choice and availability like acetic acid, lactic acid, vinegar etc.

Ingredients

1kg	Freshly dressed meat
200g	Ginger
50g	Garlic
500g	Tamarind
30g	Mustard seed
1g	Nutmeg or mace
100g	Anise
50g	Cumin
10g	Cinnamon
250ml	Mustard oil
200ml	Vinegar
20g red	Chilli
120 ppm	Sodium nitrite

Salt as desired

Procedure

1. Make the pieces of meat into a size of 1-1/2 inches and clean them with water and wipe off by using clean cloth.
2. Make a paste of ginger and garlic with little vinegar and extract the tamarind juice by boiling and pressing.
3. Fry the meat pieces in 100 ml mustard oil till brown colour appears.
4. Add ginger and garlic paste and fry further for 2 minutes.
5. Add tamarind juice, spices, salt and continue cooking.
6. Add vinegar and continue cooking for 5 minutes.
7. Remove the vessel from fire and allow the ingredients to cool.
8. Heat the remaining oil to smoke point.
9. Place the cooled meat pickle hygienically in a sterilized glass jar or PET bottles.
10. Pour the heated and cooled oil in this jar.
11. Close the lid and store the meat pickle at room temperature.

Surimi

Surimi literally means "fish puree or slurry" and referring to a fish-based food product intended to mimic the texture and colour of the meat of lobster, crab and other shellfish. It is typically made from white-fleshed fish such as Pollock or hake that has been pulverized to a paste and attains a rubbery texture when cooked. The term is also commonly applied to food products made from lean meat prepared in a similar process. Examples of surimi products are chikuwa, crab stick, fish ball, hanpen, kamaboko, tsukune, tsumire and yong tau foo etc.

History

Surimi has been made for centuries by the Japanese and is thought to date as far back as 1100 A.D. The process for making surimi was developed in many areas of East Asia over 900 years ago. In Japan, it is used in the making of kamaboko or cured surimi products. Surimi industrial technology was developed by Japan in the early 1960s for the growth of surimi industry. The successful growth of the industry was based on the Alaska Pollock or walleye Pollock. Subsequently, production of Alaska Pollock surimi declined and was supplemented by surimi production using species other than Alaska Pollock. Currently, 2-3 million tons of fish around the world, amounting to 2-3 percent of the world fisheries supply, are used for the production of surimi and surimi-based products. The United States of America and Japan are major producers of surimi and surimi-based products. Thailand has become an important producer. China's role as producer is increasing. Many newcomers to the surimi industry have emerged including Vietnam, Chile, Faroe Island, France and Malaysia.

Fish Surimi

For surimi production fish is skinned, boned, repeatedly rinsed to eliminate fishiness and pigment. It is then ground into a paste. Depending on the desired texture and flavour of the surimi product, the gelatinous paste is mixed with differing proportions of additives such as starch, egg white, salt, vegetable, humectants, sorbitol, sugar, soy protein, seasoning and chemical enhancers such as transglutaminases and monosodium glutamate (MSG). This odourless white paste is then mixed with a flavour concentrate made from real shellfish, the solution from boiled shells or artificial flavourings. The paste is then formed, cooked and cut into the various shapes of the seafood it's imitating. Fish parts commonly used are crab legs, lobster chunks, shrimp and scallops. Lastly, surimi is coloured to complete its transformation from fish to shellfish. It can be kept unopened in the refrigerator for up to 2 months and in the

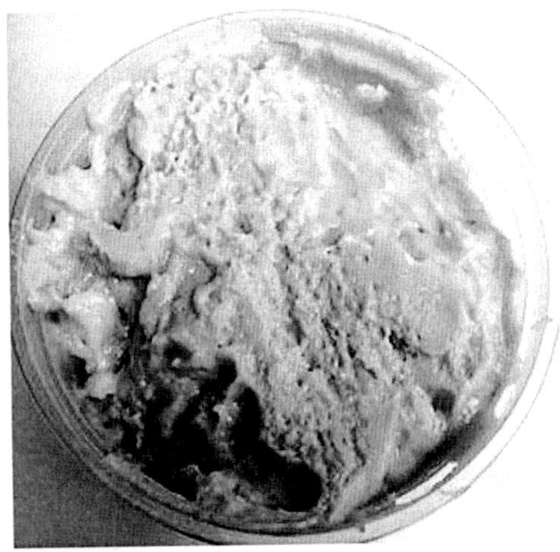

Surimi finish (*Source:* answer.com)

freezer for up to 6 months. Once opened its shelf life remains only 3 days.

Composition of fish surimi

Components	% contribution
Water	76
Protein	15
Carbohydrate	6.85
Fat	0.9
Cholesterol	0.03

Fishes used to make surimi are Milk fish (*Chanos chanos*), Swordfish (*Xiphias gladius*), Tilapia (*Oreochromis mossambicus, Oreochromis niloticus*), Big-head pennah croaker (*Pennahia macrocephalus*), Golden threadfin bream (*Nemipterus virgatus*), Cod (Gadus morhua), Bigeyes (*Priacanthus arenatus*), Pacific whiting (*Merluccius*), Alaska Pollock (*Theragra chalcogramma*) and Various shark species.

Meat Surimi

Meat surimi is less common product in western countries and Japan but pork surimi is a common product found in Chinese foods. The process of making pork surimi is similar to making fish surimi except that leaner cuts of meat are used and rinsing is not required. Pork surimi balls have similar texture as fish balls on cooking but are much firmer and denser than fish surimi. Pork surimi is also mixed with flour and water for better quality. Beef surimi can also be shaped into a ball to make beef balls. Surimi processing technology can also be used for making turkey products. It is used to make turkey burgers, turkey sausage, turkey pastrami, turkey franks, turkey loafs and turkey salami.

Smoked Fish

The basic purpose of smoking fish is its preservation but smoking also imparts typical smoked colour and flavour in the fish. In most of the time curing is prerequisite for fish smoking.

Brining

In common method of brining the fish, fishes are layered skin side down in container. Then salt is sprinkled over the fishes followed by spreading dark brown sugar over the fish. Repeat the process of layering fish and brining until the container is ¾ full of fish. This will facilitate expansion of fluid from the fishes. Storage is normally done in cool places or in refrigeration. After 24 hours fishes are examined for taste and readiness for smoking.

Smoking

After pulling out the fishes from brine, rinsing is done under tap water in a container. These fishes are then placed in smoker by skin side down. Smoke is then generated with wood and fishes are exposed to smoke for about 25 to 30 minutes. Then these fishes are cool down for 15 to 20 minutes. This process of smoking and cooling is repeated several times till the development of desired colour and taste. Care should be taken that fish should not cook. The steps involved in brining and smoking of fishes may be summarized as:

1. Brine the fish with basic brine solution containing ½ cup non-iodized salt, ½ cup sugar and 1 quart water. The fishes are placed in this brine in such a manner that brine should cover whole of the fishes. After mixing with brine fishes are placed in cool place or refrigeration for about 6-8 hrs in case of fishes less than 1 inch in thickness but in case of thick fishes (more than 1 inch thickness), fishes are kept for about 8 to 12 hours.

2. Remove brined fishes and rinse each piece under cold water. After rinsing make them dry with the help of dry cotton cloth and then allow to air dry for about one hour. After one hour we can observe glazed film over the fishes. This glazed film formation is called Pellicle which is a normal and desired characteristic of brining.

3. When fishes showing stickiness then place them in smoke house maintained at 93.3°C for 2 hours.

Smoked Fish in Soy Sauce and Wine Brine

For this purpose fillet of fishes are used along with other ingredients like sugar, non-ionized salt, soy sauce, water, onion and garlic powder, pepper and white wine. Make the brine of all ingredients mentioned above and soak the fishes in it for more than eight hours. Cover whole fishes in brine and refrigerate them. After completion of brining these fishes are exposed in smokehouse where smoke is generated by the combustion of hickory wood, alder wood or a mixture of 2/3 Apple and 1/3 Cherry wood. Smoking time is depends on size of fishes and type of smoke used.

Honey-Cured Smoked Salmon

The ingredients used in brine preparation for honey-cured smoked salmon are water, salt (½ cup), honey (¾ cup), golden rum (¼ cup), lemon juice (¼ cup), cloves (10), spices berries (10) and bay leaf (1). For making brine all ingredients are mixed. Salmon (1 large fillet) is placed in brine by skin side up in a non-reactive dish. Leave these fishes for about 2 hours in brine. Then rinse the salmon in fresh water and pat dry with paper towels. Place them on a drying rack and allow to air dry for about 1 hour. Keep the smoke salmon skin side down for about 1-2 hours at 71.1°C.

Smoked Fish Dip

For making smoked fish dip, crumbled smoked fish (1½ cups), light cream cheese (1 cup), finely minced onion (¼ cup), finely chopped celery and fresh parsley (1tsf each), sweet pickle relish (3 tsf), lemon juice (½ tsf), Worcestershire sauce (1 tsf) and cayenne, salt and pepper in desired quantity is required. Milk is added in smoked fish in a medium bowl and chill them for 30-60 minutes with the covered lid. Add the cream cheese, onion, celery, parsley, relish, lemon juice, Worcestershire sauce and cayenne, salt and pepper in a desired quantity with stirring. Cover and chill for 2 to 3 hours until flavour development.

Smoked Salmon Cakes

For making smoked salmon cake, smoked salmon, sweet pickle relish (¼ cup), bread crumbs (½ cup) and red bell pepper (1) are finely chopped in a bowl chopper. Then soy sauce (1tsf), mayonnaise (1/3 cup), slightly beaten eggs (2), dried herbs (1tsf), minced fresh dill (2tsf), curry (1tsf) and fresh ground black pepper (1tsf) are mixed with this mixture. Make 3 inches patties from this blend. Then sallow fry these patties in butter over medium to high heat. When foam subside arrange cakes and cook with periodic turning till brown colour develops.

Smoked Salmon Omelets

For the preparation of smoked salmon omlets eggs (12), salt (1tsf) and ground black pepper (½tsf) are first blended in bowl. Butter is placed (2tsf) in non-stick over medium heat and then egg mixture is put into skillet. Cook these eggs until egg softens. Place ¼ of the salmon on half of the omelet. Sprinkle 1 tablespoon onion and 1 teaspoon capers and place 2 tablespoons cream cheese on top. Fold omelet in half and slid out onto plate.

Smoked Salmon Mousse

Milk (250 ml) is heated to near boiling with one small peeled onion, eight peppercorns and 3 bay leaves. Leave it for 30 minutes then strain. Melt butter (1tsf) in a saucepan, add flour, mix to a roux then make into a white sauce with warmed strained milk. Dissolve 3 teaspoons gelatin in 3 tablespoons boiling water. Chop smoked salmon (200g) and mix together with mayonnaise (½ cup) gelatin, parsley (1 cup) and chives (½ cup). Whip cream and fold in. Whisk up egg whites and fold in. Add salt and fine black pepper in desired quantity. Pour mix into moulds and refrigerate overnight. Product is ready now for use.

Wok-Smoked Fish

Ingredients

Basic ingredient: 1kg (about ½ inch thick firm) white fish fillets such as sea bass or red snapper.

Marinade mixture: Marinade mixture contains 2 teaspoons minced ginger, ¼ cup rice wine, 3 tablespoons regular soy sauce, 3 tablespoons dark soy sauce, ½ teaspoon liquid smoke, 2 teaspoons sugar, ½ teaspoon Chinese five-spice and ½ teaspoon ground toasted Sichuan peppercorns.

Smoking Mixture: The ingredients of smoking mixture are ½ cup packed brown sugar, 1/3 cup uncooked long-grain rice ,1/3 cup black or oolong tea leaves and Julienned honeydew melon and cantaloupe for garnish.

Procedure: Make 3-inch square pieces of fish by cutting the fish crosswise. Then mix marinade ingredients in a bowl and leave it for 10 minutes. Add smoking mixture ingredients and spread evenly in a foil-lined wok. Place Fish on rack and place wok over high heat. When mixture begins to smoke, cover wok with a foil-lined lid and reduce heat to medium-low for about 7 to 8 minutes. Remove the product from heat and allow cooling with lid for 5 minutes.

Sweet Smoked Salmon

Salmon fillets are cut into 3 inches chunks with skin intact. Add the salt and keep in refrigeration for 12 to 14 hours Rinse the fish under cold water to remove all salt. Marinate the fish in the mixture of soy sauce (1 cup), 2 cups brown sugar, 1 cup honey, 2 tablespoons ground black pepper for about 24 to 36 hours. Place the fish in the smoke house with skin side down and smoke should be barkless. Smoking should be done in smokehouse at 71.1°C for 6 hours.

Smoked Red Snapper

Prepare the brine by dissolving enough salt in the cold water to float an egg. Add the sugar and the granulated garlic. Brine the fish for one hour. Then use frozen red snapper and put the frozen fish in the brine for about 2½ hours. Combine the olive oil, brown sugar, garlic and pepper to make a rub and rub it into the fish well. Oil the skin side lightly, so it won't stick to the smoking racks. Smoke the fish at 107.2°C for 60-75 minutes depending on thickness. Paint the fish with warmed maple syrup as a glaze. Allow to smoke and turn the fish periodically. Remove the product from smoke after colour and flavour development.

Reformed and Restructured Meat

In production of products such as restructured steaks, shrimp shapes, formed poultry parts, meat loaves, sectioned and formed roasts, turkey and chicken rolls and fish blocks, polyphosphates solubilize the protein that binds the pieces together and aids in moisture retention. Many meat analogues contain soy protein. Phosphates may be beneficial to improve yield and final product characteristics. The detail about this product manufacture is given in chapter-8.

Intermediate Moisture Meat (IMM)

Intermediate moisture meat is a product normally contains moisture of about 20-50% and also has the ability to maintain texture and juiciness on rehydration. These products are shelf stable at room temperature and have water activity around 0.6 to 0.85. The compounds generally used to reduce the water activity are known as humectants. These are low molecular weight compounds like glycerols, propylene glycol, sodium chloride, sorbitol, sucrose, dextrose, corn syrup. The drawback of these meat is the development of fungal growth so potassium sorbate, sodium benzoate, propylene glycol should be added in these compounds. The techniques used for production of IMM are moist infusion or desorption, dry infusion or adsorption and component blending. Whatever technique is applied the basic aim is to reduce water activity, retardation of microbial and fungal growth and improvement of sensory attributes. The examples of IMM are sweet and sour pork.

The products prepared from meat, fish, poultry and game animals are numerous. The discussion of all these products is not possible in this text book. The products which are prepared from animal and fish tissues gives variety to the products and satisfy the consumers need. Only need is to exploit some technologies for their preparation and quality control.

References

1. Briskey, E.J. (1964). Etiological status and associated studies of pale, soft, exudative porcine musculature. Adv. Food Res. 13, 89.
2. Forrest, J.C., Aberle, E.D., Hedrick, H.B., Judge, M.D. and Merkel, R.A. (1969). Structure and Composition of Muscle and Associated tissues. In: Principles of Meat Science, W.H. Freeman and Company, San Francisco, pp 27-89.
3. Hamm, R. (1960). Biochemistry of meat hydration. Adv. Food Res. 10:355.
4. Hedrick, H.B., Aberle, E.D., Forrest, J.C., Judge, M.D. and Merkel, R.A. (1994).Principles of Meat Science, 3rd ed., Kendall/Hunt Publishing Company, Dubuque, Iowa.
5. Jay, J.J. (1986). Modern Food Microbiology, 4th ed., Van Nostrand Reinhold, AVI, New York, New York.
6. Kierant, B.H., Johnson, J.A. and Siedler, A.J. (1964). A summary of nutrient content of meat. Am. Meat Inst. Found. Bull. No. 47.
7. Newbold, R.P. (1966). Changes associated with rigor mortis. In "The Physiologyand Biochemistry of Muscle as Food" (E.J. Briskey, R.G. Cassens and J.C.Trautman, eds.), pp. 213-224. Univ. of Wisconsin Press, Madison.
8. Pearson, A.M., and Gillett, T.A. (1997). In: Processed Meats. 3rd ed. CBS Publishers & Distributors, New Delhi. Sun X. D. (2009). Utilization of restructuring technology in the production of meat products: a review. Informa World, 7 (2):153-162.
9. Sharma, B.D. (1999). Structure, composition and nutritive value of meat tissues. In: Meat and Meat Products Technology (Including Poultry Products Technology), Jaypee Brothers Medical Publishers (P) Ltd, New Delhi. pp 8-22.
10. Benoit V.G. and Chateau, D. (2007). World Surimi Market. Globefish Research Programme, Volume 89.

□□□□

11 Physico-Chemical and Microbiological Quality of Meat and Aquatic Food and Food Products

Physico-chemical and microbiological quality of meat and aquatic food and food products gives its overall safety and quality status as a food. The physico-chemical and microbiological qualities of raw material have great importance on the product development. It also affects the shelf life of the raw material as well as final product.

Fresh meat is a type of meat which has not been subjected to any processing whereas raw meat is a fresh meat which has undergone freezing. The qualities of fresh meat are important as far as merchandiser, purchaser and consumers are concerned and it is also important for adaptability in further processing. The important quality parameters of fresh meat are:

1. Meat colour.
2. Water holding capacity.
3. Marbling.
4. Quantum of connective tissue.
5. Firmness.
6. pH
7. Tenderness or shear force value
8. Emulsion stability.
9. Texture and fiber size

1. Meat Colour

Meat colour is a total visual perception which can be defined in terms of Hue, Chroma and Value on the basis of myoglobin content and its chemical state. Hue means primary colour or type of colour; for example red, white etc. Chroma means intensity of colour. Value means overall brightness or reflectance of the colour. Meat colour is actually overall impression seen by the eyes. The colour of meat varies with the animal species, sex, age, and among different muscles of same species. The typical colour of meat in different animal species is:

Beef	- Bright cherry red colour
Buffalo meat	- Dark red
Veal	- Pale grey to greyish red
Chevon	- Light red
Mutton	- Light red to brick red colour
Pork	- Brownish pink
Poultry	- Grey white to dull red
Horse meat	- Dark red with bluish tinge
Camel meat	- Red
Dog meat	- Dark red
Rabbit meat	- Pale grey to grey red
Venison	- Dark red to brownish red

The colour of meat is predominantly dependant on the meat pigment myoglobin. Myoglobin constitutes about 80-90 % of total meat pigments. Role of haemoglobin in meat colour is almost negligible in properly bled muscles whereas, catalase and cytochrome enzymes are of little consequences in meat colour. Colour of meat is also dependant on oxidation state of the iron within heme ring.

Myoglobin molecule contains globin (protein portion) and heme (iron containing) ring. It is ¼ of size of structurally similar haemoglobin molecule. In normal intact meat, iron in the heme ring of myoglobin exists in reduced form (Fe2+) and due to this reduced form meat shows purple colour. This reduced form of myoglobin might be due to normal enzyme activity that is called Electron transport chain. Upon cutting or grinding meat comes in contact of air or oxygen and changes its colour. This colour change phenomenon may be of two types:

a. If the exposure of air or oxygen to the meat is in small quantity as in case of partial vacuum or a sealed semipermeable package then it forms brown colour due to oxidation of iron portion of myoglobin and formation of met myoglobin. The formation of brown colour is not a desirable characteristic because of low merchandise value and association with long term stored meat.

b. If the exposure of meat with air or oxygen becomes full then reduced myoglobin react with molecular oxygen and forms oxymyoglobin (relatively stable pigment) within 30-45 minutes after exposure to air. This oxymyoglobin is responsible for development of bright red colour (bloom) in fresh meat which is a desirable characteristic.

So the package for fresh meat should have high oxygen and low water permeability. Cellophane, PVC (polyvinyl chloride) and PE (poly ethylene) films may serve this purpose.

Facts Related to Meat Colour

i. The myoglobin contents of more active species are higher than passive species i.e Game animals have darker muscles than domestic animals.

ii. The more active parts of the body within the species contains more myoglobin than passive parts i.e. muscles of breast in poultry is lighter than muscles of leg and thigh.

iii. The pale colour of veal carcass is due to less myoglobin content as compared to mature animals.

iv. The muscles of uncastrated male contain more myoglobin than females and castrated males of respective age.

v. In general beef and mutton contain more myoglobin as compared to pork, veal, fish and poultry.

2. *Water Holding Capacity (WHC)*

WHC is an ability of meat to hold water during application of external forces i.e. cutting, heating, grinding, pressing etc. Water is an universal solvent and constitute about 76% of fresh meat. In meat water molecule carry +ve and –ve charges and on that basis water exists in three different forms:

a. *Free water*: water molecule held by capillary forces on the surface make up free water. This water can be removed by application of even minor physical force.

b. *Immobilised water*: The middle layer of water molecules remains in contact with proteins and forms Immobilised water. A large part of which can be removed by application of severe physical conditions.

c. *Bound water*: 4-5% of water molecules are so tightly bound to the charged hydrophilic groups in muscle protein that they do not allow this bound water to escape by application of any physical force.

Role of Water Holding Capacity

i. In fresh meat it is responsible for colour, texture and firmness whereas, in cooked meat for juiciness and tenderness.

ii. It has a direct effect on shrinkage of meat during storage i.e. meat with high WHC exhibit less shrinkage during storage than meat with low WHC.

iii. It helps in deciding the method of processing and save cooking energy.

iv. It has direct effect on yield of meat products.

Terms related to weight loss during storage are entirely dependant on the water holding capacity of the meat. The terms related to weight loss are shrink and weep. Shrink is loss of meat weight during storage while Weep is production of visible meat juice.

3. Marbling

Marbling refers to the intramuscular fat which can be visibly detected when the muscle surface is cut.

Role of Marbling

i. It contributes to the firmness after fat solidification.

ii. It has merchandising value that's by it is prominently figures in USDA quality grades.

iii. It helps in maintenance of certain retail cuts in handling of chilled meat i.e. chops and steaks.

iv. It enables meat to bear higher cooking temperature during thermal processing.

v. Marbling decides the juiciness and flavour of meat products. Moderately marbled meat yields a juicy and flavourful product whereas, little marbling yield dry and flavourless product. But excess marbling is not desirable.

4. Quantum of Connective Tissue (C.T.) or Texture

The amount of connective tissue has a direct effect on textural characteristics. More active muscles in the animal body tend to deposit more connective tissue to gain strength i.e. biceps femoris has a coarse texture and loin eye muscle has tenderness. But it is a noticeable point that quantum of C.T./unit muscle does not increase with age and is not responsible for toughness of meat in older animals. In fact, it is increase in muscle fibre diameter and consequent increase in muscle fibre bundles which account for the coarse texture of such meat.

Significance of Texture

i. Cutting of meat is mainly based on texture i.e. coarse with tender etc.

ii. It decides the cooking procedure.

iii. It derives maximum palatability pleasure.

5. *Firmness*

Firmness is a state of 'setting up' of carcase during chilling.

Factors Deciding Firmness of Meat

i. During carcass chilling, firmness increases due to loss of extensibility associated with the completion of rigor mortis.

ii. Firmness is also dependant on the solidification of fat within and surrounding the muscles.

iii. Firmness of meat is dependent on the length of sarcomere; if it is very short then it shows high degree of overlap of filaments and very tight and dense microstructure.

In general meat with a good degree of firmness yields comparatively better quality processed meat product. It can be measured with the help of shear force apparatus or penetrometer.

Role of Firmness

In carcase setting, fabrication, ageing, processing, slicing and product display.

6. *pH of Meat*

Freshly slaughtered cattle and buffalo have an average pH of 6.4 to 6.8 and in some cases up to 7.2. Then after pH falls rapidly to attain ultimate pH (5.6). In case where it does not fall normally or falls rapidly below ultimate pH then leads to the conditions like PSE and DFD meat. In PSE, pH falls very rapidly while in DFD, it falls very little within 48 hours of slaughter. If pH of meat remains near 6.4 or above it may lead to deteriorative changes very rapidly. The pH of meat of different animals ranges from 5.1 to 6.2 in beef, 5.3 to 6.9 in pork and 5.4 to 6.7 in lamb meat.

7. *Shear Force Value or Tenderness*

Shear force value is a measurement of tenderness of the meat and meat products. For shear force value evaluation, meat or meat products are cut or shear by using Warner Bratzler Shear Press (a mechanized shear device). Now a day automatic texture analyzers are also available to analyse the texture of meat and meat products. Tenderness of meat is an important factor in the quality of meat that makes the meat palatable and acceptable by the consumers. Meat of younger animals is tenderer than meat of older animals due to less dense connective tissues in younger ones. The meat of younger animals is also broken down during the heat treatment. More tender meats and meat products are more liked by the consumers due to its palatability, juiciness and less mechanical force of teeth requirement during mastication.

8. Emulsion Stability

Emulsion stability is the capacity of meat emulsion to hold the meat juice and its quality characteristics during cooking in water or any other heat treatment. Myofibrillar proteins are good emulsifying agents and contribute much more in emulsion stability. These proteins are especially actin and myosin which are insoluble in water and soluble in salt solutions. Several factors are responsible for good emulsion stability like temperature during emulsification, fat particle size, amount and type of soluble proteins, pH, rigor state of meat and viscosity of the emulsion. It is also considered that more stable emulsion is formed at higher pH value. As far as emulsion stability is concerned prerigor meat is superior than post rigor meat because extraction of salt soluble protein is 50% greater in prerigor meat emulsion. The amount of fat emulsified per unit of protein is called emulsification capacity.

9. Texture and Fiber Size

The size of muscle fiber is proportionate to the size of the fiber bundle and it increases with the chronological age of animals. The fiber grouping on perimyseal connective tissue (muscle bundle) is positively associated with the coarseness of muscle fibers. It also depends on the fiber type (red or white), species and breed of animals, post natal development etc. Texture is an overall impression of the muscle fibers in the muscle (course/ firm). Increase in thickness of connective strand and size of muscle fibers contributes to coarseness. Coarseness in muscle texture may also be due to softness of exudative muscle.

The chemical quality and the composition of meat and meat products is given in detail in the chapter-4. So it is not relevant to discuss same thing again.

Factors Affecting Physico-Chemical and Microbiological Qualities of Meat Foods

In normal condition and well rested animals meat appears normal in colour and qualities. Certain factors which are greatly affecting physico-chemical and microbiological qualities of the meat, meat products, aquatic foods and food products are discussed below:

A. Pre-Slaughter Factors

a. Environmental Factors

Environmental factors like extreme temperature, humidity, light, sound and space are certain factors affecting meat characteristics in various ways. Their effect is also variable depending upon the type of species, weight, age, sex, inherent stress resistance and emotional state of meat animals.

1. In case of extreme temperature body conserves heat, shivering leads to reduction in body glycogen levels and in high temperature metabolic reactions speed up to cope up from body heat and ATP is splitted. These all factors induces stress to the meat animals.
2. The humidity should be optimum for meat animals otherwise animals come in stress because humidity influences the severity of temperature.
3. Extreme light, sound and inadequate space creates stress to the animals particularly due to secretion of epinephrine or norepinephrine which leads to the fatigue condition. This condition greatly affects meat quality post mortem.
4. The animals are of three types normal, stress susceptible and stress resistant. In stress susceptible animals heat stroke, shock and circulatory collapse are the common consequences. In pigs, stress susceptible animals develop condition known as porcine stress syndrome which exhibits extreme muscularity, anxious behaviour,

muscle tremors and reddening of skin. Stress susceptible animals have rapid glycolysis rate and produce PSE and DFD meat. However, in stress resistant animals glycolysis rate is slow which leads to high pH and meat of dry or sticky texture with excellent water binding capacity. In stress resistant beef, pork and lamb dark cutting meat condition is observed which shows unattractive dark, firm, dry appearance and favourable pH for bacterial growth.

b. Hereditary and Animal Production Factors

1. Heritability of stress susceptible and stress resistant animals is the important factor to consider for quality assessment of meat. Beside, animals breed and strain is also important for quantity and quality meat production.

2. Physico-chemical qualities of meat tissue are not much influenced by these factors. Only chemical composition of the muscle can be altered by these means.

3. Transportation handling of meat animals is an important factor for quality meat production. Care must be taken to avoid stress to the animals during transportation. During this process, glycogen depletion is a normal phenomenon. So to avoid it, starchy feeds and sugars should be given to the animals.

4. Immobilization process greatly influences the properties and composition of muscles and glycogen level in these muscles.

5. Bleeding process has great impact on the microbiological quality and shelf life of meat and meat products.

B. Post-Slaughter Factors

1. Post mortem changes are greatly influenced by the temperature at which carcase are held. The enzymatic changes which takes place in meat are also temperature sensitive.

2. The conditions like thaw rigor and cold shortening produces tough meat than normal rigor. Thaw rigor is a severe type of rigor mortis develops when prerigor meat is thaw. In this condition 60-80% physical shortening of the original muscles takes place. If prerigor

meat is directly exposed to above 0°C but below 15 to16°C then cold shortening occurs. It is less severe shortening than thaw rigor. It is mainly due to release of calcium ions which leads to the muscle rigidity. Shortening of muscles is indirectly proportional to the tenderness. As the shortening increases, tenderness decreases.

3. Certain processing steps like scalding (in pigs and poultry), dehairing, skinning and evisceration have direct impact on the quality of meat.

4. Carcase suspension for tension induction in the muscles reduces the chances of cold shortening thus produces more tender meat.

5. The time interval between slaughtering and processing affects physical properties of the finished product.

Physico-Chemical Properties of Aquatic Food and Food Products

Fresh fishes are bright, their eyes are full and shinning with clear, transparent pupils and gills are bright and pink in colour with intact scales. Few hours later of catching, fish becomes rigid with slimmy greyish exudates, gills become greyish slimmy, eyes become concave in appearance with milky pupils and scales may be detached easily. Spoilage after rigor mortis development leads to easy pitting, flesh separation from bones and perforation of the abdominal cavity.

Aquatic foods contain unmatched nutritional qualities. Proteins obtained from sea foods are best at the nutritional point of view as it is easily digestible, contains all essential amino acids and have hypocholesterolemic properties. Lipid contents found in aquatic foods serve energy purpose, polyunsaturated fatty acids of fishes is supposed to lower the body cholesterol, eicosapentaenoic and docosahexaenoic acids play vital role in functioning of nervous system and blood clotting. Carbohydrate content in the fishes is almost nil while it is 0.5% in crustaceans and in significant amount in molluscan shellfish (mostly in form of glycogen). Crustaceans are higher in free amino acid contents and catheptic like enzymes while molluscan shellfish are lower in total nitrogen quantity in their flesh.

Fresh slaughtered fish meat is soft, pliable and elastic in texture. On the commencement of rigor mortis fish meat becomes stiff and inflexible and on completion it again turns to soft and pliable.

Chemical composition of fishes and other aquatic foods

Contents	Quantity (%)	Special features
Water	60-80	Highest (90%) in Bombay duck (*Harpondon nehereus*).
Protein	15-24	Finfish and shellfish contains 8 to 15%while it is 5 to 14% in some shellfishes like oyster.
Lipids	0.2 to 60-65	Lean muscles contains about 0.5 to 1% phospholipids.
Ash (Minerals)	0.4 - 2	-
Sodium	30-134 mg/100g	
Potassium	19-502 mg/100g	
Calcium	19-881 mg/100g	
Magnesium	68-550 mg/100g	
Iron	1-5.6 mg/100g	
Chlorine	3-761 mg/100g	
Iodine	0-2.73 mg/100g	
Vitamins	-	Good source of Vitamins especially-Fat soluble vitamins- Vitamin-A, D&E Water soluble Vitamins- Riboflavin, Nicotinic acid, Pyridoxine, Cyano-cobalamin, Pantothenic acid& Biotin
Carbohydrates	0.1-7	Carbohydrate is found mainly in glycogen form. Fresh fish contains 0.1 to 1% glycogen while its range in some molluscs like clam or mussel is 1 to 7%.
Non- protein nitrogenous(NPN) compounds	9-35	In teleosts 9 -18%, in molluscs& crustaceans 20-25% and in elasmobranchs 30-35%
Free amino acids	0.5-2% of muscle weight	
Nucleotides		-
Peptides	Insignificant quantity	
Guanidino-compound		
Betains	300-700mg%	
Urea		
Quaternary ammonium	400-1000 mg%	
compounds	5 mg% 1%	

Source: Balachandran, 2001. In: Post-harvest technology of Fish and Fish Products

Microbiological Quality of Meat and Aquatic Food and Food Products

Meat and sea foods are highly perishable foods and are very much vulnerable to the microbial spoilage owing to their intrinsic and extrinsic factors. Intrinsic factors like high moisture content, near neutral pH, substantial quantities of nutrients and high microbial load makes meat and sea food more perishable. While extrinsic factors like storage temperature, relative humidity, initial microbial load further aid to the spoilage.

Meat and Meat Products

C. Microbial Quality of Fresh Meat

Freshly slaughtered carcases of animals and fishes contain very few or almost negligible number of organisms. At the time of slaughter or just after, number of sources contribute towards microbial contamination of meat and meat products such as soil, water, feed, manure, intestinal contents of animals and through knives, workers, cloths, hands during slaughtering operations, skinning, cutting etc.

A number of organisms are responsible for meat and meat products deterioration like *Pseudomonas* species, *Achromobacter* species, *Microbacterium thermosphactum, Lactobacter* species and some mould species like *Cladosporium, Thamnidium* or *Mucor* etc. The contamination of meat and its products may lead to deterioration and depicts slime formation, taint or malodour formation, tainted sour, stale and putrid. The slime formation normally occurs above the total count of 10^7 to 10^8 per square cm.

Organism	Responsible for Changes
Pseudomonas species	Off odour and flavour.
Achromobacter species, *Microbacterium thermosphactum*	Spoilage in processed meat.
Lactobacteriaceae species	Spoilage of vacuum packaged cuts or ground meat.
Mould species like *Cladosporium, Thamnidium* or *Mucor*	Spoilage of beef sides or quarters during prolong storage at 0°C.

For the control of microbial contamination in fresh meat, control of moisture, pH and microbial load are the important factors to be controlled. For that purpose pH of the fresh meat should be below 6.0 because pH above 6.0 favours the growth of spoilage organisms. Surface moisture is controlled by maintaining suitable relative humidity and air speeds in the cooling chambers. Relative humidity in between 90 to 95% and air speed about 40,000 cubic feet per minute retards the growth of spoilage organisms. Other considerable point in fresh meat spoilage control is growth of Psychrophiles because they grow at refrigeration temperature. For this purpose meat should be stored at -1.1°C to +1.7°C. For the control of micro-organisms at meat surface ozone or ultraviolet rays are used in holding chambers of meat but it initiates oxidation.

D. Microbial Quality of Cooked and Cured Meat Products

Meat products are cured and cooked to impart meat colour, flavour, aroma taste and palatability. Cured products like ham and bacon, cooked products like cooked sausages also get spoiled during its processing, packaging or storage.

Cured meat products: The products like ham and bacon are used in form of processed, boiled, sliced, packaged, heat pasteurized or sterilized products. Among them pasteurized or sterilized products are more stable than others. Commercially sterile canned foods like canned ham and luncheon meat is rarely spoiled or do not spoil due to low level of spore formers and their sensitization by heat, salt and nitrite.

Cured meat type	Spoilage organisms
Sliced ham and bacon	Souring due to *Streptococcus faecium, S. faecalis* and *Microbacterium thermosphactum*
Pasteurized canned products	*Bacillus* sps., *Clostridium* sps., *Enterococci, Streptococci* and heat resistant lactic acid bacteria
Refrigerated canned products	Streptococcus sps.

Fresh and cooked sausages: The spoilage in sausages mainly occurs due to faulty processing, packaging or storage. In fresh uncooked sausages putrefaction or souring is most widely observed while in cooked sausages greening and sliming are the main changes has been seen. The main spoilage observed in sausages is greening. It is a combined reaction of ferrous state of iron in the porphyrin ring of (pink in colour) nitrosohemachrome (transformed from nitrosohaemochromogen produced in cured meat colour development from nitrite) and hydrogen per oxide produced by bacterial activities in sausages. The result product is verdoheme or choleglobin which is green in colour.

Type of sausage	Type of spoilage	Organisms responsible
Fresh uncooked sausages	Putrefaction	*Achromobacter* and *Pseudomonas*
	Souring	*Microbacterium thermosphactum,M. faecium and Streptococcus faecalis*
Cooked sausages	Irregular green spots on surface	*Lactobacteriaceae, Leuconostoc, Strepetococci* and *Pediococci*
	Green cores	*Lactobacillus* sps.
	Narrow green rings within the product	Due to enzyme liberation of certain organisms but actual cause is not well known
Cooked sausages	Sliming	Yeast, *Leuconostoc, Lactobacillus sps.* and *Microbacterium thermosphactum*

To avoid the spoilage of cured and cooked meat products there are number of precautions has to be taken. Some of these are; cooling of carcases to an internal temperature of 1.7°C, treatment with pickle solution maintained at -3.3 to 2.2°C, meat products should be stored frozen and thawing should be done at 4.4°C, refrigeration temperature must be maintained during whole storage, cooking of the products should be done at internal temperature of 71.1°C and sanitation, hygienic procedures must be followed during whole process of slaughtering, processing, packaging, preservation and marketing.

Poultry Meat and Meat Products

The source of poultry contamination is soil, water, defeathuring, pinning knives, personnel, intestines, scalding, washing etc. Normally bacterial count above 10^7 per squire cm produces off odour and above 10^8causes slime formation in poultry meat. The organisms causes spoilage in poultry meat is generally belongs to *Pseudomonas* group like *P. fragi, P.putida, P. ambigua, P. fluorescens* but the species of *Xanthomonas* are also causes spoilage in poultry meat. To minimize these count good sanitary and hygienic conditions should be maintained and meat should also be stored at frozen or chilled condition below 7.2°C.

Egg and Egg Products

It is again a fact that freshly laid egg is almost sterile and only 1% of the naturally cleaned eggs is spoiled. The bacteria most commonly found in freshly laid egg is *Lactobacteriaceae* but it does not cause spoilage of eggs. Normally 10^2 to 10^3 per square cm bacterial count is found in eggs which varies as per the cleanliness of cages.

Shelled eggs quality: Shelled egg contains naturally protective layer called cuticle which effectively seals the egg pores and helps in retaining contents of egg. It also acts as a natural barrier against microbial invasion. Native protein of egg is called egg white but it does not support the growth of microbes while nitrogenous material present in egg favours microbial growth. The components of eggs prevent the invasion of microbes are:

Egg component	Location in egg	Protective mechanism
Lysozyme	Egg albumin	Lysis gram +ve bacteria
Avidin	Egg albumin	Sequesters with biotin and making it unavailable to organisms needs for their growth
Egg albumin protein	Egg albumin	Sequesters with riboflavin and Vitamin-B3 making them unavailable to organisms needs for their growth
Conalbumin	Portion of egg albumin that is not crystallized	Most effective bacterial inhibitor. It sequesters with iron which is essential for the growth of *Pseudomonas*.

Spoilage of shelled eggs and their causative agent

Spoilage condition	Changes observed	Causative agents
Green rots	Egg white becomes green in colour which fluorescent under UV light. In later stage yolk disintegrates and mixes with white. Sweet or fruity odours.	*Pseudomonas fluorescens*
Colourless rots	Encrusted or disintegrated yolk with no odour but sometimes fruity odour.	*Pseudomonas* & *Achromobacter*
Red or pink rots	Red or pink pigmentation without fluorescent. Egg white sometimes liquefied with spots of brown, pink or red. Pinkish coagulum may appear in the yolk	*Pseudomonas*
Black rots	Egg white becomes liquefied; yolk becomes coagulated and turns black. Egg gives faecal, putrid or hydrogen sulphide odour	*Proteus melanoveogenes* & *Pseudomonas* sps.
Miscellaneous rots	Miscellaneous type rot is seen	*Pseudomonas, Serratia, Alcaligenes* etc.
Fungal rots	Coagulation or liquefaction of eggs with musty odour. Moulds initially develops on surface then it penetrates the shell and grow inside and causes changes.	Moulds of *Penecillium, Mucor,Cladosporium* and *Sporotrichum*

To prevent the growth of micro-organisms on shelled egg water used for washing should be mixed with disinfectants. Eggs laying cages should be clean. The storage of eggs should be done at -1.1°C to 0°C under the relative humidity of 80 to 82%.

Liquid egg products quality: Dried or frozen egg liquid products contain 10^4 to 10^5 organisms per ml. Principle organisms contaminate the liquid eggs are *Flavobacterium, Alcaligenes, Proteus, Pseudomonas* and *Escherichia*. To lower down the count of *Salmonella* organisms as well as total count egg liquid should be pasteurized at 60°C to 62.8°C for 1-4 minutes. Temperature near 4.4°C should be maintained during whole processing of egg liquid.

Fish and other Aquatic Foods

Fish and other aquatic foods are also sterile at the time of freshly caught and slaughtered. They get contaminated through slime, gills, intestines, water, ice, equipments, personnel and pens.

Fresh aquatic foods quality: The most commonly infected micro-organisms are Psychrophilic and Psychrotrophic bacteria. Organisms commonly found in gills and slime of fresh fish and shrimp are *Pseudomonas, Achromobacter, Vibrio, Flavobacterium, Micrococci* and *Corynebacterium.* Some organisms are mainly found in warm waters viz. *Bacilli* and others are in intestines of aquatic foods viz. *Clostridium welchii, C. sporogenes, C. tetani and C. botulinum* (Type-E). Among them *Pseudomonas* and *Achromobacter* are the main genera causes spoilage in aquatic foods. Among the *Pseudomonas* species 20 to 25% are of *P.fragi* types found in fish spoilage but hydrogen sulphide production in Atlantic cod and haddock is due to *P. putrefaciens.* For spoilage of aquatic foods bacterial counts should exceeds above 10^7 to 10^8 per gram in case of *Pseudomonas* and 10^8 to 10^9 per gram in case of *Achromobacter*. The signs of spoilage in aquatic foods are Bilgy odour due to hydrogen sulphide production by anaerobic bacteria and sweet, fishy, musty, amonical, sour or putrid odour due to aerobic bacteria. Fishy odour is mainly due to the production of trimethylamine by the action of enzyme triamineoxidase from trimethylamine oxide found in fish muscle.

Shelf life of fishes in best handling methods and storage at 0°C

Fishes	pH	Shelf life (in days)
Cod and haddock	6.5-7.0	15
Halibut	5.8 -6.8	19-24
Indian Mackerel	-	18-20
Fish fillets and steaks	-	7

To prevent the spoilage of aquatic foods, preservation in ice should be done in a manner that the layer of ice should come in between the container and fishes. Preservation in boxes prevents the mechanical damage to the fishes. It is also necessary to prevent the spoilage that the fishes or shrimps or other aquatic foods should be stored just after catch.

Cured aquatic foods quality: The initial quality of aquatic food is important for processing. Spoilage in cured fishes and other sea foods depends on the extent of salting and also on mode of salting. The organisms responsible for cured sea food spoilage may be summarized as:

Types of sea food	Organisms responsible for spoilage	Peculiar signs of spoilage, if any
Lightly salted and lightly smoked	Pseudomonas and Micrococci	-
Heavily salted and heavily smoked	Less affected by bacteria but more vulnerable to mould growth	-
Hot smoked fishes	Micrococci and Clostridia	-
Heavily salted fishes	Halotolerant Micrococci and Yeast	Type of deterioration named 'Pink' develops in which slime, softening of fish occurs
Salted dry sea foods	Moulds of genera Sporendonema and Oospora	Small brown, black or fawn coloured spots develops

Meat and meat products, egg and egg products and aquatic foods are the nutritious, precious and essential food items for human beings. They can not only satisfy the human hunger but also supplements essential nutrients like protein (amino acids),fat (fatty acids), minerals, vitamins and certain other nutrients. They provide the choice to the consumers with good palatability and compatibility. But these food items are perishable in nature so due care is required during processing, packaging and preservation. In meat and meat products including poultry meat *Salmonella* is a main threat, *Staphylococcus* may develop through human contacts and environments while *Clostridium* comes through intestines and surfaces. In aquatic food and food products *Salmonella* is not a threat but it may occur in frogs. The best way to minimize the contamination is to adopt the sanitary and hygienic measures.

Standard microbiological profile of meat food products including sea foods (counts/g)

Meat food product type	Total plate count	Coliforms	*E. coli*	*Staphylococcus*	*Salmonella*	*Clostridium*
Raw meat	10^5-10^7	Absent in 0.01-0.1g	10-100	Absent in 50g	Absent	-
Chilled and frozen meat	10^3	100	100	100	Absent in 25g	30
Precooked sausages	Not more than 10^3	Absent in 0.1g	Absent	Absent	Absent	Absent
Cured ham	Less than 10^3	-	-	-	-	-
Cooked baked meat products	Not more than 10^5	Absent in 0.01g	Not demonstrable	-	-	-
Fish & shellfish	$5x10^4$-10^6	0.7-$1.6x10^3$	Not more than 10^2	-	-	-
Frozen sea foods	Not more than 10^5	Not more than 20	Not more than 10^2	-	-	-
Oysters	Not more than $5x10^4$	$1.6x10^4$	-	-	-	-

(*Source*: Sahoo *et al*., 1993)

References

1. Balachandran, K.K. (2001). Biochemistry and Nutrition. In: Post-Harvest Technology of Fish and Fish Products, Daya Publishing House, Delhi : 1-27.
2. Forrest, J.C., Aberle, E.D., Hedrick, H.B., Judge, M.D. and Merkel (1998). Properties of fresh meat. In: Principles of Meat Science, W.H. Freeman and Company, San Francisco.175-183.
3. Gracey, J., Collins, D.S. and Huey, R. (1999). Food poisioning and meat microbiology. In: Meat Hygiene, 10th ed.W.B. Saunders Company, London: 353.
4. Kumar, A. and Singh, Y. (2007). Fish, their physical and bacteriological quality. In: Universal Meat Hygiene in Public Health Care by Vijendra Singh, Ist ed., International Book Distributing Company, Lucknow: 267-276.
5. Sahoo, J., Samoon, A.H. and Yadav, K.N. (1993). Standards formulation and quality control aspects of Indian meat industry-a perspective review. The Journal of Remount & Veterinary Corps, Vol. XXXII (4):223-224.
6. Savagaon, K.A. (1978). Microbiology of meat, fish and poultry. Indian Food Packer. XXXII (5):50-57.

□□□□

12 Basics of Sensory Evaluation of Meat Products

Sensory evaluation is a scientific method of evaluating foods including meat products that applies principles of experimental design and statistical analysis through the use of human senses like sight, smell, taste, touch and hearing. It is also called organoleptic evaluation in which we measure, analyse and interpret reactions to those characteristics of materials as they are perceived by the human senses. These attributes can be perceived well by the human sense organs as compared to instruments available for this purpose. It is a fact that no single instrument is able to assess all the attributes of meat products. With the help of these instruments we can very well evaluate the single quality attribute of meat product i.e. shear force instrument or penetrometer is good for knowing the texture and refractometer is for colour interpretation.

Importance of Sensory Evaluation

1. It helps to visualize parameters of the product which are better than any other product.
2. It opens up an opportunity for improving the product by making aware about lacunae in the product.
3. It is a useful tool for new product development.
4. It can be used for monitoring of product performance against its competitors in the market.

5. It can be used as a consumer acceptability index to determine the consumer's preference for a particular product.
6. It assist in determining the shelf life of the product and suitability of packaging material.
7. It gives an idea about raw material specifications and it may also be helpful in reducing the cost of products.
8. It is useful for research and product analysis.
9. It can be used to describe the correct procedures for temperature control, coring, shearing and serving samples to panels.

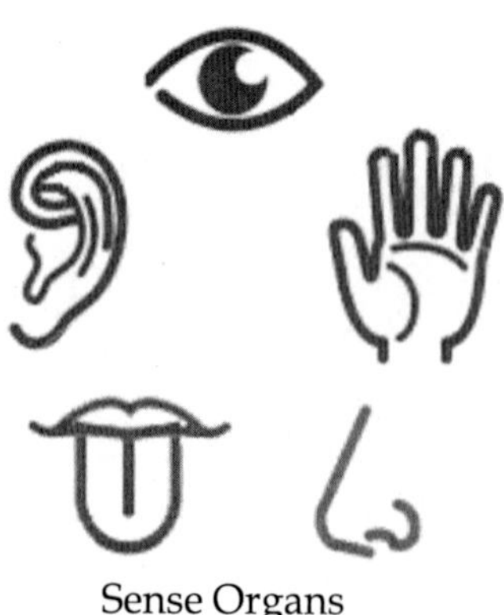

Sense Organs

Sensory Attributes

The important attributes to be evaluated in sensory evaluation are colour and appearance, texture and consistency, smell and taste, mouth feel and overall acceptability.

Colour and Appearance

Colour is an impression of light on the meat pigment myoglobin and expressed in terms of hue (primary colour), chroma (intensity) and value (brightness) in the meat products whereas; appearance is the overall impression of meat colour, size and shape, surface texture and clarity of the product. Colour is also an indication of freshness of meat and meat products. Meat deriving from different species of animals may have different colours on the basis of myoglobin contents in the particular meat. In general natural colour of fresh meat, except poultry meat, is in the shades of red colour. In judging meat colour, some experience is needed to be able to distinguish between the colours which is typical for a specific treatment or which is typical for specific freshness. Remarkable changes in the meat colour occur when fresh meat has been boiled or cooked. It loses its red colour almost entire and turns to grey (on pressure cooking and boiling) or brown(in roasting, broiling or canning). The reason for this is the destruction of the myoglobin through heat treatment. On the other hand, it has long been known that after pickling (curing) fresh meat with curing ingredients (nitrite) the meat colour remains red during longer storage periods, after ripening, drying and even after intensive heat treatment. Obviously the original meat colour has not been conserved, but a chemical reaction has taken place during the curing process transforming the unstable pigment of the fresh meat into a stable red pigment. This is the typical colour shown in sausages of all types, raw and cooked hams, corned beef, etc.

Processed meat, on the other hand, can roughly be evaluated by its appearance according to the different raw materials of which the product is composed and where the use of some components is exaggerated (for instance too many particles of visible fat or connective tissue, etc.). Special product treatments (for instance chilling, freezing, cooking, curing, smoking, drying) or the kind and quality of portioning and packaging (casings, plastic bags, cans) will be recognized by evaluating the appearance.

Texture and Consistency (Tenderness and Juiciness)

Texture and consistency, including juiciness, are an important criterion for the assessment of eating quality of meat. For perception of these attributes touch, sight and hearing are the main senses. In other words we can say that texture is a collective response of degree of teeth sink, meat fragmentation and chewing residues. Meat prepared for the consumer should be tender and juicy. Meat tenderness depends on the animal species from which the meat originates. Lamb, pork and poultry meat are sufficiently tender after slaughter, but beef requires a certain period of maturation to achieve optimal eating quality. These quality attributes of meat can also be upgraded by ripening, especially in case of beef and similar meats. It should be cooked to become sufficiently tender, but cooking should not be too intense otherwise the meat becomes dry, hard and with no juiciness.

Texture is a complex sensation manifestation of the structure or inner makeup of the product. It can be explained on the basis of textural qualities of meat products.

Mechanical properties : It is a reaction to stress and can be measured kinaesthetically. Examples are :

1. *Hardness :* It is a resistance against deformation of meat products i.e. firmness and hardness.
2. *Cohesiveness :* It is a degree of sample deformation i.e. cohesive, chewy and fracturable (crispy or crunchy).
3. *Adhesiveness :* It is a force required to remove sample from surface i.e. sticky and non sticky.
4. *Denseness :* It is a compactness of the product i.e. dense and light.
5. *Springiness :* It is a return to original shape after deformation i.e. springy/rubbery and resistant.

Geometric properties : These are the perception of particles (size, shape, orientation) and can be perceived by tactile means. Examples are :

1. *Smoothness :* It is an absence of all particles.
2. *Gritty :* It is due to presence of small hard particles.
3. *Grainy :* It is due to small particles.
4. *Chalky or powdery :* It is due to fine particle film.
5. *Fibrous :* It is due to long stringy particles.
6. *Lumpy :* It is due to large even pieces of particles.

Moisture properties : These textural properties of meat products are due to perception of water, oil and fat and can be measured by tactile means. Examples are :

1. *Moistness :* It is because of wetness and oiliness.
2. *Moisture released :* It is because of exudation of wetness and oiliness.
3. *Juicy :* It is because of moisture release from meat products.
4. *Oily :* It is because of liquid fat.
5. *Greasy :* It is because of solid fat.

The texture is of less importance in meat products, such as cured or canned products, sausages, etc., because they are either made of comminuted meat and/or meat which has undergone heat treatment or long maturation periods and will therefore generally be tender. On the other hand, inadequate processing methods (too intensive cooking, curing, comminuting) may cause losses in the desired consistency and juiciness, and the best way to check this is by chewing.

The simple way to check the consistency of foods is by chewing. Although this test seems easy, in practice it is rather complicated. Taste panellists need experience, particularly when the different samples have to be ranked, for example which sample is the toughest, the second toughest or the tenderest.

Smell and Taste (Aroma and Flavour)

These characteristics are related to each other to a certain extent because they have to be evaluated together by the oral and olfactory senses for the reliable determination of a product's flavour. Experience is required to become acquainted with the typical flavour (smell and taste) of foods. Only four basic taste components—sweet, sour, bitter and salty—will be perceived by the taste buds. These receptors are small papillae located in certain areas of the tongue and upper palate. Whereas, smell is sensed by the regio- olfactoria which lies at the top inside the nose. The smell of fresh meat should be slightly acidic, increasing in relation to the duration of the ripening period because of the formation of acids such as lactic acid. On the other hand, meat in decomposition generates an increasingly unpleasant odour owing to substances originating from the bacterial degradation of the meat proteins, such as sulphur compounds, mercaptans etc.

The freshness of meat is generally indicated by its smell together with its appearance and colour. Sorting out deteriorated meat is mandatory from the point of view of the product's palatability. It is also important because of the fact that high bacterial contamination of meat in decomposition could be accompanied by food-poisoning bacteria (pathogens), which have a deleterious impact on consumers' health. On the other hand, the best fresh meat can also be heavily contaminated with food-poisoning bacteria because these micro-organisms do not cause organoleptic alterations by destruction of meat proteins. Food poisoning can therefore only be avoided by proper hygienic meat handling. The flavour of fresh meat can also be checked putting small samples (approx. 10 pieces of 1 cm^3 each) in preheated water of 80°C for about five minutes (boiling test). The odour of the cooking broth and the taste of the warm meat samples will indicate whether the meat was fresh or in deterioration or subject to undesired influences, for instance rancidity of the meat fat, any typical meat flavour due to the feed and the sex (boar taint) of the animal or treatment with veterinary drugs shortly before slaughter.

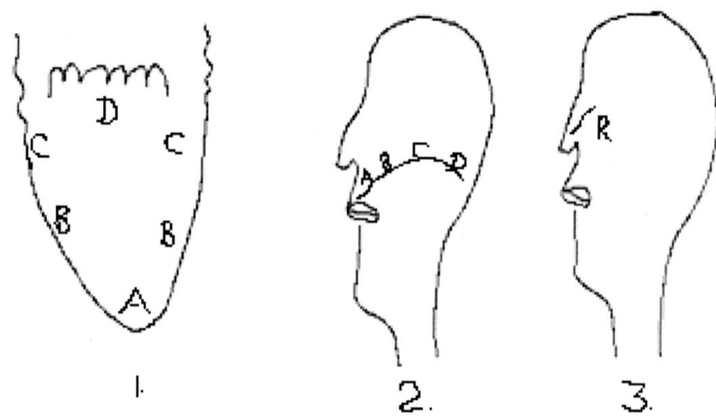

1. Location of taste papillae on tongue -A. Sweet B. Salty C. Sour D. Bitter
2. Location of taste papillae on palate-A. Sweet B. Salty C. Sour D. Bitter
3. Location of regio-olfactoria inside the upper part of nose.

When processing the meat, the smell and taste of the meat products can differ a great deal owing to heat treatment and the use of salt, spices and food additives. Every meat product has its typical smell and taste (metallic and astringent flavour of fresh beef, sweet and bland flavour of pork, sweet and flat in case of veal, typical piggy odour in boar and pigs etc.) and the test person should know about it. Changes in these qualities indicate the use of improper raw materials or a deterioration of the meat product during storage.

The overall flavour consists of smell and taste produced by the meat components, influenced and covered by spices and those compounds produced by ripening or heat treatment. Flavour test panellists should be aware of these special cases. Panellists should not smoke or eat spicy meals before starting the test and should rinse their mouth frequently with warm water during the test.

Mouth Feel or Moth Coating

It is an overall impression of meat residues remains in the mouth after swallowing and chewing of meat products. It is determined by binding ability of meat proteins with fat globulins in the meat products. It is a good quality attribute especially in frankfurters, sausages, patties etc.

Overall Acceptability

It is an overall acceptability status of any meat food product but it is not an average of all sensory attributes, it may be affected by certain attributes and may not be affected by others. In this attribute we see how a particular meat product impressed taste panellists in totality.

Sensory Evaluation by Taste Panels

The evaluation of meat food products are having two main aims, either it will be aimed to product development or consumer oriented. So on that basis we can classify the taste panel.

Consumer Panel

This panel is conducted for gathering information about likes and dislikes of consumers about the product. The panellists may be labourers, workers and may not have any training or qualification but they must be from the population in which we want to launch the product. In this panel method we choose about 100 persons randomly from the targeted population. This sensory evaluation may be done in local markets, community centres, and panchayats or in any social amenity. In this taste panel we introduced the panellists about the product and their preferences can be assessed in ranking test or hedonic scale. By this way we can assess the future market of a product.

Specialised Panel

Specialised panel is essential when we want to develop any product with a new formulation or we want to alter the existing product. This panel consist of trained and semi trained panellists who can easily identify the sensory attributes even in the similar products. The number of panellists may vary depending upon the specialised test. These panellists are selected on the basis of health status, willingness, availability, sensitivity, selectivity, capability, appetite and dependability. After that these panellists are invited to an orientation programme in which they are tested for recognition test and threshold test for four basic tastes i.e. sweet, salty, sour and bitter. After that they are giving some shot of training about the meat products and then again tested for serial dilution test till perfection. Then they are exposed to a broad and comprehensive frame of references for each product. They are introduced with a scaling method which can be taught effectively and can be treated statistically. They are alos exposed to use the panel data effectively to study the products in depth and provide detailed product analysis to management.

Important Considerations for Conducting Taste Panel

1. Sensory evaluation laboratory should be a separate unit and must be maintained at a temperature of 20±2°C with relative humidity of 70-75%.
2. There should be a provision of partition, sitting, writing, mouth rinsing, hand wash, thermostatistically controlled heating device with sufficient facility for natural and artificial light.
3. The ideal time for sensory evaluation is late morning or late afternoon or at least one and half hours after lunch.
4. Panellists should not be allowed to have food with high spices, smoking, use of liquors, sucking candies etc. at least before 30 minutes of evaluation.
5. As a general rule testing sample should be sufficient enough for two bites in case of solid product and 15 ml for liquids.

6. Number of samples may vary as per the testing procedure but maximum limit for testing samples in a session should not be more than six samples with six attributes otherwise sensory receptors become fatigue.
7. There should be a control sample along with treatments and always use a code for products to be tested.
8. The temperature of meat samples may vary as per the product type but in most of the communited meat products it should be at 40-60°C.

Various Methods Used for Sensory Evaluations by Taste Panels

1. Discriminatory sensory evaluation

It determines how products perceived and significance of difference can be identified. It requires trained panellists for discriminating the products. Examples are – recognition test, threshold test, and difference test.

2. Descriptive sensory evaluation

It determines the specific differences and how extreme are those differences. It requires trained panellists. Examples are– ranking test, Linear score card.

3. Specialised sensory evaluation

These are the specific tests used for detection of special attribute in a product and require expertise in the sensory evaluation field. Examples are-flavour profile test, texture profile test etc.

Discriminatory Sensory Evaluation

i. Recognition test

It is a qualitative test in which we judge the taste recognition ability of a person for four basic tastes. For this purpose dilute aqueous solutions of sucrose, sodium chloride, citric acid and caffeine are presented randomly to the panel members and they have to identify these tests. By this test we can identify the taste blind persons at a very initial stage.

ii. Threshold test

It is a quantative test in which different concentrations of aqueous solutions of sucrose, sodium chloride, citric acid and caffeine are presented to the panellists in increasing concentrations. On that basis concentration threshold of each panellist may be determined but retasting is always avoided.

iii. Difference test

In this test difference between two meat samples are recognised on the basis of concentration thresholds of panellists. Examples of difference tests are Triangle test, Duo- Trio test and Paired comparison test.

a. *Triangle test* : Panellists receive three coded samples. In this test two samples are same and one is different. Panellists are asked to identify the odd sample. This discriminatory testing method is often used as a tool in quality assurance programs to ensure that samples from different production lots are same or different. Triangle tests are also used in product development studies to determine the effect of various ingredient substitutions or changes in processes on product quality.

b. *Duo-Trio test* : In this test, three samples are presented : one sample is labelled "R" (reference) and the other two are also coded. One of the coded samples is identical to "R" and the other coded sample is different to "R". Panellists are asked to identify the correct sample. In this test choice is always 50%. Both Triangle and Duo-Trio tests may be used to screen panellists for their ability to repeatably select a specific trait when tasting products for flavour. However, Duo-Trio test is often used instead of the Triangle test for this purpose because the former method requires less tasting.

c. *Paired - comparison test* : A pair of coded samples are presented for comparison on the basis of some specified characteristic (saltiness, sweetness etc.) This method is similar to the triangle test, but it requires fewer samples and less tasting in comparision to previous one. However, statistical efficiency is not as great as paired-comparison test but it is similar to the triangle test.

Descriptive Sensory Evaluation

i. *Ranking test* : This test is an extension of paired- comparison test. In this test panellists are to be given three or more coded samples and asked to rank samples for intensity of some specific characteristic. Ranking tests are often used to screen one or two "best samples' from a group of samples rather than to thoroughly test all samples. However, no indication of the magnitude of difference between samples is obtained because samples are only evaluated in relationship to each other.

ii. *Scale tests* : Many types of scales or scoring systems are used for preference evaluations. These may include structured word scales or graphics. In structured scales a scale of 7 to 10 points is recommended because panellists tend to avoid using the end points on the scale. To use of less than 7 point scale may not allow the panellists to show the degree of variation. More of a word-descriptive scale becomes the most critical feature. It may be appropriate to involve the panel defining word descriptions and numerical scores to be assigned to these words. Remember, the panel results must be interpretable and accurately reflect what was objectively measured.

a. *Hedonic scale* : The word "hedonic" is of Greek origin and relates to degree or magnitudes of like or dislike.

b. *Rank preference* : when more than 4 or 5 samples are served in a ranking test, the difficulty for the panellists to rank products is increased. More re-testing is generally done in order to assure the correct positioning of the rankings.

c. *Paired preference test* : This is the most simple and oldest method for the panel. The panel is asked to indicate which sample they preferred and why they choose the preferred sample. In all preference testing at least one sample (control) with a known hedonic value (scale of like or dislike) should be included. Samples may be ranked from most to least desirable even when all samples are considered to be of questionable desirability. A known sample provides a reference point upon which to result is based.

Specialised Sensory Evaluation

It involves discrimination of qualitative and quantitative traits of a sample by use of a small (5-100 member) trained panel. Such techniques are flavour profile, textural profile and QDA (quantitative descriptive analysis).

i. *Flavour profile test :* It is descriptive sensory evaluation method in which four or five panellists are make their consensus in the characterisation of individual components of odour and flavour in the sequence of their perception. It is a useful test in monitoring of competitive meat products quality, shelf life, quality control, effects of processing on the product, new product development, effects of ingredients in the product and packaging effect on products quality.

ii. *Texture profile test:* It is a descriptive method in which six to nine specialised and trained panellists are used their senses for systemic measurements of textural dimensions of meat products i.e. mechanical, geometric, fat and moisture and their degree on which they are present. They judge that how teeth sink in the meat, how it breaks into the fragments and condition of left over residues after swallowing the meat tissues. It is useful test for new product development, product improvement, product matching, process modification, quality control of products and in shelf life study.

iii. *Quantitative descriptive analysis :* Descriptive analysis requires at least three evaluative processes. First, discrimination of the trait; second, description of the trait; and third, quantifying the trait. The steps of discrimination and description of traits are qualitative. The language used is developed through careful training and practice with the panel. This requires panellists to develop a common vocabulary which catalogues various sensory stimuli with appropriate language. Descriptive analysis is a complex cognitive process which requires more mental acuity than sharp taste or olfactory senses. Discrimination among stimuli is only part of the qualitative process. The third step in descriptive analysis is to quantify the traits as to how strong they are. Two products may be quite similar in their qualitative components but differ overall because of the relative intensities of these characteristics. Descriptive analysis is the only sensory method that deals with the total picture or profile of a food product. It may be used to suggest or interpret instrumental methods or other sensory test information or to be used as a research guideline tool, or as a method of quality assurance or quality control.

References

1. ASTM Committee E-18 (1968). Manual on Sensory Testing Methods STP 434.Am.Soc. for Testing and Material, Philadelphia, PA.
2. Bratzler, L.J. (1985). Palatability characteristics of meat. CSIRO Food Research quarterly, 45: 23-36.
3. Forrest, J.C., Aberle, E.D., Hedrick, H.B., Judge, M.D. and Merkel, R.A. (1969). Structure and Composition of Muscle and Associated tissues. In: Principles of Meat Science, W.H. Freeman and Company, San Francisco, pp 27-89.
4. Harries, J.M. (1976). Taste panel techniques and statistics. In: Conference Proceedings held at Research Institute for Animal Husbandry. Schoonoord, Zeist, Netherland,pp 309-317 (cited from FSTA, 9:S1712).
5. IFT (1981). Sensory evaluation guide for testing food and beverage products. Institute of Food Technologist, Sensory Evaluation Division Food Technology, 35(11):50-59.
6. Jellinek,G.(1985). In: Sensory evaluation of food theory and practice. Ellis Horward Ltd. Chichester England and VCH Gmbh FDR Germany.
7. Science Direct.com
8. Sharma, B.D. (1999). Eating quality and sensory evaluation of meat products. In: Meat and Meat Products Technology (Including Poultry Products Technology). Japee Brothers Medical Publishers (P) Ltd. New Delhi. 82-87.
9. Sharma, B.D., Wani, S.A. and Sharma, N. (1996). Sensory Evaluation Manual for Meat and Meat products. Publication and Information Centre, Indian Veterinary Research Institute, Izatnagar.

□□□□

13 Nutritive Value, Preservation, Packaging of Egg and Egg Products

Eggs are considered as Nature's original functional food because they are abundant source of nutrients like vitamins and minerals. It contains valuable nutrients from the high-quality protein to significant levels of beneficial vitamins, antioxidants and other healthful compounds. The protein of eggs is considered as highest quality protein as compared to other animal protein sources which is readily available and most inexpensive. Eggs are good source of all well balanced nutrients for persons of all age groups. Egg is a unique combination nutrient like it is rich in protein and low in calorie. The nutrients concentration in eggs is dependent on breed, strain, species, feed, age, season, storage and processing methods.

The nutritional value of eggs lies chiefly in their proteins of good biological value; an average-sized egg (60 g) provides approximately 7 g of proteins. These proteins are rich in essential amino acids with a very good balance between these amino acids. So the egg protein can be regarded as a reference protein. On comparison we can say that 2 eggs provide as much protein as 100 g of meat or 100 g of fish. The energy value for an average egg (60 g) is approximately 376 Kj (90 kcal). The lipid content is 7 g, most of these lipids being contained in the yolk. Among the total fatty acids 2/3rd of these are unsaturated. Egg also contains 180 mg of cholesterol and rich in vitamins (A, D, E) and trace elements (iron and zinc).

Structure of Typical Poultry Egg

Structure wise egg is a typical food consisting of four typical structures i.e. shell, shell membrane, albumen and yolk. *Shell* is outer most layer of egg mainly made up of calcium carbonate and makes 11% of the volume of egg. It is a first line of defense consisting of keratin, spongy or calcareous layer and mammary layer form outer to inner. Keratin seals the pores and prevents the bacterial invasion in the egg. However, it facilitates the evaporation of moisture and CO_2 from the pores. The *shell membrane* is also consisting of three distinct layers namely outer and inner shell membrane and air cell. Air cell is mainly located on the broad end of the egg. Shell membrane also acts as a natural barrier for bacterial entry into the egg particularly lysozyme play an important role in this function. Another structure of egg is *albumin* which consist 58% of the total egg volume and is mainly made up of water (80%) and protein. It also contains carbohydrate but in very limited quantity (0.5%). The major proteins found in egg are ovalbumin (54%), conalbumin (13%), ovomucoid (11%), lysozyme or globulin G_1, G_2, G_3 (10%), ovomucin (1.5%), flavoprotein (0.8%), ovoinhibitor (0.1%), avidin (0.05%) etc. Structure wise egg albumin consists of four distinct layers such as outer thin and thick layers, inner thin and thick layers. The final egg structure is *yolk* which accounts 31% of total egg weight. It is fat rich part of the egg and contains 32% lipid (mainly triglycerides 65%, phospholipids 28% and cholesterol around 5%). Egg yolk also contains 16% proteins, 1% ash and 0.5% carbohydrates. Egg yolk also has four district part started from inner side, germinal disc, latebra, light and dark yolk material and vitelline membrane.

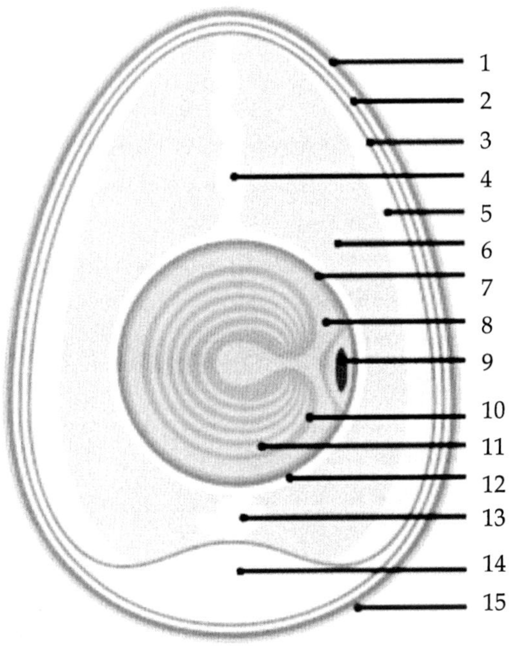

1. Eggshell
2. Outer membrane
3. Inner membrane
4. Chalaza
5. Exterior albumen
6. Middle albumen
7. Vitelline membrane
8. Nucleus of pander
9. Germinal disc (nucleus)
10. Yellow yolk
11. White yolk
12. Internal albumen
13. Chalaza
14. Air cell
15. Cuticula

Structure of egg (*Source*: wikipedia.com)

Nutritional Value of Eggs

The nutritional value of eggs and the contribution that they make to the diet is illustrated in tables. The data on the nutritional content of a single egg is based on a medium egg and all percentage composition figures relate to the contents, excluding the shell.

1. *Energy value of eggs:* A medium egg has an energy value of 78 kilocalories (324 kilojoules) and the consumption of one egg daily would contribute only around 3% of the average energy requirement of an adult man, 4% for an adult woman. With their significant protein, vitamin and mineral content and relatively low saturated fat content, eggs are a valuable component in a healthy diet.

2. *Proteins*: Eggs are an excellent source of protein. Egg protein is of high biological value as it contains all the essential amino acids needed by the human body. Eggs therefore complement other food

proteins of lower biological value by providing the amino acids that are in short supply in those foods. 12.5% of the weight of the egg is protein and it is found in both the yolk and the albumen. Although protein is more concentrated around the yolk, there is in fact more protein in the albumen. On the evaluation scale most commonly used for assessing protein, egg is at the highest point, 100, and is used as the reference standard against which all other foods are assessed. One large egg contains 6 grams of protein. The protein is almost equally split between the egg white and the egg yolk. The protein in an egg contains all the essential amino acids used for growth and development. Egg Whites are an excellent source of biologically valued protein because they provide the only protein which is instantly absorbed by the human body.

Essential amino acids of protein in eggs is a complete source of 22 essential amino acids. Essential amino acids are those amino acid which cannot be synthesized by human body but they are absolutely essential for the human body. These amino acids, therefore, need to be supplied by the food. Egg provides the body with all the nine essential amino acids. Therefore eggs are a good source of protein. Both the egg white and the egg yolk contain protein and an egg provides all the essential amino acids necessary for growth and development. In addition, the protein quality contained in an egg is far higher than the protein quality that obtained from any other food. Although, eggs are part of a healthy food diet, it is interesting to note that the nutritional requirements of eggs can vary from men, women and children.

3. *Vitamins*: Eggs contain most of the recognised vitamins with the exception of vitamin C. The egg is a good source of all the B vitamins. It is a particularly rich source of vitamins B_{12} and riboflavin (vitamin B_2) and a useful source of folate. The egg is also a good source of the fat-soluble vitamins A and D and provides vitamin E in some quantity.

4. *Minerals*: Eggs contain many of the minerals that the human body requires for health. In particular eggs are an excellent source of iodine, required to make the thyroid hormone and phosphorus,

required for bone health. The egg is a significant source of selenium, an important antioxidant and provides some zinc, important for wound healing, growth and fighting infection. Eggs also contain iron, the vital ingredient of red blood cells, although the availability of this iron to the body is still being investigated.

5. *Fat*: Fat contributes to 11.2% of the egg content. The fat of an egg is found almost entirely in the yolk and in less than 0.05% in the albumen. Most of an egg's total fatty acid (approximately 47%) composition is monounsaturated. About a further 18% is polyunsaturated and only 34% is saturated.

6. *Cholesterol*: Eggs also contain cholesterol and lecithin which are fat-like substances that are essential to the structure and function of all cells in the body. However, these substances are not dietary essentials and human body is able to synthesize them. Cholesterol helps to maintain the flexibility and permeability of cell membranes and is also a raw material for the fatty lubricants that help to keep the skin supple. Cholesterol is essential for the production of sex hormones, cortisol, vitamin D and bile salts.

Gross chemical composition of a fresh raw egg

S.No.	Food ingredients	Whole egg (weight 50g)	Egg white (weight 33g)	Egg yolk (weight 17g)
1.	Energy (in calories)	81.50	16.83	59.16
2.	Water (%)	73.70	87.60	51.10
3.	Protein (%)	12.9	10.9	16.0
4.	Fat (%)	11.5	trace	30.58
5.	Ash (%)	1.0	0.7	1.1
6.	Carbohydrate (%)	0.9	0.8	0.58

(*Source*: Watt and Merril, 1963)

Nutritional value of chicken egg per 100 g (1 large egg contains 33g egg white and 17 g yolk) (*Source*: USDA database)

Sl. No.	Nutrients	Egg white	Egg yolk
1.	Energy	48 kcal	317 kcal
2.	Carbohydrates	0.73 g	3.59 g
3.	Fat	0.17 g	26.54 g
4.	Protein	10.90 g	15.86 g
5.	Tryptophan	0.125 g	0.177 g
6.	Threonine	0.449 g	0.687 g
7.	Isoleucine	0.661 g	0.866 g
8.	Leucine	1.016 g	1.399 g
9.	Lysine	0.806 g	1.217 g
10.	Methionine	0.399 g	0.378 g
11.	Cystine	0.287 g	0.264 g
12.	Phenylalanine	0.686 g	0.681 g
13.	Tyrosine	0.457 g	0.678 g
14.	Valine	0.809 g	0.949 g
15.	Arginine	0.648 g	1.099 g
16.	Histidine	0.290 g	0.416 g
17.	Alanine	0.704 g	0.836 g
18.	Aspartic acid	1.220 g	1.550 g
19.	Glutamic acid	1.550 g	1.970 g
20.	Glycine	0.413 g	0.488 g
21.	Proline	0.435 g	0.646 g
22.	Serine	0.798 g	1.326 g
23.	Water	87.57 g	52.31 g
24.	Vitamin-A equiv.	0 μg (0%)	381 μg (42%)
25.	Thiamine (Vit.B_1)	0.004 mg (0%)	0.176 mg (14%)
26.	Riboflavin (Vit.B_2)	0.439 mg (29%)	0.528 mg (35%)
27.	Pantothenic acid (Vit. B_5)	0.190 mg (4%)	2.990 mg (60%)
28.	Folate (Vit.B_9)	4 μg (1%)	146 μg (37%)
29.	Calcium	7 mg (1%)	129 mg (13%)
30.	Iron	0.08 mg (1%)	2.73 mg (22%)
31.	Magnesium	11 mg (3%)	5 mg (1%)
32.	Phosphorus	15 mg (2%)	390 mg (56%)
33.	Potassium	163 mg (3%)	109 mg (2%)
34.	Zinc	0.03 mg (0%)	2.30 mg (23%)
35.	Choline	1.1 mg	682.3 mg
36.	Cholesterol	0 mg	1234 mg

Daily requirements of an individual with respect to value per 100g of egg

S.No.	Name of ingredients	Daily need of an Indian individual	Value of a egg(per 100g of edible portion)
1.	Energy (in calories)	2500-3000	160
2.	Protein(in gm)	45-55	12.5
3.	Calcium	0.4-0.5 g	54 mg
5.	Iron (in mg)	20-25	2.3
6.	Vitamin-A(in I.U.)	5000	1180
7.	Vitamin-D(in I.U.)	200	36.2
8.	Thiamine (in mg)	1.2-2.0	0.11
9.	Riboflavin (in mg)	1.2-2.2	0.30
10.	Nicotinic acid(in mg)	17-25	-
11.	Folic acid(in mcg)	50-100	0.029 mg
12.	Vitamin-B12(in mcg)	0.5-1.0	1.08
13.	Ascorbic acid(in mg)	30-50	-

(*Source* : Gopalan *et al.* 1971)

Preservation of Eggs

Preservation of eggs is a practice to prevent spoilage. Spoilage is normally occurs due to the entrance of air carrying germs through the shells. Normally the shell has a surface coating of mucilaginous matter which prevents for a time the entrance of these harmful organisms into the egg. But if this coating is removed or softened by washing or otherwise the keeping quality of the egg is much reduced. These facts explain why many methods of preservation have not been entirely successful and suggest that the methods employed should be based upon the idea of protecting and rendering more effective the natural coating of the shell so that air bearing the germs that cause decomposition may be completely excluded.

Eggs are often packed in lime, salt or other products or put in cold storage for further use but such eggs are very far from being perfect when they come upon the market. It is considered that water glass more closely conforms to the requirements of a good preservative than any of the substances commonly employed. 10% solution of water glass can be used for preservation of eggs so effectively. By this way three and one-half months old eggs still appeared to be perfectly fresh. In water glass preserved eggs, yolk retained its normal position and in taste they are not to be distinguished from fresh, unpacked stored eggs. Among the preservative methods like coating of the eggs with Vaseline, preservation in limewater and water glass it is concluded that varnishing the eggs with Vaseline takes considerable time and treating with limewater is likely to give the eggs a limy flavour.

Preservation of Shelled Eggs

1. *Coating with paraffin*: Eggs can be preserved for further use by coating them with paraffin when eggs are perfectly fresh. As the spores of fungi get into eggs almost as soon as they are laid so it is necessary to rub every egg with chloroform or wrap within few minutes. If only a trace of the chloroform enters the shell the development of such germs as may have gained access to freshly laid eggs is prevented. The paraffin coating prevents contamination from germ-laden air and no fungi can grow within the egg thus it retains their freshness and natural taste.

2. *Lime water preservation*: Take a litre of boiled water and add one kg of quick lime in it. Cool down the water to a room temperature. Add five litre of cold water and 225g of sodium chloride in it and allow the mixture to settle down. Then decant the solution and immerse the eggs in clear solution for about 16 to 18 hours. Dipping of the eggs should be in a manner that it stands about 10 inches deep over the last layer of eggs. In this method a thin layer of calcium is deposited on the shell which partially seals the pores. Eggs treated with lime water can be stored for 3 to 4 weeks at room temperature.

3. *Beeswax preservation*: Melt one kg of clear beeswax in a porcelain dish over a gentle fire and stir in two litre of olive oil. Let the solution of wax in oil cool somewhat and then dip the fresh eggs one by one into it so as to coat every part of the shell. A momentary dip is sufficient, all excess of the mixture being wiped off with a cotton cloth. The oil is absorbed in the shell and wax will hermetically close all the pores.

4. *Reinhard method*: The Reinhard method is said to cause such chemical changes in the surface of the eggshell that it is closed up

perfectly air-tight and an admittance of air is entirely prevented even in case of long-continued storing. In this method, eggs are for a short time exposed to the direct action of sulphuric acid whereby the surface of the eggshell which consists chiefly of lime carbonate is transformed into lime sulphate. The dense texture of the surface thus produced a complete protection against the access of the outside air which admits very long time storage of the egg without the contents of the egg suffering any disadvantageous changes regarding taste and odour. The egg does not require any special treatment to prevent cracking on boiling, etc. Some consumers are having objections on the ground that sulphuric acid is a dangerous poison that might, on occasion, penetrate the shell.

5. *Preservation in boric acid and salicylic acid*: Take about half a dozen eggs and place them in a netting (water is chilled below boiling point, even for an instant), into a boiling solution of boric acid, withdraw immediately and pack. Alternatively put up in oil carrying 2 per cent or 3 per cent of salicylic acid. Eggs treated in this way provide same taste after six months, absolutely as fresh as they were when first put up. In this method eggs should be as fresh as possible and should be thoroughly clean before dipping. The philosophy of the process is that the dipping in boiling boric acid solution not only kills all bacteria existing on or in the shell and membrane but also reinforces these latter by a very thin layer of coagulated albumen. However, packaging in salicylated oil prevents the admission of fresh germs from the atmosphere. Salicylic acid is objected to on the same grounds as sulphuric acid.

6. *Preservation in sodium silicate*: Dissolve sodium silicate in boiling water to the consistency of about 1 part of the silicate to 3 parts water. In this preservation method eggs should be as fresh as possible and must be thoroughly clean. They should be immersed in solution in such a manner that every part of each egg is covered with the liquid then removed and let dry. If the solution is kept at or near the boiling temperature, the preservative effect is said to be much more certain and to last longer.

7. *Oil coating*: In this process eggs are immersed in good grade mineral oil. By this way thin layer is formed on the surface of shell and thereby seals the pores. This treatment should be given within few hours of egg laying. Oil must be colourless, viscous and free from florescent materials. For oil coating mineral oil is preferred because it is less susceptible to oxidative rancidity during storage. Vegetable oil like groundnut oil mixed with 0.0125% Butyl hydroxyl toluene (BHT) can also be used for this purpose because it is a good sealing agent.

8. *Water glass preservation*: For the preparation of water glass one part of sodium silicate is added in 10 parts of water. In this solution eggs are immersed overnight which deposits a thin precipitate of silica on the eggshell. Silica imparts antiseptic property but does not contribute to any foreign odour or taste to the eggs.

9. *Flash heat treatment*: In this method eggs are filled in wire basket and immersed in hot water maintained at 71°C for about 2 to 3 seconds. In this process bacteria present on shell surface are destroyed and thin film of albumin present beneath the shell membrane is coagulated. It also seals the shell from internal side.

10. *Thermostabilization*: In this process eggs are immersed in hot water maintained at 49°C for 35 minutes or 54°C for 15 minutes or 56°C for 10 minutes or 60°C for 5 minutes. This process stabilizes thick albumin of eggs. In this process egg retains its quality for a longer period of time than untreated eggs.

11. *Cold storage preservation*: For the short term storage of eggs, storage temperature should be 12.5 °C to 13.5 °C with relative humidity of 70 to 80% while for long term storage eggs are stored at -10 °C with 80 to 90% relative humidity. Relative humidity is an important consideration for cold storage preservation because at optimum level it retards evaporation without danger of mould growth. Oil treatment prior to cold storage enhances storage life of eggs.

Preservation of Egg Products

Egg products are referred to eggs that are removed from their shells for processing. The processing of egg products includes breaking of eggs, filtering, mixing, stabilizing, blending, pasteurizing, cooling, freezing or drying and packaging. Egg products include whole eggs, whites, yolks and various blends with or without non-egg ingredients that are processed and pasteurized and may be available in liquid, frozen and dried forms.

Dried Egg Mix

It is a blend of dried whole eggs, non-fat dry milk, soybean oil and a small amount of salt. It contains very little amount of moisture. To reconstitute, blend 2 tablespoons of Dried Egg Mix with ¼ cup water to make the equivalent of one large whole egg. Dried egg mix is packaged in 6-ounce pouches, equivalent to about 6 eggs each. Dried egg mix was initially developed for the military during 1930's. Dried Egg Mix should be stored at less than 10°C, preferably in the refrigerator (at 4.4°C or below). After opening of the product it should be used within 7 to 10 days.

Egg Mix

A similar product called all purpose egg mix that contains a greater proportion of eggs. It is reconstituted by mixing one part egg mix with two parts of water (by weight). It is packaged in 10-pound bags. Safe storage and handling is necessary for all egg products to prevent bacterial contamination. Egg mix can be stored up to a year in a good quality frozen under storage set at -17.7 °C or lower. After thawing, refreezing is not allowed in this system.

Liquid Egg Products

Egg liquids act as an excellent media for growth of various microbial agents including pathogens. Therefore, special attention should be paid to prevent the entry of these organisms while handling egg liquids. So to conserve the quality of egg liquids holding room should be maintained at temperature of 12.8°C for one week storage and 7.2°C for more than a week storage. Washing wit a proper detergent sanitizer also helps in reducing the microbial load. Egg liquid products can also be preserved with 10% salt level at 18.3°C or lower for less than a month while for longer storage it should be held at 7.2°C.

Egg liquid products like plain egg white, yolk, whole egg or a variety of blends of yolk and white can be preserved in freezing by addition of salt and sucrose at 10% level to control its gelation. Other ingredients used for this purpose are glycerine, syrup, gums, sodium meta phosphate, triethyl citrate etc. yolk starts freezing at temperature -1°C.

Pasteurization is the another method of liquid egg preservation in which time temperature combination recommended are 60°C for 3.5 minutes or 64.5°C for 2.5 minutes. Other techniques applied for liquid egg pasteurization are lactic acid albumin sulphate (pH 7.0) process, heat plus hydrogen per oxide process, heat plus vacuum process. In routine practice high temperature short time (HTST) pasteurization system is adopted.

Unopened Dried Egg Products and Egg White Solids

Unopened dried egg products and egg white solids can be stored at room temperature as long as they are kept cool and dry. After opening it requires refrigeration storage.

Reconstituted Egg Products

Reconstituted egg products should be used immediately or it can be stored under refrigeration for further use.

Dried Egg Powders

Dried egg powders like whole egg powder, egg yolk powder, egg albumin powder etc. are most convenient and economical form of eggs for transportation, storage and recipe formulation. The preservation of dried egg powders can be achieved without any additives. Microbiological deterioration is arrested by removal of moisture below the level of 5%. Dried egg products should be stored in a cool and dry place. They should not be stored along with other items with strong odour. The shelf life of egg powder depends on temperature of storage.

Long storage at higher temperature (35°C) causes degradation of protein. It also affects some functional properties of the products. Storage of dried egg products below 25° C ensures shelf life up to a year. For reconstitution of these products following methods are adopted:

1. *Whole Egg Powder:* by addition of 3 parts of water to 1 part of powder by weight and mix to obtain uniform consistency.
2. *Egg Yolk Powder:* by addition of 1.1 parts of water to 1 part of powder by weight and mix to obtain uniform consistency.
3. *Egg Albumen Powder:* by addition of 7 parts of water to 1 part of the powder by weight and mix to obtain uniform consistency.

Beside all these systems some chemical can also be used in preservation of egg products. These are mainly ethylene oxide and propylene oxide. Some gaseous products can also be tried but they have not been given authentication by the regulatory authorities.

Packaging of Egg and Egg Products

Nature has given the egg a natural package - the shell. Despite its relative strength, the egg is an extremely fragile product and even with the best handling methods, serious losses can result from shell damage. Economical marketing generally requires that eggs be protected by the adoption of specialized packaging and handling procedures.

Requirements for Egg Packaging and Transportation

For the packaging of shelled eggs, retention of shell of eggs is an important factor. It can be protected by providing elaborate cushioning facility to protect it from shock and compressive stress in trade marketing. The other requirements for egg packaging are:

1. Package or containers should have a capacity to protect the eggs against mechanical damage.
2. Handling should be done with all possible measures to protect it.
3. Package should not alter the egg quality during exposure to normal weather conditions.

4. Package should provide protection during transportation and handling.
5. Insulated refrigerated trucks or vans can be used for long term transportation of eggs.
6. In case of unavailability of insulation vans, eggs should be transported in cooler parts of the day or in night time.

Functions of Packaging

Packaging is an important component in delivering quality eggs to buyers. It embraces both the art and science of preparing products for storage, transport and eventually sale. Packaging protects the eggs from micro-organisms such as bacteria, natural predators, loss of moisture, tainting, temperatures that cause deterioration and possible crushing while being handled, stored or transported. Proper handling and storage helps in control moisture loss but appropriate packaging may also help to prevent it. Eggs also need to breathe hence the packaging material used must allow for the entrance of oxygen. The material used must be clean and odourless so as to prevent possible contamination and tainting. Authentic egg packaging materials can be reused but careful attention must be paid to possible damage, odours and cleanliness. The packaging must be made to withstand handling, storage and transport methods of the most diverse kind and to protect the eggs against temperatures that cause deterioration and humidity. Finally, consumers like to see what they are buying, especially if it concerns fresh produce. An egg package should be designed so that the customers not only recognize the product as such but can also see the eggs during purchase. Many factors must be taken into consideration for packaging eggs. It is important to obtain information regarding the necessary requirements for a particular market such as quality maintenance, storage facilities, type of transport, distance to be travelled, climatic conditions, time involved and costs.

Packaging of Shell Eggs and Egg Products

There are many different types of egg packages which vary both in design and packaging materials used for egg packaging. Normally three or four methods are adopted for packaging of shell eggs. Eggs are mainly packaged and transported with intact shell. Egg products can also be transported in modified atmosphere packaging, shrink film packaging and vacuum packaging. But the transportation of egg products is limited due to convenience of egg products preparations. These products like pastry, cake etc. can be transported in plastic or paperboard boxes under refrigeration for short term transport. The systems adopted for shelled eggs packaging may be described as:

Packaging system first: In certain underdeveloped areas eggs are still packaged in clean and odourless rice husks, wheat chaff or chopped straw or in a firm walled basket or crates. It greatly decreases the risk of shell damage. It is also be possible to pack eggs in a simple basket. The basket has no cushioning material such as straw and therefore damage to the eggs may occur more easily. This kind of packaging may be fit for short distance transport.

Packaging system second: A very common form of packaging is the filler flats or trays. The fillers are then placed in boxes or cases. Filler trays are made up of wood pulp moulded to accommodate the eggs. They are constructed so that they can be stacked one on top of the other and can also be placed in boxes ready for transport. Filler trays also offer a convenient method for counting the eggs in each box, without having to count every single egg. Usually the standard egg tray carries 36 eggs. Therefore, if a box holds five trays, for example, the box has a total of 180 eggs (36 x 5 = 180). Standards egg filler is having the dimensions of 29.2 cm length x 20.2 cm width x 5.9 cm depth with 36 individual cells and each cell have 4.52 cm x 4.52 cm x 5.9 cm dimension.

The cases used may be made of sawn wood; however, they are more commonly made of cardboard. When using cardboard cases, special care must be taken in stacking so that excessive weight is not placed on a case at the bottom of a stack. Fillers can also be made of plastics. The advantages of using plastic egg fillers are that they can be reused and are washable. The fillers can be covered with plastic coverings and be used as packages for final sale to the buyer. More importantly, however, plastic transparent fillers allow for the inspection of eggs without handling or touching the eggs.

Packaging system third: Eggs can also be packed in packages that are smaller and specific for retail sale. Each package can hold from two to twelve eggs. These cases can be made of paperboard or moulded wood pulp or can be made of plastics. It is also possible to pack eggs in small paperboard cases and cover them with plastic film. Egg cases have also been developed from polystyrene. The advantages of using polystyrene are superior cushioning and protection against odours and moisture. The package is also resistant to fungus and mould growth.

The use of small cases is restricted by availability and cost considerations. However, small cases are good for retailers and customers. They are easy for the retailers to handle and customers are able to inspect the eggs.

Packaging system fourth: In some places eggs are also packaged in tray over wrapped with shrink films. It is a good method for display of eggs for marketing. The use of shrink film over wrapped are limited to certain places due to addition of cost.

Labelling

Labels are a source of important information for the wholesaler, retailer and consumer and not just pieces of paper stuck onto cartons or boxes. The important facts on the label contain information for buyers concerning the eggs, their size and weight and quality/grade description - AA, A or B. Labels may also indicate the producer when the eggs were laid, how to store them and their expiration date. Persuading the buyer to purchase the product without tasting, smelling or touching is another function of labelling.

Labels can be either printed directly on cartons or attached to the cartons. The cost of labelling must be taken into consideration. Simple methods of labelling are available such as stencil or stamp as can be seen below.

Costs of Packaging

When calculating the cost of packaging, expenses must be considered for packaging materials, labelling, labour, additional working capital required, changing existing facilities and packaging machinery.

Transportation of Eggs

For the successful transport of shell eggs three essential requirements must be met.

1. The containers and packaging materials must be capable to protect the eggs against mechanical damage.
2. Care should be taken at all stages of handling and transport. Workers handling eggs should be instructed so that they appreciate the need for careful handling. The provision of convenient loading platforms at packaging stations, loading depots and railing stations and handling aids such as hand trucks and lifts are of great help.
3. The eggs must be protected at all times against exposure to temperatures that causes deterioration in quality as well as contamination, especially tainting.

The permissible range of temperatures during loading and transport depends on the local climatic conditions and the duration of journey. Care is needed to avoid excessive shaking, especially where roads are bad. Egg containers should be stacked tightly and tied down securely to minimize movement. Covers should be used to protect them from the heat of the sun, rain and extreme cold where applicable. Where bicycles are used, a device such as a special carrier suspended on springs may be helpful.

Recommended temperatures for loading and transport

Conditions	Transport over 2 or 3 days	Transport over 5 or 6 days
Maximum on loading	+6° C	+3° C
Recommended for transport	-1° to + 3° C	-1° to + 1° C
Acceptable for transport	1° to + 6° C	1° to + 3° C

Source: FAO corporate document repository and Panda, 1990.

A basic prerequisite for all long-distance transport is that arrangements be made for proper reception, handling and storage at the end of the journey. This is especially important where large lots are delivered to a relatively small market. Without access to suitable storage facilities, the eggs may have to be marketed quickly under adverse climatic conditions, which may cause substantial quality deterioration and price losses.

Delivery of high quality eggs over long distances, especially in hot climates, generally calls for refrigeration. Requirements for the successful operation of refrigerated transport equipment are rather rigid and met with certain factors like efficiency and durability of insulation, adequacy and reliability of the cooling mechanism and adequate circulation of air within the vehicle or container so that variations of temperature are slight.

References

1. Chesi of books.com
2. eufic.com
3. FAO corporate document repository.
4. Gopalan, C., Ramashastri, B.V. and Balasubramanian, S.C. (1971). Nutritive Value of Indian foods. NIN (ICMR) Bull.
5. Hasler, C.M. (2000). The changing face of functional foods. Journal of the American College of Nutrition. 19: 499S-506S.
6. Mayr, G. and Kaemmerer, H. (1959). Fumigation with ethyl oxide. Food Manuf., 34: 169.
7. Mercuri, A.J., Thomson, J.E., Rowen, J.D., and Norris, K.H. (1957). Use of the automatic green rot detector to improve quality of liquid egg. Food Technol., 11: 374-377.
8. Panda, P.C. (1976). Formation, structure, food value and chemical composition of eggs. In: Text Book On Egg and Poultry Technology.Vikas Publishing House Pvt. Ltd., New Delhi, pp 9-46.
9. Panda, P.C. (1976). Packaging and marketing. In: Text Book On Egg and Poultry Technology. Vikas Publishing House Pvt. Ltd., New Delhi, pp 9-46.
10. Watt, B.K. and Merrill, A.L. (1963). Composition of foods-raw, processed, prepared, U.S.D.A. Handbook No.8.U.S. Govt. Printing Office, Washington, D.C.
11. Wikipedia.com

□□□□

14 Laws Governing National / International Trade in Meat and Meat Products

Meat and meat products industry is a sunrise industry in India having huge potential for upliftment of agricultural economy. India is the second largest food producer in world but the contribution of meat industry is still confined to localized handlers. So to uplift industry basic infrastructure, food chains, food security and safety along with standards and laws formulation and their implementations is today's need. Standards are carefully drawn specifications with respect to a food product. These standards are mainly of three types i.e. government, trade and research standards. Government standards are formulated by the government of India or state government and also have the power to implement these standards while trade standards are implied by the individual company. Research standards are formulated on the basis of comparative study of the products by the researchers. Laws are the legislations enforced by the organisations either government or by autonomous bodies made under the constitutional acts of the country. At present numerous standards and laws are in existence in individual country or at international level. The need is to harmonize them as per the industry and trade requirement.

Domestic Organizations Involved in Standards and Laws Formulation

For the formulation, enforcement and control of standards and legislations at domestic level various organizations are of prime value. Some of these are:

1. Export Import Policy of India

On the basis of WTO Agreement, the Export and Import Policy (EXIM) of India is drawn up for a period of five years, with some desired changes by the Ministry of commerce. Many export promotion measures have been adopted into the EXIM policy including the grant of special import licenses for firms having ISO certification. Before 1990s India's imports was subjected to different types of import licenses which was later dismantled and converted to quantitative restrictions (QRs). Although the removal of quantitative restrictions was started in India on unilateral basis during early 90s, most of the QRs were removed during 1997-2001 as a part of dispute settlement proceeding of the WTO. At present, the imports of all commodities can be carried out under Open General License (OGL) or 'free' list. EXIM policy 2002 announces food safety standards which also covers agricultural products. At present only 3 or 4 items are subjected to export restriction. Export Promotion Councils, certain Commodity Boards and Export Development Authorities and Export Promotion zones has been given a special status in the EXIM Policy. They grant membership to exporters based on which the exporters become eligible to get certain licenses and benefits, like duty free advance licenses for inputs for export production and benefits of deemed exports. Other relevant incentives include duty concession on import of capital goods used for export production, duty free imports for 100 per cent export oriented units (EOUs) and units in export processing zones (EPIs). Some fast track mechanisms for import clearances and additional benefits for export and trading houses showing export performance beyond a certain threshold.

2. Export (Quality Control and Inspection) Act, 1963

Under this act exportable commodities are notified for compulsory pre-shipment inspection. The inspection of products is carried out by the offices situated near the production site and at the ports of shipment. However, recently government exempted agriculture and food products, fruit products, fish and fishery products from compulsory pre-shipment inspections.

3. Export Promotion Institutions

The emphasis on export promotion has been laid down by government since late 1960s. In this connection Export Promotion Councils and Authorities has been established which is playing a twofold role for the product promotion. The first role is as nodal agencies for disbursement of export subsidies and second role as the nodal point for interaction between the Industry and the government. Some of these agencies are Marine Product Export Development Authority (MPEDA) and Agriculture Produce Export Development Authority (APEDA).

APEDA

The Agricultural and Processed Food Products Export Development Authority (APEDA) was established under the Ministry of Commerce and Industry, Government of India by the Agricultural and Processed Food Products Export Development Authority act 1985. It replaced the Processed Food Export Promotion Council and came into force from 13th February, 1986. The motto of its establishment was to develop the agricultural commodities and processed foods, and to promote their exports. APEDA is also aiming the maximize foreign exchange earnings through increased agro exports; to provide better income to the farmers through higher unit value realization and to create employment opportunities in rural areas by encouraging value added exports of farm produce. Its head quarter is at New Delhi with the regional offices at Mumbai, Hyderabad, Bangluru, Kolkata and Guwahati. It also has 13 virtual offices at Thiruvananthapuram (Kerala), Bhubaneshwar (Orissa), Srinagar (J&K), Chandigarh, Imphal (Manipur), Agartala (Tripura), Kohima (Nagaland), Chennai (Tamil Nadu), Raipur

(Chattisgarh), Ahmedabad (Gujarat), Bhopal (Madhya Pradesh), Lucknow (Uttar Pradesh) and Panaji (Goa).

Under the notification of Directorate General of Foreign Trade, Ministry of Commerce and Industry, Government of India, each and every exporter of meat must be registered their abattoir or meat processing plant under APEDA before start of the business. In first schedule of APEDA about 14 products are mentioned including meat and meat products and poultry and poultry products whose development and promotion of export is the responsibility of APEDA. For export of meat Government of India nominated following agencies to provide the health certificates i.e. all state Directorates of Animal Husbandry, Export Inspection Agencies, Directorate of Marketing and Inspections, Deonar Abattoir, Mumbai (only for chilled sheep and goat meat) etc. At present around 49 abattoirs and meat processing plants are registered under APEDA.

As per APEDA's classification the number of exporters registered

Food	2003-04	2004-05	2005-06
Processed Fruits & Vegetables	548	597	527
Other Processed Food	550	555	511
Meat & Dairy Products	520	577	522
Total	1618	1729	1560

Aim

i. Registration, promotion in production and export marketing of scheduled products.

ii. Quality assurance of the scheduled products through inspection at production, processing, storage and transport level.

iii. Setting of standards and specifications for scheduled products.

iv. Assistance for purchase of specialized transport units for meat, horticulture and floriculture sector.

v. Assistance to Exporters/ Producers /Growers/ Co-operative Organizations and Federations.

vi. Establishment of Infrastructure Facilities by APEDA or any other Government or Public Sector authority like Airport Authority of India or Port Trust.

vii. For generating relevant research and development by APEDA through research institutions for common benefit of the trade and industry.

viii. Preparation of quality assurance manuals, guidelines, documents, standards, pesticide management program and National and International standardization activities.

ix. Assistance to exporters and producers for installing quality management, quality assurance and quality control systems such as ISO 9000, ISO 14000, HACCP, TQM etc including consultancy, quality improvement and certification for these system.

x. Assistance to exporters, producers, growers, service providers, co-operative organizations etc. for purchase of Intermediate Packaging Material for domestic transportation of produce.

xi. APEDA also facilitates trainings to the exporters on various aspects of scheduled products.

MPEDA

Marine Products Export Development Authority (MPEDA) was constituted in 1972 under the Marine Products Export Development Authority Act 1972 (No.13 of 1972) by Ministry of Commerce, Govt. of India. MPEDA acts as a nodal agency for the regulation, development and promotion of marine product exports. Its aim is to cover fisheries of all kinds, increasing exports, specifying standards, processing, marketing, extension and training in various aspects of the industry. MPEDA functions under the Ministry of Commerce, Government of India and acts as a coordinating agency with different Central and State Government establishments engaged in fishery production and allied activities. The basic aims of MPEDA include:

i. Export promotion of capture and culture fisheries.

ii. To promote various market promotion programmes for projecting resource potential, product diversification, quality assurance and liberal incentives for investments and joint ventures.

iii. Training and education of fish farmers and entrepreneurs.

iv. Provides assistance for modernisation of seafood processing units.

v. MPEDA ensures the highest standards for seafood's exported from India. It works in close association with Export Inspection Council of India and other Indian and International quality control organizations.

vi. Assistance is given to registered processors to set up quality control laboratories and modern pre-processing plants throughout the country to meet the ISO 9000 quality standards. The HACCP cell in MPEDA offers advise on matters connected with EC Directives.

vii. MPEDA advises Government of India on matters connected with deep sea fishing. It undertakes techno-economic and financial appraisal of projects for production of value added marine products. Entrepreneurs and professionals get pre investment advices from MPEDA.

viii. MPEDA co-ordinates the visit of delegates from other countries or from international bodies like FAO, INFOFISH, UNDP, World Bank etc.

ix. MPEDA participates in specialised international food and trade fairs, organises buyer-seller meets in major seafood markets overseas and sponsors visit of Indian delegates and individual sales teams to foreign markets.

x. The prestigious biennial India seafood Trade Fair organized by MPEDA brings overseas buyers, sellers and other interested sectors of the industry under one umbrella.

xi. MPEDA has Overseas Trade Promotion Offices in Tokyo and New York. They ensure hassle free trade, liaising with government agencies, trade missions, seafood trade and industry associations and organising direct market promotion activities. In Europe, in Brussels, the India Trade Centre promotes seafood trade interests.

xii. MPEDA collects and compiles statistics of marine products exported through various ports in India. It monitors the overseas market situations and exchange rate fluctuations. The details are published in the weekly bulletin PRIME. Every month MPEDA collects compiles and analyses export data from all processing plants. Port-wise, grade-wise/variety-wise, information is available.

MPEDA had organized four INDAQUA expositions in 1993, 1995, 2007 and 2009 at Chennai, which had a deep impact on coastal aquaculture in the country. In aquaculture, India is the largest producer after China. During the year 2006-07 the exports of marine products from the country stood at over 612,000 MT, with a value of US$ 1,853 million. Shrimp continued to be the mainstay of seafood exports, contributing more than 54% in terms of value. Increase production of brackish water species to at least one million MT by the year 2017. MPEDA proposes to achieve implement mission mode programmes in Gujarat, Maharashtra and Orissa. 50,500 ha in Gujarat, 27,500 ha in Maharashtra and 20,350 ha in Orissa is being targeted. This is expected to generate at least 5 million additional job opportunities in the country besides the increased export earnings, which are projected at US$6 billion in place of current exports US$1.6 billion.

4. Standard Setting Bodies

The Bureau of Indian Standards (BIS) is the main standard setting body in India for all domestic market requirements. It sets voluntary standards that can be acquired to indicate the quality of the product by the use of "ISI" mark. However, BIS is also the guiding organisation behind most of the mandatory standards set by Government agencies. Notably, BIS is also the enquiry point of India under the WTO Agreement on Technical Barriers to Trade.

Bureau of Indian Standards (BIS)

National standardization activity started in India in 1947 with the establishment of the Indian Standards Institution (ISI) as a society under the Societies Registration Act 1860, to prepare and promote the adoption of national standards. In 1952, the Institution was also given the responsibility of operating a certification marking scheme under an Act of Parliament. In 1986 the national authorities made a review of the structure and status of ISI and assessed the impact made by it on the national economic development and the technological growth of various sectors of Indian industry. The Government of India felt that a new thrust had to be given to standardization and quality control activities and that a national strategy had to be evolved for giving appropriate recognition and importance to standards and for integrating them with the growth and development of production and exports in different sectors. The Government of India therefore decided to create a statutory organization as the national standards body which was named as the Bureau of Indian Standards (BIS) with adequate autonomy as well as flexibility in its operations to achieve harmonious development of the activities of standardization, certification marking and connected matters. The Bureau of Indian Standards Act was passed by the Parliament in 1986 and BIS came into being on 1 April 1987. It has its headquarter at Manak Bhawan, New Delhi with a network of regional offices at Mumbai, Kolkata, Chandigarh and Chennai and branch offices at Ahmedabad, Bangalore, Bhopal, Bhubneshwar, Guwahati, Hyderabad, Jaipur, Kanpur, Patna and Trivandrum.

Structure of BIS: BIS is a corporate body consisting of members from Central and State Governments, Industry, Scientific and Research Institutions and the Minister of Civil Supplies, Consumer Affairs and Public Distribution is the president of BIS and has administrative control over it. It is assisted by Executive Committee in which Secretary to the Ministry and Director General BIS are the ex-officio members. Its functioning bodies are Executive Committee and Advisory Committees which are engaged in dealing with finance, certification, standards, formulations, laboratories and planning.

For the formulation of standards on meat and meat products ISI constituted meat and meat products sectional committee (AFDC 18) under the Agricultural and Food Products Division Council in 1958 to prepare Indian Standards for meat industry. In this committee research scientists, technologists, manufacturers, Government agencies and consumers are the member participants. BIS committee provides familiar monogram 'ISI' after thorough examination of the products.

Functions of BIS

i. Formulation and publication of Indian standards on products, commodities, materials and processes.

ii. Promotion for adoption and implementation of these standards throughout the country.

iii. Certification of various articles and processes.

iv. Establishment, maintenance and recognition of laboratories for standardization and quality control.

v. Conduction of research for standards formulations.

vi. To provide information, documentation and other relevant services to consumers.

vii. Conduction of conferences, seminars and symposia to make aware of the consumers regarding standards and quality control measures.

viii. Provides guidance and consultancy services on standards and quality control measures.

ix. Harmonises standards and quality control activities in the country.

x. Provides guidance and recognition of quality assurance system in manufacturing and processing units.

xi. Publications of handbooks, guides and other special publications on Indian Standards.

BIS Standards for Indian Meat Industry

Standards for Abattoir and Sale of Meat

IS: 4393-1979	Basic requirement for an abattoir (Ist revision)
IS: 7053-1973	Basic requirements for stall for sale of meat of small animals

IS: 8700-1977	Basic requirements for stall for sale of meat of large animals

Standards for Ante-Mortem and Post Mortem Examination of Meat Animals

IS: 1982-1971	Code of practice for ante-mortem and post mortem inspection of meat animals
IS: 6559-1972	Code of practice for ante-mortem and post mortem inspection of poultry

Standards for Meat Plant Hygiene

IS: 8182-1976	Code of hygienic conditions for processed meat products
IS: 8182-1976	Code of hygienic conditions for processing plant

Specifications for Meat Processing Equipments

IS: 3545-1982	Specifications for meat choppers
IS: 6628-1972	Specifications for slide rails used in abattoir
IS: 7891-1975	Specifications for inedible offals trolleys
IS: 6782-1972	Specifications for hog gambrels
IS: 7909-1975	Specifications for electrical stunning tongs for pigs
IS: 994-1964	Specifications for butchers knives and fish knives
IS: 6696-1972	Specifications for egg washing machine

Specifications for meat, eggs and fish

IS: 2536-1963	Specifications for mutton and chevon-fresh, chilled and frozen
IS: 2537-1963	Specifications for beef and buffalo meat-fresh, chilled and frozen
IS: 1723-1973	Specifications for pork
IS: 2536-1963	Specifications for dressed chicken

IS: 7049-1973	Code of handling, processing, quality evaluation and storage of poultry
IS: 9810-1981	Methods for evaluation of quality of chicken eggs
IS: 6557-1972	Code of practice for cold storage of shell eggs
IS: 10763-1983	Specifications for frozen minced fish meat
IS: 8076-1976	Specifications for frozen cuttle fish and squid

Specifications for Meat, Egg and Fish Products

IS: 8539-1977	Terminology for meat products and meat animal including poultry

Mutton and Chevon Products

IS: 3044-1973	Specifications for curried and canned mutton and chevon

Beef and Buffalo Meat Products

IS: 11746-1986	Specifications for canned Luncheon beef
IS: 11747-1986	Specifications for canned corned beef
IS: 11771-1986	Specifications for beef soup stock

Pork Products

IS: 2474-1979	Specifications for smoked bacon
IS: 2476-1963	Specifications for ham
IS: 3060-1979	Specifications for canned pork sausages
IS: 3061-1979	Specifications for fresh pork sausages

Chicken Products

IS: 5558-1970	Specifications for chicken essence
IS: 10697-1983	Specifications for chicken canned in brine

Egg Products

IS: 4723-1978	Specifications for egg powder
IS: 10382-1982	Specifications for edible egg albumen powder
IS: 6557-1972	Specifications for non edible albumin flakes

Fish Products

IS: 10760-1983	Specifications for fish muscles canned in oil
IS: 10761-1983	Specifications for sardine canned in curry

Specifications for Slaughter House By-Products

IS: 8895-1978	Guidelines for handling, storage and transport of slaughterhouse by-products
IS: 1981-1978	Specifications for animal casings
IS: 4054-1966	Specifications for neats foot oil

Specifications for Proximate Analysis of Meat and Meat Products

IS: 5960	Methods of test for meat and meat products

Specifications for Meat Food Packaging

IS: 7688	Code of practice for labelling of pre-packaged food
IS: 10146-1982	Specifications for polyethylene as a packaging material
IS: 10151-1982	Specifications for poly vinyl chloride as a packaging material

Specifications for Sensory Evaluation of Foods Including Animal Products

IS: 10642-1983	General guidelines for consumer sensory evaluation of foods and beverages
IS: 6273	Guidelines for sensory evaluation of foods

Specifications for Food Microbiology

IS: 5404-1984	Methods of drawing and handling of samples for microbiological analysis
IS: 6854-1973	Methods for sampling and testing of ingredients used in media for microbiological study
IS: 10232-1982	Guidelines for preparation of dilutions for microbiological study of foods
IS: 5402-1969	Methods for total plate count in foods
IS: 5401-1969	Methods for detection and estimation of coliform in foods
IS: 5887-1976	Methods for detection of bacteria responsible for food poisoning
	Part-I for *E.coli* count
	Part-II for *Staphylococcus aureus* and faecal *Streptococci*
	Part-III for *Salmonella* and *Shigella*
	Part-IV for *Chlostridium welchii, C. botulinum,* and *Bacillus cereus*
IS: 5403-1969	Method for yeast and mould counts in foods

Specifications for Food Preservatives and Chemicals used in Meat Processing

IS: 4753-1968	Specifications for good grade potassium nitrate
IS: 5957-1969	Specifications for good grade potassium nitrite
IS: 9505-1980	Specifications for good grade monosodium-L glutamate
IS: 5342-1969	Specifications for good grade ascorbic acid
IS: 5344-1969	Specifications for good grade butylated hydroxyl toluene
IS: 3543-1966	Specification for papain

5. Enforcement Bodies

The Export Inspection Council (EIC) is the chief enforcement body for exports. The EIC was set up by the Government of India in order to ensure sound development of export trade of India through quality control and inspection. The EIC and its associated agencies are responsible for:

i. Notification of commodities which are subjected to quality control and/or inspection prior to export and to establish standards of quality for such notified commodities.

ii. To specify the type of quality control and/or inspection to be applied to such commodities.

iii. To promote the export for international trade of a notified commodity as per the standard specifications.

iv. Certification of quality of export commodities through installation of quality assurance systems in the exporting units as well as consignment-wise inspection.

v. Certification of quality of food items for export through installation of Food Safety Management Systems in the food processing units as per international standards.

vi. Issue of certificates of origin to exporters under various preferential tariff schemes for export products.

vii. Laboratory testing.

viii. Training and technical assistance to the industry in installation of Quality and Safety Management Systems based on principles of Hazard Analysis Critical Control Point (HACCP), ISO-9000 and other related areas.

6. Ministry of Food Processing Industries (MoFPI)

Though the private, public and co-operative sectors are to play their rightful role in the progress of the industry, the 'Ministry of Food Processing Industries' is the nodal agency for developing a strong and vibrant food processing sector in the country. It acts as a catalyst and facilitator for attracting domestic and foreign investments towards developing large integrated processing capacities; providing technical guidance and advice to the industry; as well as creating conducive environment for its growth. It covers the products of fruits and vegetables, dairy, milk, poultry, fishery, consumer food, grains, non-molasses based alcoholic drinks, aerated water and soft drinks. The objectives of the Ministry are to:-

i. Utilize and make value addition to agricultural produce for enhancement of income of farmers.

ii. Minimize wastage at all stages in the food processing chain by the development of infrastructure for storage, transportation and processing of agro-food produce.

iii. Induct modern technology into the sector from both domestic and external sources.

iv. Use efficiently agricultural residues and by-products of the primary agricultural produce as well as of the processed industry.

v. Encourage R&D in food processing for product and process development and improved packaging.

vi. Provide policy support, promotional initiatives and physical facilities to promote value added exports.

vii. Promote rationalisation of tariffs and duties relating to food processing sector.

viii. Create the critical infrastructure to fill the gaps in the supply chain from farm to consumer.

The MoFPI being the nodal point, actively interfaces with various Ministries of the Government of India and State Governments. For export consignments, MFPI interacts with APEDA, MPEDA and EIC all these of the Ministry of Commerce and other industry associations. Thus, the coordination for effectively addressing the export obligations is performed by MFPI in between food parks and agri-export zones. MFPI is deeply involved in updating the Codex norms. In fact, MFPI is the Chairman of following five Shadow Committees of Codex

Committees: Food Additives and Contaminants; Food Labelling; Processed Fruits and Vegetables; Cocoa and Chocolate Products and Mineral Water.

7. National Meat and Poultry Processing Board (NMPPB) India

The National Meat and Poultry Processing Board (NMPPB) have been set up to ensure safe meat and poultry meat production with no environmental hazard. The basic aims of NMPPB are:

i. Production of hygienic, safe and wholesome meat and meat products.

ii. Harmonization of domestic standards with international standards.

iii. Develop uniform and effective meat quality testing systems in the country.

iv. To address the environmental pollution issue arising out of the present conditions in the meat industry.

Functions of NMPPB

i. Helping the industry in setting up/modernization of abattoirs by providing technical consultancy for production of hygienic meat and meat products and for utilization of slaughterhouse wastes to prepare animal by-products with value addition.

ii. Setting up quality control laboratories and analytical laboratories for meat and meat products to meet the required domestic and international market standards.

iii. Promotion and training of meat producers and entrepreneurs to adopt Good Manufacturing Practices (GMP), Hazard Analysis and Critical Control Points (HACCP), ISO-22000 in meat production.

iv. Setting up a mechanism for implementation of the existing regulations and laws in India on meat and meat production, processing and marketing.

v. To undertake market surveys and help the industry to create market intelligence, data base and its dissemination on regular basis for improvement of the meat sector.

vi. To provide help for research and for setting up training institutions to train workers, technicians, managers in meat and meat processing industry.

vii. To help industry to establish infrastructure for backward and forward linkages for trace-ability of meat/poultry meat processing sector of India.

viii. Work as a Central/National hub to address issues related to Meat and Poultry processing sector for its systematic and proper development.

NMPPB is a body having great deal with the management of meat industry wastes which is very much neglected in our country. Utilization of animal waste materials and by-products into value added products may solve the problem of environmental pollution and health hazards. It may also be helpful in generation of employment to the rural peoples.

Rules and Regulations on Product Standards

The Ministry of Food and Consumer Affairs is the main Government agency dealing with product standards for consumption in the domestic market. Although each Ministry/Department has its own system of framing and notifying product standards. State Governments also have their own systems of adoption of standards, notably in the area of weights and measures. For the products, main rules and regulations are contained in the Prevention of Food Adulteration Act, Export Quality Control and Inspection Act and the regulations for spice quality. Today imported goods seem to get even better than national treatment as they are seldom subjected to the same enforcement procedures as the domestic units producing.

1. *Prevention of Food Adulteration Act (PFA, 1954):* It is the basic statute to protect consumers against supply of adulterated food. The Central Committee for Food Standards 'under the Directorate General & Health Services, Ministry of Health and Family Welfare has specified the standards.

2. *Export (Quality Control and Inspection) Act, 1963*: It is operated by the Export Inspection Council and under this act many exportable commodities have been notified for compulsory pre-shipment inspection unless specifically requested by the importer not to do so.

3. *Standard of Weights and Measures (Packaged Commodities) Rules, 1977*: These standards lay down certain obligations for all commodities in packaged form with respect to their quality declaration. The Directorate of Weights and Measures under the Ministry of Food and Civil Supplies operates these rules.

Legislation/ act	Governing bodies
Meat Food Product Order 1973	Ministry of Agriculture
Agricultural Produce (Grading and Marking) Act	Ministry of Rural Development: Directorate of Marketing and Inspection (DMI)
Prevention of Food Adulteration Act 1954	Ministry of Health & Family Welfare
Export (Quality Control & Inspections) Act 1963	Ministry of Commerce
Standards of Weights & Measures Act	Ministry of Civil Supplies, Consumer Affairs and Public Distribution
Standards of Weights & Measures (Enforcement) Act	Ministry of Civil Supplies, Consumer Affairs and Public Distribution
Bureau of Indian Standards (BIS) Act 1986	Ministry of Civil Supplies, Consumer Affairs and Public Distribution
Aquaculture Authority Notification 1997 & 2002	Ministry of Environment and Forests
Environment (Protection) Act 1986, Environment (Protection) Third Amendment Rules, 2002	Ministry of Environment and Forests

8. Meat Food Products Order (MFPO), 1973

MFPO was promulgated under section 3 of the Essential Commodities Act, 1955 , it aims to ensure supply of wholesome meat food products to the consumers. It deals with quality control of meat food products from processing to finished product by way of ante-mortem and post-mortem inspection of meat animals so as to ensure hygienic conditions of processing of meat food products. It was earlier implemented by Directorate of Marketing and Inspection (DMI), but its administration has been transferred to the Ministry of Agriculture. The sanitary, hygienic, packing, marking and labelling requirements are specified in separate Schedules of the Order. To keep pace with recent developments in the manufacturing of meat food products and to hormonize the MFPO standards with PFA, Codex, EU, FDA and other international food standards, the Ministry has taken the initiative to review the existing MFPO, 1973 which aims to suggest amendment in the meat products standards based on the scientific development and modernization of the meat and meat processing industries and the rules governing them. The actual order came in force from the 15.07.1975. The Principal Order was published by Department of Agriculture, Ministry of Agriculture in the Gazette of India Extraordinary Part-II, section 3, sub-section (ii) vide S.O.No.176(E) dt.28.3.1973 and later, the subject was transferred to the Ministry of Food Processing Industries vide S.O. No.452(E) dt.2. 4. 2004.

Structure wise MFPO is constitutional body having MFPO advisory committee and the tenure of the committee is renewed at an interval of every two years. Central Government, by Order, published in the Official Gazette, constitute a Committee called Meat Food Products Advisory Committee which is consist of the Joint Secretary to the Government of India in the Ministry of Food Processing Industries who shall be the Chairman thereof and the following members, namely:

(a) Animal Husbandry Commissioner, Government of India or his nominee.

(b) Director General of Health Services, Government of India or his nominee.

(c) Director, Indian Veterinary Research Institute, Izzatnagar, U.P. or his nominee.

(d) Executive Director, Food and Nutrition Board, Department of Women & Child Development, Government of India or his nominee.

(e) Director, Central Food Technological Research Institute, Mysore or his Nominee.

(f) Two officers of the Department of Animal Husbandry or Veterinary Services of State Governments to be nominated by the Central Government.

(g) Two persons among the manufacturers to be nominated by the Central Government.

(h) An officer of the Ministry of Food Processing Industries to be nominated by the licensing authority who shall act as the Secretary of the Committee.

A member of the Committee shall hold office for the period for which the Committee has been constituted: Provided that a member may resign his office by notice in writing given to the Chairman of the Committee.

The main objectives of the MFPO, 1973 are to regulate production and sale of meat food products through licensing of manufacturers, enforcement of sanitary and hygienic conditions prescribed for production of wholesome meat food products, exercise on strict quality control at all stages of production of meat food products, fish products including chilled poultry etc. Under the provision of MFPO all manufacturers of meat food products engaged in the business of manufacturing, packing, repacking, relabeling meat food products meant for sale are licensed but excluding those manufacturers who manufactures such products for consumption on the spot like a restaurant, hotel, boarding house, snack bar, eating house or any other similar establishment.

Categories of MFPO

MFPO is categorised into three main categories based on the raw material utilization by the processor in their meat processing plant.

Category 'A'

Category 'A' deals with the Manufacturers who make meat food products exclusively from meat of animal(s) slaughtered and dressed in his factory. The licensing fee is depending upon the quantity of meat processed as if the quantity of meat food products manufactured is more than 150 tonnes per annum then Rs.5, 000/-per annum fee is charged, if the quantity of meat food products manufactured less than 150 tons per annum then Rs.2, 500/ will be the licence fee.

Category 'B'

Category 'B' deals with the manufacturer who makes meat food products exclusively from meat of animal(s) slaughtered and dressed in a recognised slaughter house including a slaughter house maintained by Category 'A' licensee. The fee schedule is decided on the same basis as in category 'A' viz. if the quantity of meat food products manufactured is more than 150 tons per annum; Rs 2, 500/-, If the quantity of meat food products manufactured is less than 150 tons per annum Rs.1, 000/-

Category 'C'

This category deals with the manufactures that are purchasing the meat from other sources. The manufacturer who makes meat food products exclusively from poultry and/or pig meat at places where authorised slaughter houses do not exist are comes under this category. Fish products shall also be covered under this category. The licensing fee in this category is Rs.1, 000/-

Schedules of MFPO

'Schedule' means a Schedule appended to MFPO. It deals with the licence provisions and their renewal, sanitary, hygienic and packaging issues related to meat food products. MFPO contains four schedules depending on the meat food products requirements.

First Schedule

First schedule normally comes under clauses 4 (2) and 5 (2) of the MFPO. It deals with application for licence/renewal of licence under the Meat Food Products Order, 1973. It has mainly three forms viz. form A, B and C.

Form A: Its provision is given in clause 4 (2) and 5 (2)) of the MFPO. It contains Name and address of the applicant, name of the managing director, director, proprietor, partner etc., address of factory, source of raw material like animals slaughtered in the factory premises or purchased directly from approved public slaughter houses or from other sources and type of the product manufacturer wants to produce. In addition it should have the following information like installed capacity per shift of 8 hours, existing licence No. if any, total value of meat food products manufactured during the previous year and a declaration statement.

Form B: Its provision is given in clause 6 of MFPO. Form B contains the licence issued by competent authority. It should have the information like Licence No. M.F.P.O, category, name and address of the Licensee, address of the factory, source of raw meat, details of animals authorized to slaughter and their meat for processing and the type of licence *i.e.* validation and renewal.

Form C: Provision of Form C is given in Clause 10 of the MFPO. It deals with the information related to packaging of the meat food products like name and address of the licensee, address of the factory, M.F.P.O. Licence No., Category, statement showing the quantities of meat food products manufactured during the year and value, serial no., name of the meat food product, size of can or bottle, sale price per kilogram, quantity manufactured in kilograms, value in rupees, quantity exported, ports of export, country to which exported, rate per kilogram c.i.f./f.o.b., value and declaration by licensee.

Second Schedule

Second schedule covers the duties mentioned in Clause 9 (2) of the MFPO. It deals with Sanitary and other requirements to be complied with by a licensee.

Under this schedule, all parts of the factory shall always be kept clean, adequately lighted and ventilated and shall be regularly cleaned, disinfected and deodorized.

1. Floorings shall be impervious and washed daily. Lime washing, colour washing or painting as the case may be, shall be done at least once in every twelve months. The floors, walls, ceilings,

partitions, parts, doors and other parts of all structures shall be of such materials, construction and finish that they can be readily and thoroughly cleaned.

2. Windows, doors and other openings suited to screening shall be fly proof. All doors shall have strong springs so that they may close automatically. The ceiling or roof shall be of permanent nature.

3. All operations in connection with the preparation or packing of meat food products shall be carried out under strict hygienic conditions.

4. There shall be efficient drainage and plumbing systems and all drains and gutters shall be properly and permanently installed.

5. The rooms and compartments where edible products are handled shall be separate and distinct from the rooms and compartments for inedible products. The equipment and the manufacturing area approved for the manufacture of meat food products shall not be used for the manufacture of any other products repugnant to the manufacturing of the meat food products except under the condition given as under:- If the licensed premises are used for the manufacture of meat food products and nonmeat food products there shall be a gap of at least one month when the change is made from marine products to meat food products and three days gap when the change is made from fruits and vegetable products to meat food products.

6. All factories shall have adequate cold storage facilities.

7. The rooms and compartments in which any meat food product is prepared or handled shall be free from dust and from odours emanating from dressing rooms, toilet rooms, catch basins, hide cellars, casing rooms and livestock pens.

8. All practicable precaution shall be taken to exclude flies, rats, mice and vermin from the factory. The use of poisons for any purpose in rooms or compartments where any unpacked product is stored or handled is forbidden. Entry of dogs and cats is prohibited.

9. No vessel, container or other equipment, the use of which is likely to cause metallic contamination injurious to health shall be employed in the preparation, packing or storage of meat food products. Copper or brass vessels shall always be heavily tinned and no iron or galvanised iron shall come in contact with meat food products.

10. Water used in the manufacturing shall be potable and, if required by the licensing authority, shall be examined chemically and bacteriologically by a recognised laboratory. The cost of such analysis shall be borne by the manufacturer.

11. Wherever five or more employees of either sex are employed, a sufficient number of latrines and washbasins for each sex as specified below shall be provided.

No. of workers	Number of latrines	Number of wash basins
Not exceeding 25	1	1
Exceeding 25 but not exceeding 49	2	2
Exceeding 50 but not exceeding 100	3	3
Exceeding 100 and above	5	5

12. Whenever cooking is done on open fire, chimneys shall be provided for removal of smoke and soot.

13. No person suffering from infectious or contagious diseases shall be allowed to work in the factory.

14. The factory staff should be vaccinated with commonly occurring diseases. The workers working in processing and preparation shall wear proper aprons and head wears which shall be clean.

15. Meat used for the preparation of meat food products, if it is not slaughtered in the factory, shall be obtained only from slaughter houses in which ante-mortem and post-mortem inspections have been carried out in accordance with the rules prescribed in that connection and so certified by the local authority.

16. A laboratory facility should be there to inspect and examine the meat food products before launching.

Third Schedule

Third schedule of the MFPO is governed by the Clause 9(3) of MFPO. It deals with the hygienic and other requirements for a licensee who also slaughters animals in his factory.

In addition to the conditions prescribed in the Second Schedule, every manufacturer who slaughters animals within the premises of his factory for the purpose of manufacturing meat food products shall comply with the following requirements:

1. The slaughter house attached to the factory shall have adequate separation between clean and dirty sections and shall be so organized that from the introduction of a live animal into the slaughter house up to the emergence of meat and offal classed as fit for human consumption, there shall be a continuous forward movement without any possibility of reversal, intersection or overlapping between the live animal and meat and between meat and by -products or waste.
2. The slaughter house shall have a reception area of resting ground, lairage, slaughter hall, ancillary accommodation and refrigeration room. The reception area or resting ground shall have facilities for watering and examining animals before they are sent to holding pens. Animals suspected of contagious or infectious diseases shall be segregated and kept in separate pens which shall also be provided with arrangements for watering and feeding. The resting ground must have some overhead protective shelter.
3. Lairage shall be adequate in size for the number of animals to be laired.
4. Every factory shall make separate provision in the slaughter hall for the slaughter of different species of animals and for different methods of slaughter. After every type of operation the slaughter house shall be cleaned and washed.
5. Every part of the internal surface of the walls and every part of the floor and pavement of the slaughter house shall be kept in good order and repair at all time with well washing facilities.

6. It may be ensured that dogs, cats or birds do not have access to the slaughter hall. Open areas in the factory shall be having covered by wire rope netting to prevent carrion birds from access to the slaughter hall or the factory.
7. Suitable and sufficient facilities shall be provided for the isolation of meat requiring further examination by the Meat Food Products Inspector in a suitable laboratory within the premises of the slaughter house.
8. The drainage system for blood shall either be underground with facility for easy cleaning or a portable receptacle with lid.
9. Separate space shall be provided for stunning, bleeding and dressing of the carcasses. The slaughtering of an animal shall not be done in the sight of other animals. The dressing of the carcass shall not be done on the floor.
10. Rooms and compartments in which animals are slaughtered or any product is processed or prepared shall be kept sufficiently free from steam, vapours and moisture so as to ensure clean operations.
11. Suitable and sufficient accommodation shall be provided for segregation and storage of condemned meat.
12. Suitable and sufficient facilities shall be provided for persons working in the slaughter house for changing their clothes and cleaning their hands before entering rooms used for the preparation and storage of meat.
13. Suitable and separate space shall be provided for the storage of hides and skins with the facility of separate exit.
14. Whenever the dressed meat is not used up for the preparation of meat food products and some portion has to be stored without further immediate processing, such storage shall be in a room maintained at 3.5 °C to 10 °C.
15. All the floors in lairages, slaughter halls, work rooms, hanging rooms shall be of impervious and non-slippery material.

16. Ceiling or roofs shall be constructed and finished to minimise condensation, mould development, flaking and accumulation of dirt.

17. A constant supply of clean hot water may be available in the slaughter hall during working hours.

18. The equipment and fittings in slaughter hall except for chopping blocks, cutting boards and brooms shall be of such material and of such construction as to enable them to be kept clean. The implements shall be of metal or other cleansable and durable material resistant to corrosion.

19. Suitable and sufficient facilities shall be provided in convenient places with in the slaughter house for the sterilisation of wiping clothes, knives and other equipment used in the slaughter house.

20. Suitable and sufficient receptacles furnished with comely fitted covers shall be provided for collection and removal of all garbage filth and refuse from the slaughter house at convenient time to a place away from the factory for disposal

21. All blood, manure, garbage, filth or other refuse from any animal slaughtered and the hide, fat, viscera and offal there from, shall be removed from the slaughter house within 8 hours after the completion of the slaughtering and in such a manner and by such means as will not cause nuisance at the premises or elsewhere. Every such vessel or receptacle shall be thoroughly cleaned immediately after use and shall be kept thoroughly clean when not in actual use.

22. The inner side of the skin shall not be rubbed or caused to be rubbed upon the ground within any portion of the slaughter hall. Hides and skins shall not be dragged within the slaughter hall. No gut-scraping, tripe cleaning, manufacture or preparation of meat food products, household washing or work of any nature other than is involved in the slaughter and dressing of the carcass shall be permitted in any slaughter hall except in the adjuncts to the slaughter hall intended for these products and purposes.

Fourth Schedule

Fourth schedule is a description of Clause 9(4) of MFPO. In this schedule requirements packaging, marking and labeling of containers of meat food products are described in detail. As per the schedule meat food products shall be packaged in containers having following quality characteristics:

1. Container shall be securely packed and sealed as per the detail given below:
   a. New sanitary top cans with tin plate covering can be used.
   b. Cans shall be lacquered internally and sealed hermetically after filling. The lacquer used shall be sulphur resistant and shall not be soluble in fat or brine.
   c. Cans used for filling pork luncheon meat shall be coated internally with edible gelatine, lard or lined with vegetable parchment paper before being filled.
   d. The exterior of the cans shall be free from major dents, rust, perforations and seam distortions.
   e. Cans shall be free from leaks.
   f. Bottles and jars used for packing shall be new and must be capable of being sealed hermetically.
2. Packaging material shall be clean and should be stored in a clean and sanitary manner to prevent contamination of the final product.
3. Meat food products packaged in hermetically sealed containers shall be processed to withstand spoilage under commercial conditions of storage and transport.
4. No water other than potable water shall be used for cooking or cooling of any hermetically sealed container.
5. After processing, containers shall be handled in such a manner as to avoid contamination of the product. Belts, runways and other can conveying equipment shall be maintained in clean condition and good repair.

6. Processed hermetically sealed containers shall be inspected to exclude defective containers.
7. Every manufacturer shall provide adequate facilities for the incubation of random samples of individual batches of containers.
8. The manufacturer shall cause an appropriate label to be securely affixed to each container after packing it with meat food products derived from meat which has been previously inspected and passed.
9. Specimens of all labels shall first be got approved by the licensing authority before use.
10. The following particulars shall be clearly marked on the labels such as name of the product, date of manufacture, net weight or volume of the contents at the time of packaging, name and address of the manufacturer, unauthorised use of words, picture etc. Every package of meat food product contains mono-sodium glutamate shall bear the following label: "This package of——— (product name) contains monosodium glutamate unfit for infant below 12 months". If preservative is used then write the name of preservative, in case of added flavourings then mark it and also mention the safety levels of different chemicals and additives level on the package with the actual residues present the meat food products.

Depending on the source of meat the manufacturers are licensed under category A, B & C. Presently, 279 units are licensed under MFPO as on 01.04.09. They are processing more than 170 meat food products. The most common foods are different types of ham, bacon, sausages, curried meat, meat chunks or chops, minced meat, corned meats, luncheon meats, roasted and fried meats, patties and burgers, tikkas, spreads, rolls or grills, kababs, pickles, speciality meats like mutton pulao, chicken and lamb biryani, pork vindaloo, meat paste chicken etc. and soups and pastes. Region-wise details are given below: -

Region	Category A	Category B	Category C	Total
Western Region	11	32	43	86
Southern Region	12	37	35	84
Northern Region	9	33	39	81
Eastern Region	7	6	15	28
TOTAL	39	108	132	279

Terms related to MFPO

Carcass means the dead body or any part thereof including the viscera of any animal which has been slaughtered.

Factory means any premises including the precincts thereof, wherein meat food products are manufactured or packaged for sale.

Licensee means a manufacturer to whom a licence is granted under this order.

Licensing authority means the Joint Secretary to the Government of India in the Ministry of Food Processing Industries and includes any other officer authorised by him in this behalf with the previous approval of the Central Government.

Local Authority means a municipal council, committee, corporation, panchayat, notified area committee or other authority entrusted with the regulation and licensing of slaughter houses in any local area.

Manufacturer means a person engaged in the business of manufacturing, packaging, repacking, relabelling meat food products meant for sale but shall not include a person who manufactures such products and serves on the spot for consumption in a restaurant, hotel, boarding house, snack bar, eating house or any other similar establishment.

Meat means the flesh and other edible parts of a carcass.

Meat Food Products means any article of food or any article intended for or capable of being used as a food which is derived or prepared from meat by means of drying, curing, smoking, cooking, seasoning, flavouring, freezing or following a method of processing meat akin to any of the above methods but shall not include the following products unless the manufacturer himself desires to be covered under the provisions of the said order such as:

i. Meat extracts, meat consommé and stock, meat sauces and similar products not containing fragments of meat.

ii. Whole, broken or crushed bones, meat peptones, animal gelatine, meat, powder, pork-rind powder, blood plasma, dried blood, dried blood plasma, cellular proteins, bone extracts and similar products.

iii. Fats melted down from animal tissues.

iv. Stomachs, bladders and intestines, clean and bleached, salted or dried;

v. Products containing fragments of meat, but which contain a quantity of meat or meat product not exceeding ten percent of the total weight of the final product.

vi. Patties, puffs, rolls, samosas, cutlets, koftas, kababs, chops, tikkas and soups made from mutton, chicken, goat meat, buffalo meat, beef and grilled chicken which are prepared for immediate consumption, the ampoules of chicken essence, hot-dogs and hamburgers prepared for immediate consumption which can not be stored even under refrigerated conditions.

Meat Food Products Inspector means an official veterinarian appointed by the licensing authority and includes any officer of a local authority authorised to perform the functions of the Meat Food Products Inspector under this Order. He is having the powers to inspect the premises of meat food processing, can seize the whole premise, documents and meat or meat products present in that premise and also can dispose off the meat food products and other materials.

Slaughter House means the building, premises or place which is licensed as a slaughter house by the local authority for the slaughter of animals intended for human consumption.

9. Food Safety and Standards Act, 2006

It is also known as Integrated Food Law because it consolidate the laws relating to food, establish the food safety and standards authority of India for laying down science based standards for articles of food. In addition it also regulates manufacture, storage, distribution, sale and import of food articles with a view to ensure availability of safe and wholesome food for human consumption. It also pools infrastructure, manpower and testing facilities for better standard fixation and enforcement through their proper re-deployment.

Its aim is to achieve a high degree of consumer confidence in the quality and safety of produced, processed, sold or exported food. It seeks to overcome problems like multiplicity of food laws and standard setting and enforcement agencies which creates confusion in the minds of consumers, traders, investors and manufacturers. As a result of such incentives and measures, the industry has witnessed fast growth in most of its segments. Due to this act the growth and development of meat and meat processing sector, poultry meat is the fastest growing animal protein in India. The estimated production is 1500 thousand tonnes growing at a rate of 13 per cent through 1991-2005. India exports more than 500,000 MT of meat of which major share is buffalo meat. Indian buffalo meat is witnessing strong demand in international markets due to its lean character and near organic nature. Its exports have the potential to grow significantly and hence present an opportunity for exporters in the food processing segment. India is the fifth largest exporter of bovine meat in the world. However, in order to develop necessary infrastructure for processing of meat and meat food products for domestic market as well as for export market, the Ministry is providing financial assistance by way of grant-in-aid. During the year 2007-08 (upto December 2007), it assisted nine projects for manufacture of meat and meat food products.

Moreover, the Ministry of Food Processing Industries has finalised the document regarding the Vision 2015 for the growth of Indian food processing industries which is known as the 'Integrated Strategy for Promotion of Agri-business - Vision, Strategy and Action Plan for the Food Processing Sector based on the recommendations made by the Group of Ministers (GoM) for growth of the sector. The objective of the strategy is to increase the level of processing of perishable food from 6% to 20%, value addition from 20% to 35% and share in global food trade from 1.6% to 3% by 2015. The thrust areas identified for strategic intervention are detailed mapping of food clusters, establishment of Mega Food Parks in identified SSI/ horticulture/ meat/ dairy/ marine sectors, strengthening backward and forward linkages and developing supply chain with cold chain mechanism, modernisation of Abattoirs; developing infrastructure for organized food retail market, rationalizing tax structure for the sector etc. All these efforts have given competitive edge to the food processing industry on a global platform. More and more people are consuming value-added and processed food products. The industry possess high export opportunities and its growth seeks to bring immense benefits to the economy by raising agricultural yields, enhancing productivity, creating employment and raising life-standards of a large number of people across the country, especially those in rural areas. Thus, there exists innumerable business opportunities in the diverse areas of food processing.

But, the food processing sector still remains largely untapped because of high packing costs, cultural preference of the people for fresh food, seasonalities of raw materials, lack of adequate infrastructural facilities and quality control mechanism. As a result, there is a need to diversify the sector by fully harnessing its potentialities, providing greater incentives as well as creating conducive environment for more investments and exports.

10. Food Safety and Standards Authority of India (FSSAI)

FSSAI is a science based food standard enforcement body. It is a modified version of Food Safety and Standards Act, 2006. This act is in operation since August, 2011 and it is a single window system integrating nine different food laws and eight different ministries involved in food sector. Some of the acts which were integrated under this authority are Prevention of Food adulteration act, 1954, Fruit Products order, 1955, Meat Food Products Order, 1973, Vegetable Oil Products (Control) Order, 1947, Edible Oils Packaging (Regulation) Order, 1988, Solvent Extracted Oil, De-oiled meal, and Edible Flour (Control) Order, 1967, Milk and Milk Products Order, 1992, Essential Commodity Act, 1955 etc. The major emphasis of this law is on the food safety through Good Manufacturing Practices (GMP), Good Hygiene Practices (GHP), Hazard Analysis Critical Control Points

(HACCP), Food Safety Management System etc. The salient features of this authority include:

1. It has multilevel and multidepartment control.
2. It has integrated approach and harmonization to deals with the International standards and the formulation of standards related to food safety, sanitary and phytosanitary measures at domestic level. It also deals with the novel foods, GM foods etc.
3. It has power to license the manufacture of food and commission food safety or designated officer is the authority to grant the license.
4. It is a single referral point to deals with the food safety standards, regulations and their enforcement.
5. It facilitates the self compliance of the standards and regulations in the food organization through food safety management system.
6. It also has the provisions of the penalties for various offenses.

Structure wise FSSAI has overall control of central government with the name of food authority. It also has the bodies like central advisory committee, scientific panels, scientific committees and enforcement bodies. The enforcement bodies of the acts includes central licensing authority, state licensing authority in each state/union territory through the state food safety commissioners, designated officers and food safety officers for licensing, inspection and sampling etc. The registering authority under this acts are Panchayat raj and municipal bodies. It has a provision of single license for one or more food articles and different establishments or premises in same areas. The requirements of license for petty or small food business operators are depending on their total output but their registration and adoption of food safety measures is compulsory. The small food operators having annual turnover above 12 lakhs or who is slaughtering more than 2 large animals or 10 small animals or 50 poultry must have the license to do so. However, act is not having the provision of license for livestock reares so the strict control over raw material is lacking in this standard.

Offences and penalties provisions under FSSAI

Offence	Dealing section of FSSAI	Provision of penalties
Sub standard food	Section -51	Penalty of five lakh rupees
Misleading advertisement	Section -53	Penalty of ten lakh rupees
Foods with extraneous materials	Section -54	Penalty of one lakh rupees
Disobey the directions of Food Safety Officer	Section -55	Penalty of two lakh rupees
Unhygienic or unsanitary processing and manufacturing of foods	Section -56	Penalty of one lakh rupees
Possession of adulterant	Section -57	If adulterant is injuries to health then penalty of maximum Rs ten lakhs and if not injurious than maximum of two lakh rupees
Interference with seized material	Section-60	Imprisonment upto 6 months and fine upto two lakh rupees
False information	Section-61	Imprisonment upto 3 months and fine upto two lakh rupees
Obstructing or impersonating the Food Safety Officer	Section-62	Imprisonment upto 3 months and fine upto one lakh rupees
Carrying out the business without license	Section-63	Imprisonment upto 6months and fine upto five lakh rupees

International Organizations

1. World Trade Organization (WTO)

The General Agreement on Tariffs and Trade (GATT) has been the beacon of the multilateral trading system since 1948. Through the results of the Uruguay Round of multilateral trade negotiations, the World Trade Organisation (WTO) came into existence in 1994 and came into force on 1/1/1995. Article 20 of WTO allows member countries to deviate from their obligations under the Agreement inter-alia in case of three types of trade measures. These are, measures necessary to protect human, animal or plant or life of health; measures relating to the conservation of exhaustible natural resources if such measures are made effective in conjunction with restrictions on domestic production or consumption, and measures necessary to secure compliance with laws or regulations not otherwise inconsistent with GATT rules. However, such unilateral measures have to pass a composite trade test. This trade test has three components viz. no arbitrary discrimination, no unjustifiable discrimination and no disguised trade protection. It is often called the least trade restrictiveness test. Jurisprudence has shown that the second of these measures has become the most potent tool for taking GATT compliant unilateral trade measures pursuant to environmental objectives. WTO agreement is mainly based on five principles i.e. non discrimination, reciprocity, binding and enforceable commitments, transparency and safety valves.

The Agreement on the application of sanitary and phytosanitary measures (SPS) is an elaboration of GATT rules. Under this Agreement, member countries are required to base their SPS measures on scientific principles and refrain from maintaining measures without sufficient scientific evidence. The Agreement encourages harmonisation of SPS measures and considers the standards set by three international standard setting bodies as acceptable standards. These are the Codex Alimentarius Commission, the International Office of Epizootic and the International Plant Protection Convention. The *Agreement on Technical Barriers to Trade (TBT)* allows members to apply standards (both mandatory and voluntary) for protection of human health or safety, animal or plant or life of health or the environment. This Agreement also requires sound science and fulfillment of the least trade restrictiveness test. The Agreement does not consider standards set by any particular international setting organization as acceptable. The main aim of TBT is to ensure that the regulations, standards, testing and certification procedures do not create unnecessary obstacle to trade. In practice, however, ISO standards are considered compatible unless certain trade rules and certain jurisprudentially developed practices are not followed in setting them. For example, standards based on non-product related process and production methods and those differentiating between like products may not be acceptable.

2. International Standards Organisation (ISO)

ISO is the most important of international standard setting organizations. It is a world federation of 123 national standards bodies, an international non-governmental organization, however, a majority of its members coming from the public sector. Its core business is the development, approval and promulgation of consensus based international standards. Unlike WTO, majority vote is practiced in this organization. ISO develops standards through 200 technical committees split into about 650 sub-committees and 2000 working groups. It also develops guide for standard setting. In preparing these, ISO interfaces with specific users of standards including those in the private sector. All its standards and guides are voluntary in nature. However, given its credibility as the most internationally accepted organization, ISO standards have considerable trade affects due to their wide use in international trade. Therefore, those who can afford do apply for ISO certification. ISO certification is a costly process by Indian standards. It may take anything between rupees 100,000 to 500,000 to get certified, apart from the cost of maintaining the certificate. While ISO 9000 series is the general quality certification standard of ISO, there is an environmental management standard also, viz. ISO 14000 series. India has about 5000 ISO 9000 companies. About 100 companies have taken ISO 14000 certification. ISO is a detailed quality management system in which twenty elements like management responsibility, design control, purchasing, product identification, process control, inspection and testing, corrective action, packaging; proper documentation, internal audit etc. have to be compliance by the manufacturers.

ISO-9000

ISO-9000 is a quality system which provides the series of guidance to adopt method of choice model for assurance of quality in organization. It is for the industry now to select and design an appropriate system which they would like to opt as per their need. There are various steps in ISO system to adopt the standards i.e. system designing, system documentation, implementation of documented system, internal verification of documented system, getting the system verified by reputed certification body and finally the provision of undertaking necessary to follow up actions, to sustain the achieved standard etc. These standards have various quality assurance modes which may be summarized as:

ISO-9001	:	Deals with the manufacturers having their own research and development (R&D) and assures quality design, development, production, installation and services
ISO-9002	:	Deals with the contract manufacturers not having their own R&D and assures production, installation and services
ISO-9003	:	Deals with commodity suppliers and assures final inspection and testing
ISO-9004:2000	:	Guidance for continual improvement
ISO-10005: 1995	:	Quality plan management and revision
ISO-10006: 1997	:	Guidelines for project process and products both
ISO-10007: 1995	:	Outline for complex process even after change in ingredients
ISO-10012: 1997	:	Guidelines for application of statistical process control
ISO-10013: 1995	:	Guidelines for development and maintenance of quality manual

ISO-14000

ISO 14000 is a voluntary environmental management system and helps in integration of environmental management systems of companies that trade with each other in all corners of the world. The basic aims of ISO 14000 standards include minimization of the environmental pollutions in industry through the provisions of minimization of air, water, or land pollution etc., enforcement of applicable laws, regulations and other environmentally oriented requirements and continuous improvements in these provisions. Some important ISO-14000 specifications are as under:

ISO- 14001	: Environmental management systems—Requirements with user guidance
ISO- 14004	: Environmental management systems—General guidelines including principles, systems and support techniques
ISO- 14015	: Environmental assessment of sites and organizations
ISO -14020	: ISO-14020 to 14025 deals with the environmental labels and declarations
ISO -14030	: Provisions of post production environmental assessment
ISO- 14031	: Guidelines for environmental performance evaluation
ISO- 14040	: ISO- 14040 to 14049 deals with the life cycle assessment and pre-production planning and environment goal setting
ISO -14050	: Terms and definitions
ISO -14062	: Provisions of improvements in environmental impact goals
ISO -14063	: Guidelines and examples of environmental communication
ISO -14064	: Measurement, quantification and reduction in greenhouse gas emissions.
ISO 19011	: Specifies one audit protocol for both 14000 and 9000 series standards together.

ISO-22000

ISO-22000 is a food safety management system through which international standard are designed to ensure safe food supply chain worldwide. The basic aims of this standard include the harmonization of food safety requirements at global level, facilitation and implementation of the provisions of codex alimentarius, HACCP system for food hygiene, implementation of food safety management system etc. These standards have unique characteristics like interactive communication, system management, pre-requisite programming and HACCP implementation. These standards may be summarized as:

ISO-22000: 2005 : Food safety management-General guidelines

ISO/TS-22004:2005 : Application guidelines for ISO-22000

ISO-22005:2007 : Traceability in feed and food chain

ISO/TS-22002-1:2009 : Specific pre-requisites for food manufacturing

ISO/TS-22002-3:2011 : Specific pre-requisites for farming

ISO/TS-22003 :2007 : Guidelines for audit and certification bodies

3. Codex Alimentarius Commission (CAC)

The Codex Alimentarius Commission was established in the year 1963 by the Food and Agriculture Organization (FAO) and World Health Organization (WHO). It is an UN body, compiles agreed-upon standards, guidelines and other recommendations into the Codex Alimentarius (Latin word meaning "Book of Food"). It is compilation of internationally recognized standards, codes of practices, guidelines etc. relating to foods, food production and safety. The CFC attempts to create harmonized standards. Prior to the SPS Agreement, the CFC could be adopted, applied and /or ignored at the discretion of a government. However, the CFC has now been adopted within the SPS Agreement as the benchmark. The countries not imposing standards higher than CFC standards have right to seek these standards for their imports. Codex Alimentarius has incorporated HACCP plans and principles as an integral part of the CFC. Volume V of the Food Code sets standards for number of specific fish and fish products. World Trade Organization (WTO) recognized the CAC as a reference organization for the resolution of disputes related to the food safety and consumer protection at International level. All types of the foods whether raw, processed, semi processed all are comes under the umbrella of CAC. CAC is responsible for the protection of standards on all aspects of foods such as food production, labeling, hygiene, additives, residues, biotechnologically produced foods etc. Structure wise CAC is having executive body comprising of 01 Chairman, 03 Vice-Chairman, 07 Regional Representatives, 06 Regional Coordinators followed by regional coordinating committees and secretariat of Commission. It also has 11 vertical committees including the Codex committee on meat and animal meat hygiene, codex committee on meat, milk and milk products as well as codex committee on fish and fishery products etc.

Aims

1. Consumers health protection and fair trading at global level.
2. Harmonization and co-ordination of International standards with Governmental and non Governmental organization.
3. Formulation of standards through the assistance of various organizations and Governmental agencies.
4. Publication and amendments of the existing standards after due survey at international level.

4. *Hazard Analysis Critical Control Point (HACCP)*

The Hazard Analysis Critical Control Point (HACCP) system is being increasingly used as a food safety system all over the developed world. HACCP is not the magic bullet that solves all food safety problems. It is, when properly applied, a set of preliminary steps and principles that gives a systematic method for identifying significant hazards and properly applying preventive measures so that food borne hazards are prevented, eliminated or reduced to an acceptable level. With emerging international and national agreement on HACCP principles, their application would create commonality of understanding of the development, implementation and maintenance of a food safety system. Having these commonly understood principles, many food processors, for example, require their suppliers to have a HACCP system for production of ingredients that they supply. Knowing that a source of food borne hazards can be from a particular point there will be more attention given to that for implementation of effective, documented systems that eliminate or reduce the likely occurrence of food borne hazards. Application of HACCP offers widely understood principles for identifying significant risks and their control. HACCP does not cover only pathogenic bacteria. In applying HACCP, all food borne hazards are to be considered. There are a number of hazards that can originate during production. Some examples of food borne hazards that can originate during production include Biological -*Salmonella, Campylobacter jejuni, E. coli, Listeria monocytogenes, Yersinia enterocolitica, Cryptosporidium parvum,* and *Trichinella* and some chemicals, particularly pesticides and drugs. An important definition in HACCP is the one for Critical Control Point (CCP): a point, step or procedure at which control can be applied and a food safety hazard can be prevented, eliminated or reduced to an acceptable level. Therefore, if the identified food safety hazards are to be controlled through a HACCP system, there must be a step or steps in production where control can be applied and there must be an associated preventive measure. It is essential that there be scientifically documented steps and preventive measures. If this criterion cannot be met, then a HACCP system cannot be developed. A HACCP system can only be developed through proper application of the preliminary steps and principles of HACCP. An essential prerequisite to HACCP is the adoption of Good Manufacturing Practices (GMPs). The biggest problem in HACCP Plans is the lack of true CCPs. The issue is that biological hazards are much more difficult to deal with than most of the food processing. For example, we know that proper heating times and temperatures will kill *E.coli*, therefore, this can be a CCP. However, at present not enough is known about the sources and control of *E.coli* to be able to apply preventive measures. Hence, the emphasis on Good Agricultural Practices (GAP) as a precursor to the HACCP Plans. Thus there is lack of knowledge and research at pre-processing stage. The research has not provided for reduction or elimination of these pathogens at pre-processing stage. There are possible interventions that could be considered as preventive measures on which a CCP could be based. However, these interventions need considerable research before they could be applied on a practical basis in a HACCP system for actual production. The recommended Seven-Step HACCP Plan is solely dependent on a serious review of the pre-requisite programmes made up of GAP and GMP. These seven steps or principles may be described as:

Principle 1: Identify the potential hazards associated with food production at all stages from growth, processing, manufacturing, distribution etc.

Principle 2: Determine the points/ procedures/ operational steps that can be controlled to eliminate the hazards or minimize its likelihood of occurrence.

Principle 3: Establish critical limits which must be met to ensure the CCP is under control.

Principle 4: Establish a system to monitor control of CCP by scheduled testing as observations.

Principle 5: Establish the corrective action to be taken when monitoring indicates that a particular CCP is under control.

Principle 6: Establish procedures for verification including supplementary tests and procedures to conform that the HACCP plan must be on file at the food establishment and must be made available to official inspectors on request. Forms for recording and documentation may be developed or standards forms may be used with necessary modifications.

Principle 7: Establish documentation concerning all procedures and records appropriate to these and their application.

HACCP is a very useful system in controlling the meat and meat products processing procedure. It is a overall quality management system in which we find out the threats available in the processing steps of meat food products processing. It monitors the process right from slaughter to final consumption of the product.

5. Good Manufacturing Practices or Good Hygienic Practices (GMP/GHP)

Good manufacturing practices are a coherent system of activities which assures that the products meet a set of defined quality marks. It is so important now a day because consumers are seeking quality products even in higher prices. To get the GMP achieved all the steps of product development right from farm to fork must be managed in an appropriate manner. In case of meat production all the food chains right from meat animal production, raw materials, process, post process handling, storage, transportation etc must be well managed. If the sanitary and hygienic measures are followed on all these aspects then there will be the safe meat production for human health. So the safe meat supply to consumer is the primary aim of GHP. By following GMP/GHP we can assure both quality and safety in the food chains as a result final product produced assures the quality and safety.

6. Total Quality Management (TQM)

Quality is a fitness for use as quoted by the famous personality J.M. Juran. Now quality is the reality but its achievement is very uncommon in under developed countries. As a result products particularly food products production is now stressing on the TQM. It can be achieved by the integrated approach of three directives such as: quality management throughout the food chain starting from farm to fork, strict quality control over the services in food production and finally the premises and equipments used must be of quality grade and well managed for quality food production. To achieve the TQM all the measures related to GMP/GHP, HACCP, SPS etc. must be adopted.

7. Sanitary and Phytosanitary (SPS) requirements for meat quality

SPS agreement is basically meant to harmonize the measures among the member countries. The essential harmonizing agencies are Codex Alimentarius commission (CAC), Office International des Epizootics (OIE), presently known as World Organization for Animal Health and International Plant Protection Convention. SPS measures are generally comprised of 14 essential elements such as:

a. General provisions.

b. Basic rights and obligations.

c. Harmonization.

d. Equivalence.

e. Assessment of risk.

f. Determination of appropriate level of sanitary and phytosanitary protection.

g. Adaptation to regional conditions.

h. Transparency.

i. Control.

j. Inspection and approval procedures.

k. Technical assistance.

l. Special and differential treatment.

m. Consultations

n. Dispute settlement.

To implement the strict regulations and standards on food and food products is a need of today because adulteration is now common practice all over the world. The incidences and prevalence of adulteration is much more in the developing and underdeveloped countries. So the enforcement agencies must be powerful and practical in its implementation.

References

1. BIS (1988). Year Book, Bureau of Indian Standards, Manak Bhawan, Bhadhur Shah Zafar Marg, New Delhi.
2. Jay, J.M. (1986). Modern Food Microbiology,3rd ed. CBS Publishers and Distributors, Delhi.
3. Majhi,S.C. (1975). Indian standards for meat and meat products. Proceedings of short term course on meat and meat products, Division of Livestock Products Technology, IVRI, Izatnagar.
4. Mehta, R., Saqib, M. and George, J. (2002). Addressing Sanitary and Phytosanitary Agreement: A Case Study of Select Processed Food Products in India, RIS-DP#39
5. Sahoo, J., Sahmoon, A.H. and Yadav, K.N. (1993). Standards formulation and quality control aspects of Indian meat industry-A perspective review. The Journal of Remount & Veterinary Corps. 211-225.
6. Santwani, M.T. (1975). Indian standards for met and meat products. Proceedings of short term course on meat and meat products, Division of Livestock Products Technology, IVRI, Izatnagar.

7. Sharma, B.D. (1999). Structure, composition and nutritive value of meat tissues. In: Meat and Meat Products Technology (Including Poultry Products Technology), Jaypee Brothers Medical Publishers (P) Ltd, New Delhi. pp 8-22.
8. The poultry site.com

□□□□

15 Organic Meat Food Products

Organic meat food products are choice products for health conscious people. These are the products produced mainly in most natural way without using fertilizers, pesticides and growth regulators in their feed and fodders. In addition, meat animals are also reared without growth hormones, antibiotics drugs etc. and grazing of the animals is a prerequisite in organic farming system.

The term organic farming was first time used by Lord Northbourne. The term organic farming was derived from his concept of "the farm as organism". It is a holistic, ecologically balanced approach to farming. In 1991, the European Commission formulated the first government system to regulate organic labelling. In India, standards for organic agriculture were announced in May 2001 and the National Programme on Organic Production (NPOP) is administered under the Ministry of Commerce. The concept of organic meat food products has been emphasized now a day due to animal welfare point of view, consumer's conscious ness, less residue level of chemicals, antibiotics and drugs, Bovine spongiform encephalopathy (BSE), Foot and mouth disease (FMD), genetically modified food etc.

Organic meat food products as a whole are dependent on the life stages of the livestock like its origin, feeding, housing, health, breeding, transportation and slaughter. The other factors accounting for organic foods are its production, harvesting, preservation and processing. Inspite of low growth rate of organic red meat globally, growth in dairy, egg and poultry is increasing day by day. At present 1.2 million hectares (0.6%) of Indian land is producing organic products (Willer and Kelcher, 2011).

Factors Responsible for Organic Meat Food Production

The animals reared on farm for organic meat production must have following criterion to fulfil.

1. Organic meat foods should be obtained from grass fed animals without use of synthetic chemicals, growth hormones, antibiotics and drugs other than natural ones. But the chickens of two day old, egg production from hens of two months of age, piglets of 1.5 months of age and calves of one month of age receiving colostrums or on milk diet are eligible for organic meat production.
2. The animals should breed naturally. Embryo transfer technology, hormonal treatment and use of genetically modified organisms in production of organic meat food animals are not allowed.
3. Livestock must be grown on full organic feed. The use of certain growth promoters, synthetic appetizers, additives, preservatives, urea, animal by-products, solent extracted oil cakes; pure amino acids and GMO based feed are not permissible.
4. Animals should be reared on natural medicine (homeopathy, ayurvedic medicine and acupuncture techniques are eligible), vaccines are eligible in emergency but they should not be produced from genetically engineered organisms.
5. The rearing system of the animals and birds should also be organic. Building for animal rearing should be well ventilated with natural air and light, there should be sufficient space for animals and birds, bedding material should also be organic, there should be sufficient pasture and water facilities.
6. Indian indigenous animal breeds are more resistant to diseases and can better survive in organic farming system. They also need less allopathy medicines and antibiotics.
7. The pasture based animal rearing is less costly in India as compared to developed countries.

Qualities of Organic Meat Food Products

Organic livestock products are gaining popularity due to its eco-friendly production, animal welfare oriented, safe, nutritious and of peculiar taste. However, organic carcass is less developed than other carcasses and has less fat contents. It is also lower in chemical, antibiotics and drug residues but on nutrition there is no reliable data available. The other characteristics of organic meat food products are:

1. *Carcase quality characteristics*: Carcase obtained from the animal reared organically shows less development due to more locomotive movement and uncontrolled environmental conditions of rearing. At the same time carcase is also low in fat contents and higher in muscle contents due to more body activity. In chickens, organic farming leads to more development in breast muscle percentage. The less fat is a desirable characteristic in carcase quality; it is more suitable in pork carcase with higher level of lean. On the other side, due to without use of drugs, antibiotics etc. poses great problems of disease outbreaks, their lesions on carcase and also increase likelihood of trichinae, salmonella etc.
2. *Physico-chemical quality characteristics*: The physico-chemical characteristics of meat foods obtained from organic farming has lower ultimate pH which has great effect over myofibril structure, meat colour, water binding capacity and scattering of light on such meat. The reason for higher shear force value might be due to greater motor activity in organic meat animals. These animals also have greater degree of lipid oxidation than conventional meat animals.
3. *Microbiological quality characteristics*: The meat food obtained from organic animals poses great problem of microbial contamination particularly of *E.coli, Salmonella* and *Campylobacter*. It also has higher incidences of *Trichinella* in pork meat produced by organic farming. The chances of poisoning from such meat are higher than conventional meat foods.

S.No.	Quality characteristics	Level in organic meat foods as compared to conventional meat production
1.	Moisture	Higher
2.	Fat	Lower
3.	Energy	Lower
4.	Water holding capacity (WHC)	Lower
5.	Ultimate pH	Lower
6.	Cooking loss	Higher
7.	Tenderness	Almost same
8.	Shear force value	Higher
9.	Fat profile	
	i. Saturated fatty acids	Higher
	ii. Monounsaturated fatty acids	Lower
	iii. Phospholipids	higher
	iv. Polyunsaturated fatty acids	Higher
10.	TBARS number	Higher
11.	Metal ions	Higher

4. *Organoleptic quality characteristics*: Organic meat food products are suggested to have better flavour than conventional meat foods. It also has more juiciness in their products while other organoleptic qualities remain almost unchangeable.

5. *Nutritional quality parameters*: It is supposed that organic meat foods have more nutrients than conventional meat foods. Particularly organic meat foods are rich in protein, nitrate and vitamin-C.

6. *Quality characteristics of processed meat food products*: There are very limited products produced from organic meat worldwide due to restricted use of organic herbs in these products. The other ingredients which are permissible in these products are sodium, potassium, calcium citrate and lactic acid. The examples of organic meat food products are beef, chicken, lamb and pork cuts, home cured bacons and ham, beef burgers, lamb and pork kababs, beef, lamb, rosemary, pork and herb, pork and pepper, pork and spring onion sausages etc.

Benefits of Organic Food Products

Organic meat food products have a lot of health benefits. Some of them may be summarized as:

1. It reduces the ingestion of toxic chemicals which are toxic to the human organs and produce cancer like diseases.
2. Totally avoids genetically modified organisms which are known to be responsible for transgenes production.
3. Reduces the amount of food additives and colourings through food products. Thus it reduces the health problems in adults and children like allergic reactions, headaches, asthma, growth retardation and hyperactivity.
4. Increases the amount of beneficial vitamins, minerals, essential fatty acids and antioxidants in the human body.
5. It also has the potential to lower the incidence of common conditions such as cancer, coronary heart disease, allergies and hyperactivity in children.
6. Grass fed animals producing meat foods lead to much lower amount of total fat in these foods than grain fed meats. In fact, grass-fed meat has about the same amount of fat as skinless chicken or wild. Meat food products of lower fat level and higher in lean, actually lower LDL cholesterol levels thus reduce the obesity.
7. Organic or grass-fed beef is naturally high in omega-3 fatty acids and especially important for children. It also helps in protection of these good fats from rancidity. And the natural CLA improves metabolism and protects against weight gain. Omega-3 fats also help in weight control.
8. It is highly nutritious and provides much more nutrition per gram fat. Fatty nutrients such as conjugated linolenic acid (CLA), natural beta carotene, vitamin E, and omega-3 fatty acids are significantly higher in organic than conventional fat. All together, full fat organic animal food is far less toxic, less inflammatory and more nutritious.

Draw backs of Organic Food Products

Besides huge benefits of organic meat food products it also has some limitations which hinder its growth.

1. Large space requirement for rearing the animal under organic farming.

Kind of animals and birds	Space requirement
Cattle	6.0 m^2 indoor+4.5 m^2 outdoor area
Calves	1.5 m^2 indoor+1.1m^2 outdoor area
Fattening pigs	1.3 m^2 indoor+1.0 m^2 outdoor area
Sow with piglets	7.5 m^2 indoor+5.0 m^2 outdoor area
Laying hens	1660 cm^2 indoor+4.0 m^2 outdoor area

Source: Sundrum, 2001.

2. It restricts the use of drugs, antibiotics etc which will hinder the treatment plan of the animal, processing and preservation of such meat food products becomes difficult due to ineligibility of certain ingredients in these foods like nitrite and phosphate.

3. Cost of production enhances which has ultimate effect on its total production.

Standards Applicable for Organic Meat Food Products

At present there is no single standard governing the organic foods globally. It is restricted or constricted and may vary country to country. Its implementation is also not up to a mark which is a critical point in the growth of organic food industry. There are few international standards related to organic foods which are in existence like:

1. IFOAM basic standards

2. EU regulation No. 1804/1999

3. Codex Alimentarius ALINORM 99/ 22 A

Other then these international standards various countries have their own standards like UKROFS in UK, JAS in Japan, California organic standards in state of California, USA, National standards for organic production in India etc.

Global Scenario of Organic Meat Food Products

Global market of organic food and beverages are mainly confined to developed countries like USA, UK, EU, Argentina, Brazil etc. Among these in USA, organic meat and meat products including poultry and their products are the sixth fastest growing sector. The reason behind its development in these countries is their food safety consciousness and over production of the food items. But the scenario is just reverse in developing countries including India and China where population is a great problem and their food security is much more concern than food safety. In developing countries, organic foods are mainly of agriculture produce and in very lesser amount of animal products.

Countries		Share of organic food in total food productions
USA	i.	6th growing segment of food commodity.
	ii.	5% of total domestic organic food sales.
Austria	i.	87% cattle are rearing organically.
	ii.	49% pigs and 51% poultry are rearing by this method.
	iii.	Organic meat is a main exporting commodity.
Spain	i.	52% of total beef is organic.
	ii.	28% mutton and lambs are organic.
	iii.	5% goat production is organic.
France		Organic meat shares about 3% of total organic food production.
Argentina		One million hectare of land is used for organic livestock production and producing mainly beef for export to EU.
Oceania		Contributes to half of the world organic farm land.
New Zealand		Main exporter to UK and Germany.
Japan		3rd largest market for organic food after USA and EU.

Source: Pathak *et al.* (2003)

Organic meat food products may be the export hub in future if we tackle such commodity on commercial basis. The need is to explore our livestock resources. The future development of this sector is bright and little efforts have to be made to organize our traditional practices for livestock and poultry rearing. The utmost need is to educate the consumers on various aspects of organic food of animal origin. However, poor sanitary conditions, disease existence, traceability, capacity building measures are another issues which must be taken care of in organic meat production.

References

1. Biswas, A.K., Kondaiah, N, Mendiratta, S.K. and Mandal G.P. (2004). Organic meat production: a critical review. Indian Food industry. 23, 2 : 65-67.
2. Chander, M. and Kumar S.(1999). Indigenous cattle and buffalo wealth of India: exploring its role in promoting organic farming practices. Proceeding of 4th IFOAM-Asia Scientific Conference, Tagaytay city, Philippines, Nov. 18-21.
3. Givens, H. (1999). Aims and aspirations of the organic trade association. Ecology and Farming, 27,10-11.
4. ITC (2002). Overview world markets for organic food and beverage (estimates). International Trade Centre, UNCTAD/WTO, Geneva.
5. Pathak, P.K., Chander, M. and Biswas, A.K. (2003). Organic meat: an overview. Asian-Austra. J. Anim. Sci., 16, 8: 1230-1237.
6. Sundrum, A. (2001). Organic livestock farming-A critical review. Livestock Prod. Sci., 67: 207-215.
7. Younie, D., Hamilton and Nevison,I. (1990). Sensory attributes of organic and conventional beef. Animal Production, 50,565-566.

□□□□

16 Food Products of Genetically Modified Animals and Marine Origin

Genetically modified organisms (GMOs) can be defined as organisms in which the genetic material (DNA) has been altered in a way that does not occur naturally. The technology is often called "modern biotechnology" or "gene technology", sometimes also "recombinant DNA technology" or "genetic engineering". It allows selected individual genes to be transferred from one organism into another, also between non-related species. Genetically modified (GM) foods are foods derived from genetically modified animals and marines. Genetically modified animals and marines are those in which specific changes introduced into their DNA by genetic engineering using a process of either Cisgenesis or Transgenesis. These techniques are much more precise than mutagenesis where animals and marines are exposed to radiation or chemicals to create a non-specific but stable change. Other techniques by which food animals can be modified are selective breeding and somaclonal variation. By this means desired quality of meat, egg and other animal products can be produced. But it is a common thinking that foods derived from genetically modified animals and marines are far from safe. They are likely to be contaminated by potent vaccines, immune regulators and growth hormones, as well as nucleic acids, viruses and bacteria that have the potential to create pathogens and to trigger cancer.

History

In first instance GM foods came in market in the early 1990s. These were mainly transgenic plant products: soybean, corn, canola and cotton seed oil. But animal products have also been developed in 2006. In this year pig was controversially engineered to produce omega-3 fatty acids through the expression of a roundworm gene. Then genetically-modified breed of pigs was developed that was able to absorb plant phosphorus more efficiently.

Pros and Cons of Genetically Modified Foods

Most of the genetic modification work has been done on the farm animals like cattle, sheep, pigs, chickens and goats especially in developed countries like USA, Australia, New Zealand and Japan. The basic aims behind production of GM animals are increasing meat production efficiency, improving the amount and quality of wool from sheep, altering milk composition to facilitate cheese production or reduce milk intolerance, increasing disease resistance, reducing pollution from pig manure, producing spider silk fibres in goat milk etc. The success rate of genetic modification in animals is limited to only 1-3%. Cloning is often used together with GM which also increases the losses. Deaths occur at the embryo stage and also just before and after birth. The GM and cloned animals are often oversized, weak and susceptible to disease. It is also considered that GM food is carcinogenic and produces allergy in most of the human beings. Dolly, the cloned sheep, had to be put to sleep at only 5 years of age because she had severe arthritis. Matilda, the first cloned sheep in Australia, was found dead in her field.

Overall use of GM animals is economic and meat, cheese and wool may be produced at lower cost. The future demand of animal products can be readily available. It is also possible that if efforts to make animals resistant to disease were successful, suffering would be reduced. Costs of treatment and production losses may also be reduced giving an additional economic benefit. Another greater benefit of GM animals is in the production of drugs in their milk or in meat and organs. On the horizon are fish that mature more quickly, cows that are resistant to bovine spongiform encephalopathy (mad cow disease) are some additional benefits.

Major genes and their function in meat quality

To get the desired quality meat various types of genes were controlled by the various technologies. By controlling the genes the qualities of meat like colour and texture, fat, meat purge control, flavour etc. can easily be modified. Some of the major genes responsible may be listed as:

Gene	Location	Functions	Affected animal species
1. Halothane gene	Chromosome-6	• Responsible for PSE meat. • Responsible for extensive protein degeneration. • It is also responsible for higher carcass yield and lean percentage in pigs having homozygous and heterozygous to this gene. • It has negative effect on water holding capacity and colour	Pigs
2. RN$^-$ gene	Chromosome SSC15 (*Sus scrofa*)	• Responsible for high muscle glycogen in sarcoplasmic and lysosomal components. • Related to the acid meat condition. • Produces light meat with inferior water holding capacity.	Pigs
3. Callipyge gene	Chromosome-18	• Responsible for extreme muscling in hind quarters, reduced fatness, higher feed efficiency but tough meat.	Sheep
4. REM gene	Locus-18	• Its effect is localized on rib eye muscle area or on longissimus muscle.	Sheep

Contd.

Gene	Location	Functions	Affected animal species
5. Myostatin (GDF-8)	-	• Responsible for large cross sectional area and mass at equivalent live or carcass weight. • It acts as a negative growth factor and resp onsible for inhibition of terminal differentiation of myoblasts and proliferation of myogenic cells. • Double muscled body of Belgian blue and Piedmontese cattle is the result of inactivation of this gene.	Cattle
6. Calpain and BT-47 CAST system gene		• Calpain is responsible for myofibrillar protein breakdown which is related to the meat tenderness. • CAST regulates postmortem proteolysis by the inhibition of μ and m-calpains activity.	Cattle
7. Melanocortin (MC4R) receptor gene	-	• Regulates homeostasis. • In pigs it is responsible for feed intake and carcass fatness.	Pigs
8. Insulin like growth factor-2 (IGF2)	-	• Decides muscularity.	Pigs

So by controlling these major genes meat quality can be improved. The other responsibility is its uniform development in the body muscle mass. It can be easily achieved by the DNA technology and by the exploitation of certain gene markers. To achieve the desired quality candidate gene is also having same importance.

Genetically Modified Food Animals

Genetically modified crops are most abundantly found in the market but animals are also being genetically modified for production of milk, eggs or meat for us to eat. Genetically modified food animals are mainly of two types: heritable and non-heritable. Heritable genetic modification involves genetic changes that persist in sperm and egg while non-heritable modification involves the introduction of modified genes such as vaccines into the somatic tissue of animals. As per the record Herman the bull is first genetically modified bovine was created in 1990.

a. *Heritable modified food animals*: Heritable modified animals were achieved in early 1980s by genetic modification through naked DNA injection. For their production about 1 and 20 million copies of the transgene (gene to be integrated into the animal genome) are injected into the embryo pronucleus (the nucleus before fertilization) or into the egg cytoplasm. By this way about one percent of injected embryos becoming transgenic animals. Lentivirus of the Retroviridae family is used as most efficient gene delivery vectors while others like HIV (human immunodeficiency virus), SIV (simian immunodeficiency virus) and FIV (feline immunodeficiency virus) are other examples of lentiviruses which can be used as gene delivery vectors in farm animals such as chicken, pig and cow.

   Food quality of heritable modified food animals can enriched with certain nutrients. For example transgenic clones of cattle producing milk with higher levels of beta casein and kappa casein proteins. Genetically modified 'neutraceuticals', animals and animal products can produce enhanced nutritional value. Cloned transgenic pigs have been produced rich in beneficial omega-3 fatty acids normally obtained by eating fish. Pigs expressing an *E. coli* salivary phytase produced low phosphorus manure. Phytase increases the availability of feed phosphorous and decreases its release in manure, thereby eliminating environmental pollution by phosphorus. Transgenic chickens expressing bacterial beta-galactosidase hydrolyze lactose in the intestine and to use that sugar as an energy source. Chickens fed lactose-containing foods normally develop diarrhoea while transgenic chickens can thrive on lactose containing feed such as dairy products or waste products. Early chicken embryos were transformed using the spleen necrosis retrovirus vector (SNTZ),

b. *Non-heritable modified food animals*: Non-heritable genetic modifications of food animals has a number of applications such as DNA vaccination, transgenic probiotic bacteria as vector for vaccines and growth hormones, using RNAi (RNA interference) for epigenetic modifications, and stem cell chimeric animals whose somatic tissue but not the germ cells are transgenic. In non-heritable techniques DNA plasmids and viral vectors in both vaccination and in gene therapy are used to improve meat production or quality.

   Food derived from genetically modified animals pose several kinds of health risks, whether heritable or not. These foods have not been recommended to use until risks have been assessed. In this technique non-heritable traits are includes potent synthetic antigens for vaccination and powerful immune regulators, while both heritable and non-heritable traits include growth hormones. These contaminants in foods are likely to have adverse impacts on the immune system and development of human beings, especially the young.

Transgenic Fish

Transgenic fish can be produced in confined land-locked ponds, fish pens in confined fjords or sounds or released to open seas or lakes. Fish genes are most frequently used in producing transgenic fish and these are considered as substantially equivalent to the native fish though they are unable to inter breed with the species receiving the transgene.

Transgenic Atlantic salmon was first develops by Aqua Bounty Inc. in 1999. It contains a Chinook salmon growth hormone gene driven by the ocean pout antifreeze promoter, resulting in a dramatic increase in growth rate. Transgenic Coho salmon was developed by introducing a sockeye salmon growth hormone gene driven by a sokeye metalothionen-B promoter. The transgenic animals were hemizygous for the transgene, being F1 animals from crosses between transgenic and normal animals. The transgenic salmon consistently outgrew normal animals. A rainbow trout growth hormone (rtGH) gene was used to produce transgenic carp. DNA from a cloning vector, pRSV-2 ,

Typical examples of genetically modified food animals

Type of food animals	Invention association	Benefits	Drawbacks
Featherless chicken and bird-flu resistant chicken	Scientists of Israel created a prototype with the breeding of naked neck chicken	To save the time of plucking, environmental friendly, reduce rearing cost and extremely safe.	Loss of protection against parasites, extreme weathers etc. Birds becomes vulnerable to skin injuries
Tilapia	-	Early maturity and to protect fish from mouth brooding	-
Pharmaceutical camels	Dubai scientist	To cure the genetic diseases by modifying animals to produce curative proteins in the milk.	-
Super cows	-	Cow developed which are resistant to mad cow disease, less horny and udder infection etc.	-
Popeye pigs	In popeye pig, gene of spinach has been inserted in pigs.	It is to convert the saturated fat into unsaturated fat (linoleic acid)	However, addition of vegetable gene does not like by some consumers.

was introduced by microinjection into cells at an early stage of embryo development. The recombinant plasmid contained the rtGH gene driven by the long terminal repeat (LTR) from Rous sarcoma virus (RSV) and additional apparently non-functional flanking sequences of bacterial DNA.The transgenic carp had an altered body form and higher proportion of protein to fat than the wild-type carp, and required high histidine and lysine ratios in its diet for maximum growth. Other transgenic fishes are transgenic mud loach and transgenic zebra fish.

Animal Products Produced from Genetically Modified Source

The production of meats, milk and eggs is very limited from genetically modified animals. But genetic engineering has a lot to do with the production of many animal products such as animal feed, feed additives like vitamins, amino acids, and enzymes, veterinary medicines and vaccines are produced with the help of genetically modified microorganisms. The meat and meat products produced by this technique are mainly Sausage and Ham. Many additives commonly found in sausage and ham is often produced using methods involving genetically modified microorganisms. Examples are ascorbic acid (vitamin C) is used to prevent oxidation, stabilising the colour of sausage, Glutamate is used to enhance flavour, enzymes, proteases can make meat more tender and improve aroma. They can also be used to help separate meat residues from bones. There are other additives which can be produced from GM soybeans or GM maize includes soy protein, dextrine or maltodextrine (from GM maize) as a filler or stabiliser and soy lecithin or soy mono- and diglycerides as emulsifiers.

Controversies Related to GM Foods

Technologies for genetically modifying foods offer dramatic promise for meeting some of the 21st Century's greatest challenges. Like all new technologies, they also pose some risks, both known and unknown. Controversies surrounding GM foods and crops commonly focus on human and environmental safety, labeling and consumer choice, intellectual property rights, ethics, food security, poverty reduction, and environmental conservation. The following controversies related to GM foods are of special concern:

i. It is considered that GM foods have human health impacts, like allergens, transfer of antibiotic resistance markers etc.

ii. They have potential environmental impacts like unintended transfer of transgenes through cross-pollination, loss of flora and fauna biodiversity etc.

iii. It may create the domination of world food production by a few companies and may increase dependency on industrialized nations by developing countries and biopiracy or foreign exploitation of natural resources.

iv. It may also create some ethical issues like violation of natural organisms intrinsic values, tampering with nature by mixing genes among species, objections to consuming animal genes in plants and vice versa, stress for animals etc.

v. Labelling of such foods will not be done in proper way as it is not mandatory in USA.

International Regulations for GM Foods

No specific international regulatory systems are currently in place for GM food regulations. However, several international organizations are involved in developing protocols for GMOs. The Codex Alimentarius Commission (Codex) is the joint FAO/WHO body responsible for compiling the standards, codes of practice, guidelines and recommendations that constitute the Codex Alimentarius is said international food code. Codex is developing principles for the human health risk analysis of GM foods. The premise of these principles dictates a premarket assessment, performed on a case-by-case basis and including an evaluation of both direct effects (from the inserted gene) and unintended effects (that may arise as a consequence of insertion of the new gene). Codex principles do not have a binding effect on national legislation but are referred to specifically in the Sanitary and Phytosanitary Agreement of the World Trade Organization (SPS Agreement) and can be used as a reference in case of trade disputes. The Cartagena Protocol on Biosafety (CPB), an environmental treaty legally binding for its Parties, regulates transboundary movements of living modified organisms (LMOs). GM foods are within the scope of the Protocol only if they contain LMOs that are capable of transferring or replicating genetic material. The cornerstone of the CPB is a requirement that exporters seek consent from importers before the first shipment of LMOs intended for release into the environment. The Protocol will enter into force 90 days after the 50th country has ratified it.

Now GM food is a reality and person who don't want to eat GM foods may be surprised to know that millions of tons of genetically modified organisms (GMOs) are going into producing the food we eat. The main source of GM food in animal and marine products is their feed. Because there is no regulatory agency in this concern even in European Union's GM food labelling laws, the meat, dairy products and eggs produced with GM animal feed do not have to be labelled as such, creating a complete lack of transparency. So, animal feed means GMOs are getting into the human food chain through the back door.

References

1. Brophy B, Smolenski G, Wheeler T, Wells D, L'Huillier P and Laible G. (2003). Cloned transgenic cattle produce milk with higher levels of beta-casein and kappa-casein. *Nat Biotechnol.* 21(2), 157-62.
2. Cummins J. (2003). Floating transgenic crops in a leaky triploid craft. Science in Society, 24,32
3. Devlin RH, D'Andrade M, Uh M and Biagi CA. (2004). Population effects of growth hormone transgenic coho salmon depend on food availability and genotype by environment interactions.*Proc Natl Acad Sci U S A.* 101(25), 9303-8.
4. Fiester, A. (2006). Why the omega-3 piggy should not go to market. Nature Biotechnology 24: 1472–1473.
5. Guelph (2005). Transgenic pig research: Enviropig TM an enviro programnmentally friendly breed of pigs that utilizes plant phosphorus efficiently.
6. Kang J.X. *et al.* (2007). Why the omega-3 should go to market. Nature Biotechnology 25 (5): 505–506.
7. Lai L *et al.* (2006). Generation of cloned transgenic pigs rich in omega-3 fatty acids. Nature Biotechnology 24 (4): 435–436.
8. www.genewatch.org

□□□□

COLOUR PLATES

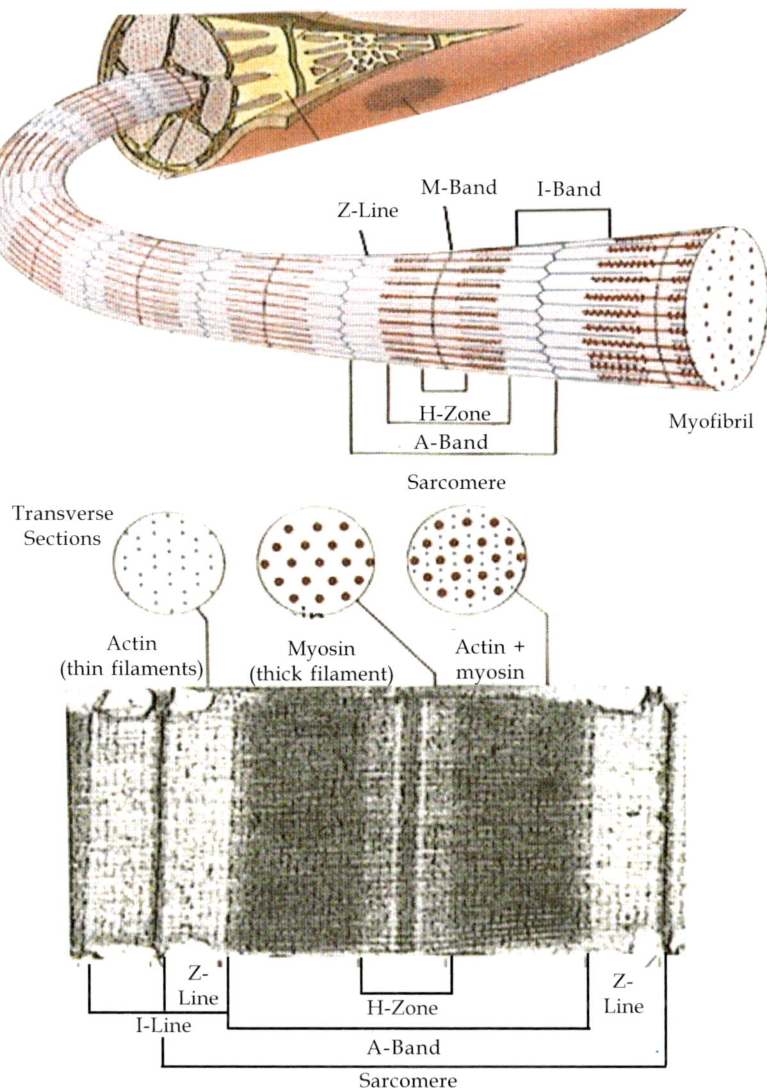

Fig. 2.4 : (*Source:* M.J. Farabee 2007) www.emc.maricopa.edu/faculty/farabee/BIOBK/BioBookMUSSKEL.html

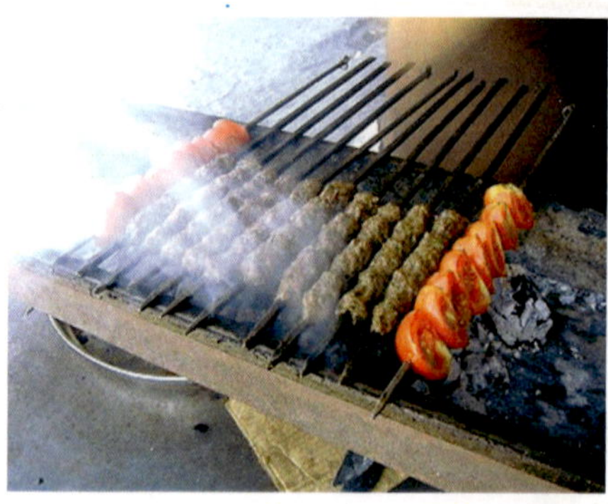

Kabab preparation
(*Source:* wikipedia.org)

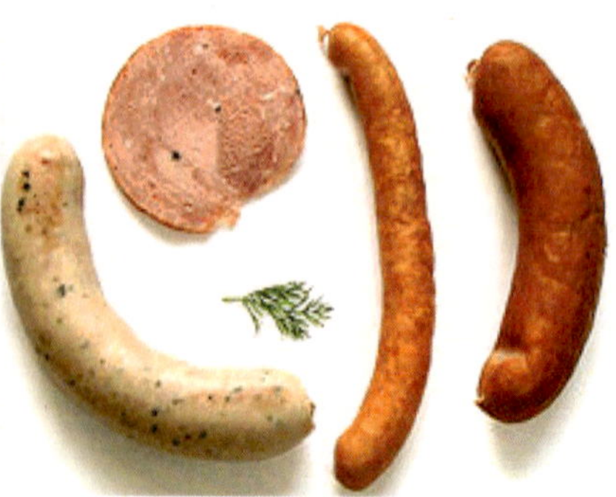

Meat sausages
(*Source:* sausage wikipedia)

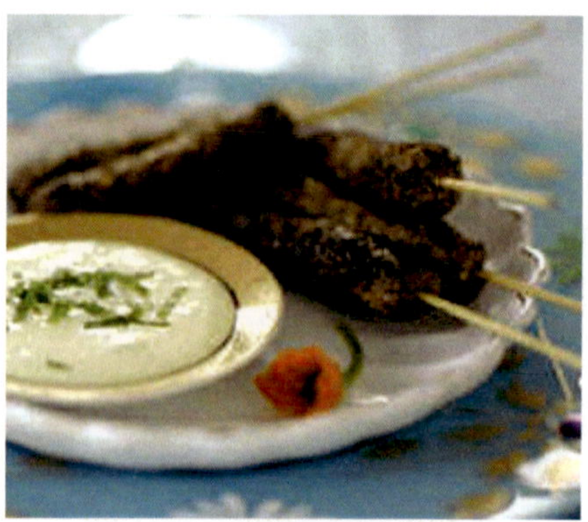

Seekh Kabab

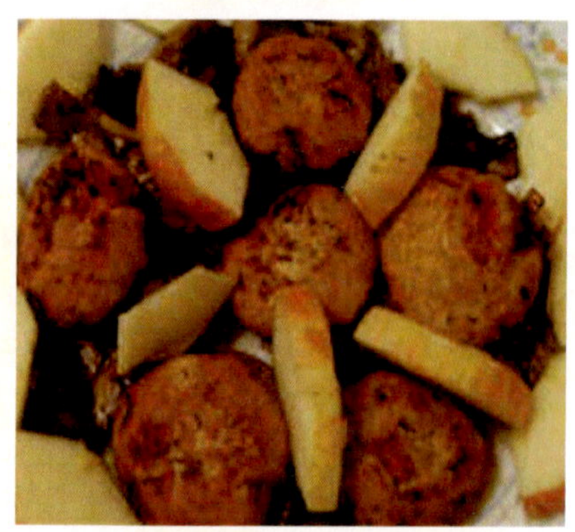

Shami Kabab

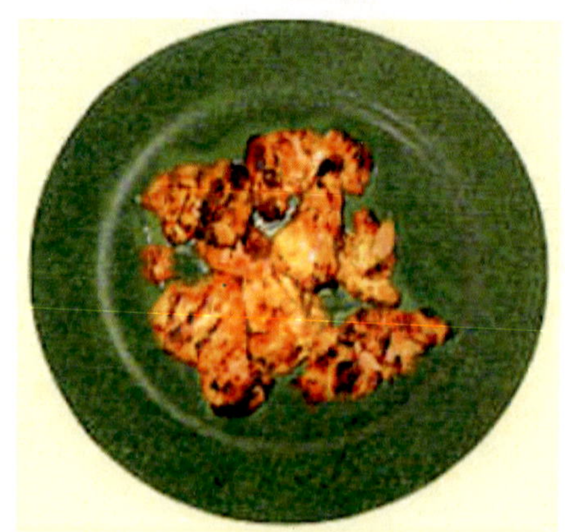

Boti Kabab

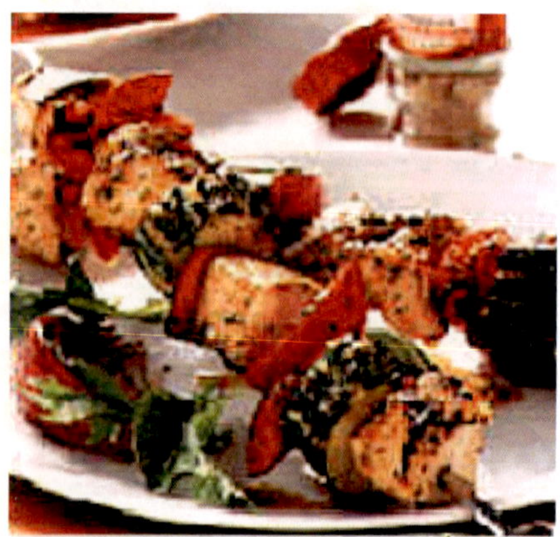

Hussaini Kabab

Different types of kababs (*Source:* Indian food co.com)

Index

Symbol

α–actinin 27, 31, 114
β-actinin 27, 32

A

Acid meat 51, 339
Acid phosphatase 114
Actin 18, 19, 21-23, 27, 29-32, 44-46, 50, 52, 82, 114, 155, 237, 297
Active packaging 177
Actomyosin 30, 31, 45, 113
Adhesiveness 254
Adipose tissue 24, 27, 34, 35
Adrenaline 52
Agar Gel Immunodiffusion Test (AGID) 74
Agar Gel Precipitation Test (AGPT) 74
Ageing of Meat 22, 46, 111, 112, 116, 117
Alcohols 100, 132, 134, 135, 177
Aluminium 141, 142, 165, 169, 175
Anatomical Methods for Carcass Differentiation 69
Animal products 100, 335, 337, 338, 341, 344
Animal proteins 33, 57, 192, 193
Antibiotics Preservation 89, 109
Antioxidants 6, 63, 96, 108, 128, 149, 177, 181, 192, 265, 333
APEDA 6, 8, 9, 285-287, 298
Apoptosis 53
Appearance 18, 23, 34, 53, 92, 118, 141, 148, 153, 169, 172, 186, 189, 191, 206, 239, 240, 252, 253, 255
Aroma 56, 100, 133-135, 183, 187, 189, 190, 192, 243, 255, 344
Artery pumping 97, 130, 131
ASCAD 11, 12
Ascorbat 74, 96, 97, 127, 128, 149, 183, 184, 207, 213
Aseptic Canning 104, 142
ATP 28-30, 39-42, 44, 45, 47, 48, 115, 120, 238
Aureomycin 109
Autooxidation of fat 88
Avidin 245, 266

B

Bacterial cultures 192
Bacteriocins 109, 110
Bacteriophages 110
Beef Bungs 206
Beeswax preservation 272
Benefits of Organic Food Products 333
BHA 108, 109, 149, 192, 221, 290
BHT 108, 109, 149, 192, 221, 274
Biltong 149, 176
Binders 153, 157, 183-187, 208
Bio-based packaging 178
Biobased Packaging Materials 170
Biological Methods 68, 73
Biomolecules used in edible packaging 181

Biopreservation 109, 110
Biosensors 178, 180
Bird- flu resistant chicken 343
BIS 9, 289-291, 300
Black pepper 191, 199, 200, 209-212, 220, 227, 228
Black rots 246
Blast Freezing 93
Blood 15, 16, 22-25, 34-36, 39, 40, 43, 47, 56, 57, 61, 65, 73, 91, 125, 193, 206, 211, 212, 240, 269, 308, 309, 313
Boilable bags 176
Bologna 212, 126, 156, 190, 191, 201-204, 206
Bone 15, 24, 25, 55, 69, 91, 118, 193, 211, 217, 219, 223, 240, 269, 313, 344
Bound water 27, 234
Bowl chopper 156, 205, 207, 227
Braising 139, 140
Braunschweiger 203, 213
Brine curing 130, 132, 189
Brine Freezing 92
Brining 225, 226
Broiling 138, 253
Bromelin 119, 149
Brown fat 24
Brown Soup Stock 218
BSE 11, 329
Bureau of Indian Standards 9, 289, 290, 300, 327

C

CAC 322, 323, 326
Callipyge gene 339
Calpain 113-116, 340
Canning 5, 88-90, 101-104, 123, 124, 141, 142, 165, 253
CANP 114
Carbohydrates 26, 28, 36, 55, 57, 63, 184, 185, 188, 241, 266, 270
Carbon dioxide 39, 134, 173, 177, 179
Carbon dioxide scavengers 177
Carbonyls 100, 134, 135
Carcass quality characteristics 331
Cardboard Package 164
Cardiac muscle 15, 23, 29, 30
Connective tissue 15, 16, 24, 25, 27, 28, 32, 34, 35, 36, 46, 47, 58, 112, 113, 115, 116, 146, 147, 206, 231, 235, 237, 253,
Carnitine 63
Carotene 48, 58, 73, 333
Carrageenan 151, 157, 181, 188
Cartilage 15, 24, 25, 33, 206
CASF 114, 115
Casings 139, 155, 201, 205-213, 253, 294
CAST system gene 340
Cathepsin B and D 114
Cation exchange chromatography 81
CBPP 11
Cellulose 81, 133, 137, 151, 163, 164, 165, 169, 170, 178, 181, 193
Cellulosic Casing 206
Chalky 254
Charque 150
Chemical methods 68, 72
Chemical Preservation 107, 110
Chili pepper 190
Chilling 51, 89, 90, 93, 120, 157, 158, 207, 208, 236, 253
Chlorine dioxide generators 177
Chloromycetin 109
Cholesterol 28, 34, 35, 56, 61, 151, 193, 224, 243, 265, 266, 269, 270, 333
Chondrocytes 24
Chunking and forming 153 CIE 77
Circulatory system 40, 41
Coated films 169
Coating with paraffin 272
Codex Alimentarius Commission 159, 318, 322, 326, 345
CAC 322, 223, 326
Coextruded films 170
Cohesiveness 188, 254
Cold shortening 48, 52, 53, 90 112, 113, 115, 119, 120, 239, 240
Cold smoke 99
Cold storage preservation 274
Collagen 24, 28, 33, 34, 46, 47, 58, 59, 112, 114, 115, 140, 181, 201, 206
Collagen Casing 206
Colour 25, 26, 32-34, 36, 39, 42, 46, 47, 49, 51, 68, 69, 73, 77, 81, 89, 92, 95-97, 99-101, 105, 110, 119, 120, 123-128, 134-137, 148, 149, 154, 172, 173, 178, 179, 183, 184, 190, 191, 203, 206, 210, 214, 222, 224, 225, 227, 228, 231, 232, 233, 234, 238, 240, 243, 244, 246, 248, 251, 252, 253, 255, 304, 331, 339, 344
Colourless rots 246

Commercial Sterility 137, 141, 142
Communition 156
Conalbumin 245, 266
Conditioning 48, 111, 112, 113, 114, 115, 116
Conjugated linoleic acid 63, 64
Connective tissue 15, 16, 24, 25, 27, 28, 32, 34, 35, 36, 46, 47, 58, 112, 113, 115, 116, 146, 147, 206, 231, 235, 237, 253
Connective tissue proper 24
Connective tissue proteins 28, 32, 46, 58
Consistency 68, 69, 124, 146, 154, 188, 189, 205, 252, 253, 255, 273, 277
Consumer panel 257
Contractile proteins 28
Controversies Related to GM Foods 344
Cooked Sausage 176, 203, 204 212, 213, 243, 244
Cooked Smoked Sausage 204
Cooking 57, 60, 80, 96, 98, 99, 105, 117, 123, 126, 127, 134, 138, 139, 140, 148, 151, 154, 169, 188, 196, 200, 202, 203, 207, 210, 217, 221, 222, 224, 234, 235, 237, 244, 253, 255, 256, 306, 310, 312, 332,
Coriander 149, 189, 195, 200, 209, 210, 212, 213, 216
Counter Immunoelectrophoresis (CIE) 77
C-protein 27, 32, 114,
Creatine phosphate 28, 44, 45, 64, 120
Creatines 63
Cumin 189, 190, 199, 216, 219, 220, 221
Cured aquatic foods quality 248
Cured meat packaging 174, 175
Cured meat products 174, 189, 243
Curing 88, 89, 94-97, 99, 121, 124, 125, 127-132, 146, 153, 154, 183, 184, 189, 202, 224, 253, 255, 312
Curing methods 97, 129
Cytochrome 28, 32, 41, 81, 82, 232

D

12-D concept 145
Daily requirements of an individual 271
Dark cutting beef 52
Dark cutting beef or lamb 52
D-Concept 104, 145
Denseness 254
Dental formula 70
Descriptive sensory evaluation 259, 261, 262
Desmin 29, 32, 46, 114
DFD 47, 49, 50, 51, 236, 239
Dietary fibre enhancer 151
Difference test 259, 260
Direct addition method 97
Discriminatory sensory evaluation 259
DNA Hybridization Technique 81
Dot-bot technique 75
Double Immunodiffusion Test (DID) 74
Draw Backs of Organic Food Products 334
Dried Egg Mix 275
Dried Egg Powders 276
Dry Sausage 102, 109, 128, 157, 201, 204, 210
Dry ageing 116
Dry curing 94, 97, 129, 130
Dry heat processing 138
Drying 89, 91, 93, 99, 102, 121, 124, 134, 146, 147-150, 191, 204, 226, 253, 275, 312
Duo-Trio test 260
D-Value 98, 144

E

Edible packaging 178, 181
Egg Albumen Powder 277, 294
Egg albumin protein 245
Egg and egg products 245, 248, 265, 277
Egg Mix 275
Egg proteins 151, 185, 187
Egg White Solids 276
Egg yolk 266, 268, 269, 270, 276, 277
Egg Yolk Powder 276, 277
Elastin 22, 24, 25, 28, 33, 34, 115
Electrical Stimulation 48, 117, 120
Electron accelerator irradiation 106
Electrophoretic methods 68, 78
ELISA 76, 77, 85
Emulsification 39, 56, 128, 237
Emulsifiers 32, 157, 184, 188, 344
Emulsifying 29, 187, 207, 237
Emulsion Stability 157, 184, 185, 231, 237
Endogenous antioxidants 63
Endomysium 16
Energy value of eggs 267
Enforcement Bodies 296, 316

Enzyme-linked Immunosorbent Assay 76
Enzymes 22, 26, 27, 32, 34, 53, 55-57, 64, 83, 88, 91, 93, 94, 97, 101, 111, 113, 114, 116, 117, 119, 120, 125, 137, 141, 152, 176, 177, 192, 232, 240, 344
Epimysium 16
Epithelial tissue 15, 23
Erythorbate 124, 128, 136, 183, 184, 207, 211, 212
Ethics of meat eating 64
Exhausting 102, 142
Export (Quality Control and Inspection) Act 9, 285, 299, 300
Export Import Policy of India 284
Export Potential of Indian Meat Industry 6
Export Promotion Institutions 285
Exsanguination 40, 41, 43, 45, 48
Extenders 157, 183, 184, 207
Extracellular fibers 24

F

F-actin 29, 31
Fast freezing 91, 92
Fat 6, 15, 17, 24, 26, 32, 34-36, 47, 48, 52, 55-61, 64, 73, 97, 101-103, 105, 108, 109, 111, 112, 132, 139, 141, 146, 148, 149, 151-153, 156, 157, 173, 184-186, 188, 190, 192, 193, 200, 201, 203, 207-215, 217, 224, 235, 236, 237, 241, 248, 253, 254, 256, 257, 262, 266- 270, 275, 309, 310, 331, 332, 333. 343, 344
Factors Affecting Post-Mortem Changes 46
Fat identification 69
Fat mimetic 151
Fat mimics 192
Fat replacers 6, 151, 192
Fat substitutes 151
Fatty acid 6, 35, 39, 57, 60, 61, 73, 95, 96, 105, 124, 125, 127, 151, 152, 177, 240, 248, 265, 269, 332, 333, 338, 341
Fatty acid profile replacers 6
Featherless chicken 343
Fennel 190
Fiber Size 231, 237
Fibrous 24, 29, 30, 31, 33, 185, 206, 212, 254
Fibrous Casing 206, 212
Ficin 119, 152, 190
Fillers 157, 184, 279
FINS 85
Firmness 51, 130, 152, 231, 234-236, 254
Fish 4-6, 25, 45, 56, 57, 60, 64, 88-90, 92-94, 97, 99, 101-103, 108-110, 128, 142, 152, 164, 174, 178, 181, 194, 217, 219, 222, 223-229, 233, 240-242, 247-249, 265, 285, 287, 288, 297, 302, 303, 322, 323, 338, 341-344
Fish and other Aquatic Foods 247
Fish products 4, 142, 181, 241, 302, 303, 322
Fish Soup 219
Fish Surimi 223, 224
Flaking and forming 153, 154
Flash 18
Process 104
Flash heat treatment 274
Flavoprotein 32, 266
Flavoproteins 32
Flavour 35, 39, 47, 56, 89, 90, 94-97, 99, 100, 105, 107, 110- 112, 116-121, 125, 126-130, 132, 133-137, 140, 142, 152, 157, 173, 174, 177-179, 181, 183-187, 189, 190-193, 201, 203, 206, 208, 210, 212, 214, 219, 223, 224, 226, 228, 235, 242, 243, 255-257, 259, 260, 262, 272, 323, 339, 344
Flavour/odour absorbers 178
Flavour profile test 259, 262
Flavourings 189, 193, 223, 311
Flexible plastic films 168
FMD 2, 11, 12, 329
Food products of genetically modified animals and marine 337
Food Safety and Standards Act 10, 313, 315
Food Safety and Standards Authority of India 10, 313, 315
Frankfurters 94, 128, 136, 137, 156, 174, 185, 190, 191, 202, 203, 206, 213, 257
Fraudulent Substitution of Meat 67
Free water 27, 95, 234
Freezing 5, 88, 89, 90-94, 105, 111, 117, 119, 253, 275, 276, 312
Freezing point 111
Fresh aquatic foods quality 247
Fresh Beef Sausages 208, 209
Fresh meat packaging 171

Fresh Pork Sausages 203, 208
Fresh Sausage 201, 203
Fresh Smoked Sausage 203
Freshness indicators 179
Frozen meat packaging 174
Frying 102, 138, 139, 198, 199, 214
FSSAI 10, 315-317
Functions of Package 161, 182
Fungal rots 246
F-Value 99, 143-146

G

G-actin 29-31
Gamma rays irradiation 105
Garlic 149, 150, 189, 191, 195, 198, 199, 200, 209, 211, 212, 221, 222, 226, 228
Gas sensors 179
Gases 100, 134, 136, 162, 165, 167-169, 173, 174
GATT 9, 317, 318
GDF-8 340
Gellan gum 188
Genetically Modified Food Animals 340, 341
Genova Salami 211
Geometric properties 254
Germinal disc 266, 267
GHP 315, 325, 326
Ginger 149, 191, 195, 198, 199, 200, 208, 209, 212, 213, 216, 219, 220, 221, 222, 228
Glass 101, 102, 140, 141, 163-166, 176, 222, 271, 272, 274
Glassine bags 176
Globulin G_1, G_2, G_3 266
Glycogen 17, 23, 28, 36, 39-43, 45, 47, 50, 51, 52, 55, 63, 72, 120, 238, 239, 240, 241, 339
GMP 192, 298, 315, 324-326
Golgi complex 22
Good Hygienic Practices 325
Good Manufacturing Practices 298, 315, 324, 325
Gostaba 5
Grainy 254
Gravy 102, 142
Greasy 69, 254
Green rots 246
Grinder 153, 201, 205, 208, 209, 210, 214, 215
Gritty 254
Ground substance 22, 24, 112, 114
Guanosine monophosphate 192
Guar gum 188

H

HACCP 4, 6, 287, 288, 296, 298, 316, 322-326
Haemoglobin 27, 32, 56, 89, 91, 232
Halothane gene 339
Halothane sensitivity gene (HAL) 49
Hamburger 59, 139, 156, 175, 176, 185, 209, 313
Hammering 117, 118
Hanging 1, 106, 117, 118, 147, 148, 281, 282, 308,
Hardness 254
Hazard Analysis Critical Control Point 298, 315, 323
HDPE laminates 176
Heat shortening 119
Heavy meromyosin 30
Hereditary 47, 51, 52, 239
Heritable modified food animals 341, 342
High Intensity Pulsed Electric Field 158
High-density polyethylene (HDPE) 166, 167, 170
Histological methods 68, 72
Hog Casing 205, 206
Homeostasis 40, 41, 43, 340,
Honey-Cured Smoked Salmon 206
Hot Dog 175, 176, 191, 212, 313
Hot processing 157
Hot smoke 99, 248
HTST 98, 276
Hurdle technology 6, 89, 158
Hussaini Kebab Recipe 200
HVP / HPP 187
Hydrocarbons 100, 133, 134, 136, 137
Hydrolised vegetable proteins 129
H-Zone 19-21

I

IGF2 340
Immobiline gels 80
Immobilised water 234
Immobilization 40, 239
Immunoblotting 80
Immunodiffusion Test 74, 77

IMP 192
Indicators 178, 179
Infusion of Calcium Chloride 117, 120
Injection curing 130
Inorganic substance 36
Insulin like growth factor-2 340
Intelligent packaging 6, 110, 178
Intermediate Moisture Meat (IMM) 157, 229
Intermediate moisture meat processing 157
International Regulations for GM Foods 345
International Standards Organisation 319
Intramuscular fat 35, 47, 73, 235
Iodine Number 73
Ionising radiations 105, 106
Ionosine monophosphate 192
Iron 28, 36, 55, 56, 58, 61, 62, 64, 96, 129, 138, 177, 232, 233, 241, 244, 245, 265, 269-271, 306
Irradiation 88, 89, 104-107
ISO 4, 318, 319
ISO-14000 320, 321
ISO-22000 298, 321, 322
ISO-9000 298, 319
Isoelectric Focusing (IEF) 80
Isoelectric point 31, 42, 50, 80, 116

J

Jellied Products 203, 204
Juiciness 39, 111, 116, 118, 128, 158, 188, 229, 234, 235, 237, 253, 255, 332
Juicy 235, 253, 254

K

Kabab 5, 193-197, 199, 200, 311, 313, 332
kGy 105, 107
Kilishi 148
Kofta 5, 157, 312, 313
Kreb cycle 42, 52

L

LAB 109
Lactate 96, 129, 175, 179
Lactic acid 28, 39-43, 45, 50, 51, 52, 95, 108, 109, 170, 179, 204, 209, 211, 221, 243, 255, 276, 332
Lactic acid bacteria 109, 243
Lamb Casing 205
Laminated films 169
Latebra 266
LDPE 166, 167, 171, 174, 214
Lenoleic acid 61
Light meromyosin 30
Lime water preservation 272
Linking 207
Lipid 17, 26, 28, 34, 152, 171, 181, 240, 241, 265, 266, 331, 332
Liquid Egg Products 246, 275
Liquid egg products quality 246
Liquid smoke 100, 136, 138 228
Liver Sausages 213
Livestock health 7, 11
Loaves 185, 192, 202-204, 229
Long bones 25, 71
Low-density polyethylene 166
Lumpy 254
Luncheon Meat 174, 175, 203, 204, 243, 310, 311
Lymph 22-25, 45
Lysozyme 245, 266

M

M rad 107
Mace 109, 191, 208, 212, 221, 434
Maltodextrins 192, 193
Marbling 35, 68, 231, 235
Massagers 155, 156
Meat 1-12, 15-20, 22-29, 32-37, 39-53, 55-65, 67, 68, 72-77, 79-85, 87-95, 97-99, 101-121, 123-158, 161-169, 171-177, 181, 183-215, 217-222, 224, 229, 231-245, 248, 249, 251-260, 262, 265, 283, 286, 290-295, 298-315, 323, 325, 326, 329-342, 344, 346
Meat ball 5, 157, 213
Meat characteristics 68, 238
Meat colour 32, 36, 47, 68, 95, 126, 128, 135, 231-233, 243, 244, 252, 253, 331
Meat curry 5
Meat export trend 8
Meat extension 157
Meat Food Products Order 8, 10, 300, 303, 315
Meat kofta 157, 213
Meat patties 156, 157, 214

Meat pickles 5
Meat rolls 5
Meat samosa 5, 157
Meat soup 218, 219
Meat Surimi 224
Meat tikka 5
Meat-Based Bioactive Compounds 63
Mechanical properties 167, 254
Melanocortin receptor gene 340
Metal Cans 165, 166
Metal Containers 141, 155, 165
Metal foil plastic laminates 176
Methods of Ageing 116, 117
Methods of Preservation 89, 129, 271
MeV 106, 107
MFPI 9, 296, 297
MFPO 300-304, 307, 310-312
Microbial Quality of Cooked and Cured Meat Products 243
Microbial Quality of Fresh Meat 242
Microbiological quality of meat and aquatic food 231, 242
Microwave heat processing 138, 140
Microwaves 105, 106, 140
Milk composition 338
Minced Meat Kebab 194, 195
Minerals 58, 61, 64, 72, 124, 241, 248, 265, 268, 333
Ministry of Food Processing Industries 9, 296, 301, 302, 312, 314
Miscellaneous rots 246
Mitochondria 17, 22, 23, 26, 27, 32, 42, 63, 81, 82
Mixers 155, 156
Modern Packaging Materials 163, 164
Modern processing technologies 123
Modified atmosphere packaging 172, 174, 279
Modified humidity packaging 172
Moist heat processing 138, 139
Moistness 254
Moisture absorbers 177
Moisture properties 254
Monosodium Glutamate 96, 97, 129, 192, 208, 223, 311
Mortadella 213
Motor end plate 17
Mouth coating 257
Mouthfeel 193, 252, 257
MPEDA 285, 287-289
M-protein 27, 31
MSG 129, 192, 213, 223
Muscle 15-36, 39-48, 50-53, 55, 56, 59-64, 69, 72, 76, 80, 90-92, 110-122, 127, 140, 146-148, 194, 195, 232-237, 239, 240, 241, 247, 294, 331, 339, 340
Muscle colour 42, 46, 51
Muscle pH 39, 42,48, 51, 119
Muscle Stretching 117, 118
Muslin Casing 206
Mustard 150, 152, 185, 189, 190, 209, 210, 221, 222
Mutton dopiyaza 5
Mutton korma 5
Myofibrillar proteins 28, 29, 31, 32, 42, 113, 115, 120, 155, 156, 158, 237
Myofibrils 29-32, 46
Myofilaments 18, 22, 23, 44,
Myoglobin 26, 32, 43, 46, 56, 72, 79, 81, 96, 127, 128, 136, 173, 232, 233, 252, 253
Myoneural junction 17, 22
Myosin 18, 19, 21-23, 27, 29-31, 44-46, 50, 52, 113, 114, 155, 156, 237
Myosin light chains 30
Myostatin 340

N

Natamycin 109
Nate-yakini 5
National Meat and Poultry Processing Board 298
Nervous tissue 15, 23
Neutral lipid 28, 34, 35
Newer Biotechnological Methods 68, 81
NFDM 186
Niacin 55, 57, 58, 62, 63, 64, 100
Nisin 109, 181
Nitrate 94-97, 124-127, 130, 131, 149, 183, 295, 332
Nitrite 6, 94, 95, 97, 99, 108, 124-128, 130, 131, 136, 146, 183, 192, 207, 209-213, 221, 243, 244, 253, 295, 334
NMPPB 298, 299
Non Specific Loaf 212
Non-heritable modified food animals 342
Normal contraction 45
Nuclei 17, 20, 22, 337
Nutmeg 189-191, 209, 210, 212, 213, 221

Nutritive value of meat 34, 55, 57, 63, 91
Nylon 142, 167, 171, 172

O

Oat bran 192, 193
Oat fiber 192, 193
Odka 148
Odour absorbers 178
OIE 11, 326
Oil coating 274
Oily 69, 254
Oleic acid 35, 60, 61, 63, 64, 73, 152, 177, 343
Onion 149, 191, 195-198, 211, 212, 217, 220, 226, 227, 332
Organ meats 64
Organic acids 100, 108, 115, 133, 134, 135, 177, 179
Organic farming 329, 330, 331, 334
Organic Meat Food Production 330
Organic meat food products 329, 331, 323-334, 335
Ovalbumin 266
Overall acceptability 252, 257
Overwrap packaging 171, 172
Ovoinhibitor 266
Ovomucin 266
Ovomucoid 266
Oxygen scavengers 177
Oxygen sensors based on flouroscence 180

P

Packaging 6, 9, 10, 22, 91, 105, 110, 116, 121, 142, 148, 161-179, 181, 208, 214, 243, 244, 248, 252, 253, 262, 265, 273, 275, 277-282, 287, 294, 297, 303, 304, 310, 311, 312, 315, 319
Packaging materials 142, 163, 164, 166, 170, 171, 172, 174, 176, 278, 280, 281
Packaging of egg and egg products 265, 277,
Packaging techniques 176
PAGE 28, 79, 85, 152
Paired - comparison test 260
Palmitic acid 60, 61
Papain 117, 119, 152, 295
Paper 140, 164, 167, 169, 175, 176, 217, 226, 279, 280, 310
Paprika 150, 189, 190, 212
Pasteurization 98, 105-107, 137, 276
Pastirma 149, 150
PCR 81-85
PCR-RFLP 83
Pepperoni 157, 190, 202, 203, 211
Perimysium 16
PFA act 67
pH 47-51
pH of Meat 47, 63, 236
Pharmaceutical camels 343
Phenols 100, 133-135
Phosphates 28, 96, 124, 127, 128, 155, 229
Phospholipids 28, 34, 35, 60, 241, 266, 332
Phosphorous 28, 36, 55, 57, 61, 62, 341
Physico-chemical and microbiological quality of meat and aquatic food 231
Phytosanitary measures 6, 9, 316, 318
Pickle curing 97
Pickles 5, 212, 221, 311
Pink rots 246
Plastic 116, 139, 141, 145, 148, 149, 154, 163, 164-166, 168, 169, 171, 172, 176, 201, 253, 279, 280
Plate Freezing 92
Poly Acrylamide Gel Electrophoresis 79
Polyamides 167, 175
Polyester 142, 168-170, 172, 174-176
Polyethylene 141, 142, 164, 166-170, 176, 181, 294
Polymerase Chain Reaction 81-83
Polypropylene 142, 167-170, 174
Polystyrene 168, 170, 171, 280
Polyvenyl chloride 167
Polyvinylidene chloride 167, 169
Popeye pigs 343
Post-Mortem Changes in Muscle Structure 45
Post-mortem heat generation 41
Post-mortem pH decline 42
Pot-roasting 139
Poultry meat and meat products 244
Powdery 254
PP 167
Preblanding 153
Pre-cooked Frozen Meat Products Packaging 175
Precooking 102, 142
Preservation packaging of egg and egg products 265

Preservation of Egg Products 275
Preservation of meat and aquatic food 87-90, 99, 105
Preslaughter 41
Pressure cooking 139, 140, 221, 253
Principles of Preservation 88
Processed meat food products 332
Processing of animal and fish products 4
Propyl gallate 108
Protein matrix 154, 155
Proteins 17, 24, 27-29, 31-33, 42, 45, 46, 49-51, 55-60, 62, 73, 76-78, 80, 81, 85, 95, 96, 99, 100, 113-116, 120, 124, 127, 129, 146, 151, 153, 155, 156, 158, 170, 181, 184-187, 192, 193, 207, 212, 234, 237, 240, 255, 256, 257, 265-268, 313, 341, 343
Proteomics 53
PSE 18, 47-49, 50, 51, 53, 115, 236, 238, 239
PVC 167, 171, 174, 175, 233,
PVDC 167, 174, 175
Pyrolysis 100, 137
Pyruvic acid 52

Q

Qualities of Organic Meat Food Products 331
Quantitative descriptive analysis 262
Quantum of Connective Tissue 231, 235
Quick Freezing of Carcass 117, 119
Qwanta 148

R

Rad 107
Radappertization 107
Radicidation 107
Radio-frequency identification tags 180
Radurization 107
Rank preference 261
Ranking test 257, 259, 261
RAPD 84
Rapka 5, 159
Recognition test 258, 259
Reconstituted Egg Products 276
Red muscle 26, 52, 60, 115
Red muscle fibers 26
Red pepper 191, 209, 216
Red rots 246
Refractive Index 73
Refrigeration 88, 89-92, 101, 105, 130, 131, 137, 172, 175, 201, 204, 206, 207, 209, 214-216, 225, 228, 243, 244, 276, 279, 282, 307
Regulatory Proteins of Myofibrils 31
Reinhard method 272
REM gene 239
Restructured Meat 153, 229,
Restructuring 153, 154
Reticulin 24, 28, 34
Retorting 103, 142
Riboflavin 55, 57, 62, 63, 64, 100, 241, 245, 268, 270, 271
Rigor mortis 30, 36, 43, 44, 45, 55, 63, 91, 113, 119, 120, 121, 236, 239-241
Rigor shortening 45
Ring Precipitation Test 74
Ripening 111, 253, 255, 257
RN^- gene 339
Roasting 98, 102, 123, 138, 139, 149, 215, 221, 253
Rounds 16, 17, 24, 29, 161, 191, 206, 208, 273

S

Sage 190
Salt 5, 6, 27, 32, 33, 89, 91, 92, 94-97, 101, 102, 108, 123, 124-126, 128-132, 146, 148-151, 153-156, 163, 183, 188, 195, 198, 199, 200, 201, 207-223, 225-228, 237, 243, 248, 255, 256, 258, 260, 269, 271, 275, 276, 313
Salt replacers 6, 151
Salting 89, 94, 123, 147, 148, 150, 200, 248
Sarcolemma 17, 20, 22, 32
Sarcomere 18-21, 32, 44, 111, 113, 236
Sarcoplasm 17, 20, 22, 23, 26, 27, 32, 49, 53, 58, 78, 114, 115, 155, 339
Sarcoplasmic proteins 32, 49, 58, 78, 115
Sarcoplasmic reticulum 17, 20, 22, 23, 53, 114
Sausage-Burger 209
Sausages 96, 99, 109, 128, 129, 135, 140, 156, 157, 176, 184, 186, 187, 190, 191, 193, 200, 201-203-213, 243, 244, 249, 253, 255, 257, 293, 311, 332
Scale test 261
SDS-PAGE 79, 85
Seaming 103, 142

Seasonings 102, 124, 148, 153, 189, 201, 207-209, 217
Sectioning and forming 154, 155
Semi Dry Sausage 204, 206, 210
Sensory Attributes 87, 110, 187, 229, 252, 257, 258
Sensory evaluation of meat products 251
Shakudi 5
Shear Force Value 231, 236, 331, 332
Sheep Casing 206, 209
Shell 57, 222, 223, 240, 241, 245, 246, 249, 266, 267, 271-274, 277, 279, 281, 293
Shell membrane 266, 274
Shelled eggs quality 245
Shrink film overwrap packaging 172
Shrink packaging 175
Significance of meat preservation 87
Simmering 139, 220
Skeletal muscle fiber 16, 17
Slow freezing 92
Smell 105, 176, 190, 251, 252, 255-257, 280
Smoke drying 99
Smoke generation process 133
Smoked Fish 224, 226, 227, 248
Smoked Fish Dip 226
Smoked Fish in Soy Sauce and Wine Brine 226
Smoked Red Snapper 228
Smoked Salmon Cakes 227
Smoked Salmon Mousse 227
Smoked Salmon Omelets 227
Smoking 88, 89, 99, 102, 123, 131-136, 169, 201-203, 205, 207, 211, 224-226, 228, 253, 258, 312
Smoothness 254
Sodium alginate 157, 188
Sodium Dodecyl Sulphate PAGE 79
Sorbate 96, 97, 128, 149, 229
Soups 169, 192, 217, 311, 313
Soy proteins 185, 186
Specialised sensory evaluation 259
Spices 94, 124, 132, 149, 189, 193, 195, 196, 198-200, 201, 207, 210, 211, 213, 214, 218, 219, 222, 226, 256-258
Spinach and Minced Meat Soup 219
Springiness 254
SPS 9, 10, 243, 244, 246, 318, 322, 326, 345
Stabilizers 157, 184, 188
Standard Setting Bodies 289, 318
Standards Applicable for Organic Meat Food Products 334
Stearic acid 60, 61, 62, 73
Steel 128, 129, 155, 165
Sterilization 98, 102-107, 137, 141-144, 146
Stewing 139
Stitch pumping 130, 131
Stout bags 176
Stretching of Carcasses 117, 118
Structure and composition of muscle 15
Structure of typical poultry egg 266
Stuffer 205, 207
Subtilin 109
Sugar 47, 94, 95, 97, 115, 124-126, 130, 131, 149, 151, 163, 184, 187, 208-210, 213, 223, 225, 228, 239, 341,
Summer Sausages 156, 191
Super cows 343
Surimi 222-224
Sweet Smoked Salmon 228
SWOT analysis of meat industry 3
Synthetic Casing 206
Synthetic fat replacers 192

T

T -tubules 17
Tabak manss 5
Tandoori Chicken 215
Taste 57, 99, 101, 105, 111, 115, 119, 125, 126, 129, 148, 158, 164, 178, 185, 190, 191, 194, 203, 225, 243, 251, 252, 255-260, 263, 272-274, 331
Taste panels 257, 259
Taurine 63
TBHQ 108, 109, 152
TDT 99, 145
Tearing and forming 153, 154
Temperature 39, 41, 43-48, 53, 88-94, 96, 98-104, 111, 113, 115, 116, 127, 132-134, 136-138, 139-146, 149, 155-157, 161, 162, 166, 167, 172, 174, 178, 179, 184, 186, 188, 193, 207-212, 214, 215, 221, 222, 229, 235, 237-239, 242-246, 252, 258, 259, 272, 273-278, 281, 282, 324
Tender cut method 118
Tenderising 111
Tenderness 29, 33, 36, 39, 44, 47, 53, 95, 111-113, 116, 117, 119-121, 125, 137, 140, 158, 203, 219, 231, 234-337, 240, 253, 332, 340
Terramycin 109
Tetracycline 109

Texture 5, 6, 16, 56, 94, 107, 117, 119, 140, 141, 151-154, 158, 174, 178, 183, 185, 186, 188, 193, 203, 222-224, 229, 231, 234, 235, 237, 239, 241, 251-253, 255, 259, 262, 273, 339,
Texture modifier 6
Texture profile test 259, 262
Thaw rigor 48, 52, 53, 91, 239, 240
Thermal death time 99, 145
Thermal Processing 89, 94, 98, 103, 104, 137, 138, 235
Thermostabilization 274
Thiamine 37, 55, 57, 62-64, 100, 105, 270, 271
Thick filament 18, 19, 21, 29, 30, 32, 113
Thin filament 18, 19, 21, 29, 31, 111, 113
Threshold test 258-260
Thuringer Blood Sausages 211
Thuringer cervelat 210
Tikka Kebab Recipe 199
Tilapia 224, 343
Time-temperature indicators 179
Tocopherols 109, 192
Total quality Management (TQM) 326
Traditional Packaging Materials 163
Traditional Spices 189
Transgenic Fish 342, 344
Transportation of Eggs 278, 281
Tray with overwrap packaging 171
Triangle test 260, 261
Triglycerides 35, 60, 151, 266
Tropomyosin 18, 27, 29, 31, 114
Troponin 18, 27, 29, 31, 46, 114
Tumblers 155, 156
Tylosin 109

U

Ultra high temperature sterilization 98
Ultrasonics 155, 156
Ultraviolet rays (UV rays) 106
Unopened Dried Egg Products 276

V

Vacuum and gas packaging 175
Vacuum packaging 105, 121, 148, 172, 175, 176, 279
Vertebrae 25, 70
Vindaloo 5, 311
Vitamin B_{12} 55, 62, 271
Vitamin B_6 37, 55, 58, 62
Vitamin D 56, 57, 63, 269, 271
Vitamin D_3 63
Vitamin-A 58, 62, 63, 73, 241, 270, 271
Vitamins 36, 37, 55, 58, 62, 64, 72, 103, 105, 124 241, 248, 265, 268, 333, 344
Vitelline membrane 266, 267

W

Water 5, 17, 26-28, 32, 34, 36, 39, 42, 45, 46, 48-51, 60, 81, 90-97, 99, 101-104, 115, 116, 121, 125-128, 130, 132-134, 137-140, 143, 146, 147, 149-151, 155-158, 161, 162, 164, 167, 172, 174, 176, 181, 184-186, 188, 189, 192, 193, 198, 202, 204, 207, 209, 212-214, 217-219, 222, 224-229, 231 233, 234, 237, 239, 241, 242, 244, 246, 247, 254, 256, 257, 266, 269-275, 277, 289, 297, 298, 306, 307, 309, 310, 320, 330-332, 339
Water binding capacity 46, 96, 127, 128, 209, 239, 331
Water glass preservation 274
Water Holding Capacity (WHC) 36, 42, 45, 46, 51, 116, 121, 126, 193, 232, 234, 332, 339,
Wet ageing 116
White fat 24, 69
White muscle 25, 26, 115
White muscle fibers 25
White pepper 191, 208, 212, 213
Whole Egg Powder 187, 276, 277
Whole Muscle Meat Kebab 194, 195
Wok-Smoked Fish 227
World Trade Organization (WTO) 317, 322, 345

X

Xanthan gum 188
X-radiation 104

Y

Yeast proteins 185, 187
Yolk 187, 246, 265, 266, 267, 268, 269, 270, 271, 275, 276, 277

Z

Zinc 28, 55, 56-58, 61, 62, 64, 265, 269, 270
Z-line 18, 19, 20, 21, 44, 49, 113, 115,
Z-line ultrastructure 19
Z-Value 98, 144, 145